Food Fraud as a Global Problem: Advanced Analytical Tools to Detect Species, Country of Origin and Adulterations

Food Fraud as a Global Problem: Advanced Analytical Tools to Detect Species, Country of Origin and Adulterations

Guest Editors

Hongyan Liu
Hongtao Lei
Boli Guo
Ren-You Gan

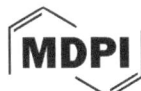

Basel • Beijing • Wuhan • Barcelona • Belgrade • Novi Sad • Cluj • Manchester

Guest Editors

Hongyan Liu
Institute of Urban Agriculture
Chinese Academy of
Agricultural Sciences
Chengdu
China

Hongtao Lei
College of Food Science
South China Agricultural
University
Guangzhou
China

Boli Guo
Institute of Food Science
and Technology
Chinese Academy of
Agricultural Sciences
Beijing
China

Ren-You Gan
Department of Food Science
and Nutrition
The Hong Kong Polytechnic
University
Hong Kong
China

Editorial Office
MDPI AG
Grosspeteranlage 5
4052 Basel, Switzerland

This is a reprint of the Special Issue, published open access by the journal *Foods* (ISSN 2304-8158), freely accessible at: www.mdpi.com/journal/foods/special_issues/food_authenticity.

For citation purposes, cite each article independently as indicated on the article page online and using the guide below:

Lastname, A.A.; Lastname, B.B. Article Title. *Journal Name* **Year**, *Volume Number*, Page Range.

ISBN 978-3-7258-3230-9 (Hbk)
ISBN 978-3-7258-3229-3 (PDF)
https://doi.org/10.3390/books978-3-7258-3229-3

© 2025 by the authors. Articles in this book are Open Access and distributed under the Creative Commons Attribution (CC BY) license. The book as a whole is distributed by MDPI under the terms and conditions of the Creative Commons Attribution-NonCommercial-NoDerivs (CC BY-NC-ND) license (https://creativecommons.org/licenses/by-nc-nd/4.0/).

Contents

About the Editors vii

Gang Zhao, Lingyu Li, Xing Shen, Ruimin Zhong, Qingping Zhong and Hongtao Lei
DNA Barcoding Unveils Novel Discoveries in Authenticating High-Value Snow Lotus Seed Food Products
Reprinted from: *Foods* 2024, 13, 2580, https://doi.org/10.3390/foods13162580 1

Feng Chen, Mengsheng Zhang, Weihua Huang, Harse Sattar and Lianbo Guo
Laser-Induced Breakdown Spectroscopy–Visible and Near-Infrared Spectroscopy Fusion Based on Deep Learning Network for Identification of Adulterated Polygonati Rhizoma
Reprinted from: *Foods* 2024, 13, 2306, https://doi.org/10.3390/foods13142306 14

Simona Schmidlová, Zdeňka Javůrková, Bohuslava Tremlová, Józef Hernik, Barbara Prus and Slavomír Marcinčák et al.
Exploring the Influence of Soil Types on the Mineral Profile of Honey: Implications for Geographical Origin Prediction
Reprinted from: *Foods* 2024, 13, 2006, https://doi.org/10.3390/foods13132006 29

Ming-Ming Chen, Qiu-Hong Liao, Li-Li Qian, Hai-Dan Zou, Yan-Long Li and Yan Song et al.
Effects of Geographical Origin and Tree Age on the Stable Isotopes and Multi-Elements of Pu-erh Tea
Reprinted from: *Foods* 2024, 13, 473, https://doi.org/10.3390/foods13030473 41

Tao Lin, Xinglian Chen, Lijuan Du, Jing Wang, Zhengxu Hu and Long Cheng et al.
Traceability Research on *Dendrobium devonianum* Based on SWATHtoMRM
Reprinted from: *Foods* 2023, 12, 3608, https://doi.org/10.3390/foods12193608 56

Sarah Currò, Stefania Balzan, Enrico Novelli and Luca Fasolato
Cuttlefish Species Authentication: Advancing Label Control through Near-Infrared Spectroscopy as Rapid, Eco-Friendly, and Robust Approach
Reprinted from: *Foods* 2023, 12, 2973, https://doi.org/10.3390/foods12152973 73

Laura Filonzi, Alessia Ardenghi, Pietro Maria Rontani, Andrea Voccia, Claudio Ferrari and Riccardo Papa et al.
Molecular Barcoding: A Tool to Guarantee Correct Seafood Labelling and Quality and Preserve the Conservation of Endangered Species
Reprinted from: *Foods* 2023, 12, 2420, https://doi.org/10.3390/foods12122420 81

Syed Abdul Wadood, Yunzhu Jiang, Jing Nie, Chunlin Li, Karyne M. Rogers and Hongyan Liu et al.
Effects of Light Shading, Fertilization, and Cultivar Type on the Stable Isotope Distribution of Hybrid Rice
Reprinted from: *Foods* 2023, 12, 1832, https://doi.org/10.3390/foods12091832 106

Grégoire Denay, Laura Preckel, Henning Petersen, Klaus Pietsch, Anne Wöhlke and Claudia Brünen-Nieweler
Benchmarking and Validation of a Bioinformatics Workflow for Meat Species Identification Using 16S rDNA Metabarcoding
Reprinted from: *Foods* 2023, 12, 968, https://doi.org/10.3390/foods12050968 121

Kapil Nichani, Steffen Uhlig, Bertrand Colson, Karina Hettwer, Kirsten Simon and Josephine Bönick et al.
Development of Non-Targeted Mass Spectrometry Method for Distinguishing Spelt and Wheat
Reprinted from: *Foods* **2022**, *12*, 141, https://doi.org/10.3390/foods12010141 . . . . **140**

About the Editors

Hongyan Liu

Dr. Liu has been engaged in food authentication, geographical traceability, and extraction of food product development for a long time. In the past five years, she has published more than 50 *SCI* papers, including 30 *SCI* papers as the first/corresponding author. She also participated in the compilation of three books and authorized eight national invention patents. She was guest editor of *Foods*, *Frontiers in Nutrition*, *Antioxidants*, and other journals.

Hongtao Lei

Dr. Hongtao Lei is a distinguished professor at South China Agricultural University (SCAU) in Guangzhou, China. He obtained his bachelor's degree in food science and engineering from Northwest Agriculture and Forestry University in 1997. He then pursued his master's studies in food chemistry at SCAU from 1997 to 2000, after which he began his academic career as an assistant lecturer at the College of Food Science at SCAU. From September 2003 to June 2006, he completed his Ph.D. research in food safety at SCAU. Dr. Lei further enriched his academic experience with a year-long postdoctoral fellowship at the Institute of Global Food Security, Queen's University Belfast, UK, from 2009 to 2010. In December 2012, he was promoted to the rank of professor in food science. Dr. Lei's research focuses on food quality and safety, molecular recognition, food authenticity, and related areas. He has led over 25 scientific research projects supported by national and local funding and has developed 18 professional standards for product quality and analytical methods. His significant contributions to the field are reflected in his publication of more than 100 peer-reviewed articles in international journals, and over 80 invention patents in the area of rapid detection. Dr. Lei's academic and teaching excellence has been widely acknowledged, earning him seven national and provincial awards. He serves as associate editors for *Chemical and Biological Technologies in Agriculture* and *Future Postharvest and Food*, and is a member of the editorial boards of more than 10 other journals such as *Foods* and *Food Chemistry Advances*. He also holds several key leadership roles, including Deputy Director of the National Teaching Steering Committee for Higher Education in Food Science and Engineering under the Ministry of Education, Deputy Chairman of the Agricultural Products Processing and Storage Engineering Committee of the Chinese Society of Agricultural Engineering, etc.

Boli Guo

Prof. Boli Guo carried out research on the theory and technology of food geographical origin traceability, and she is now the chief of the Cereal Processing and Quality Control Innovation Team at the Institute of Food Science and Technology, Chinese Academy of Agricultural Sciences. Her main research directions include the following: 1) evaluation of the material basis and processing suitability of cereal raw materials; 2) mechanism of quality formation and key processing technologies of cereal products; and 3) cereal nutrition and personalized product creation. She has successively led or participated in more than 20 projects, including key research and development plans of the state, projects of the National Natural Science Foundation of China, agricultural finance projects of the Ministry of Agriculture, and science and technology consultation projects of the Chinese Academy of Engineering. She has published over 150 academic papers; she has mainly published 5 academic monographs; she has been granted more than 20 invention patents; and she has obtained more than 30 computer software copyrights.

She won one first prize for scientific and technological progress from the Chinese Institute of Food Science and Technology, one second prize for scientific and technological progress from Shaanxi Province, and one outstanding scientific and technological innovation award from the Chinese Academy of Agricultural Sciences.

Ren-You Gan

Dr. Renyou Gan is an assistant professor and presidential young scholar at the Department of Food Science and Nutrition, Faculty of Science, the Hong Kong Polytechnic University (PolyU), Hong Kong SAR, China. He received his medical bachelor's degree from Sun Yat-sen University (SYSU) and his Ph.D. degree from the University of Hong Kong (HKU). He was previously an assistant professor at Shanghai Jiao Tong University (SJTU); a chief scientist at the Institute of Urban Agriculture (IUA), Chinese Academy of Agricultural Sciences (CAAS); a principal scientist at Singapore Institute of Food and Biotechnology Innovation (SIFBI), Agency for Science, Technology and Research (A*STAR); and an adjunct assistant professor at the Department of Food Science & Technology, National University of Singapore (NUS). His research mainly focuses on plant-based foods, food functional ingredients, probiotics, gut microbiomes, and human nutrition/health, and related work has generated more than 200 SCIE-indexed publications, including more than 130 papers as the first/corresponding author and more than 20 ESI highly cited papers. He has also filed more than 30 Chinese patents, with 20 of them awarded. According to Google Scholar, his publications have been cited more than 21,000 times, with an H-index of 74. He serves as an editorial board member of several international journals, including *iMeta* (executive associate editor), *iMetaOmics* (executive editor), *Current Research in Biotechnology* (executive editor), *Fermentation* (section editor-in-chief), *Frontiers in Nutrition* (section associate editor), and *Nutrients/Antioxidants/Foods/Antibiotics/npj Science of Food/Discover Food* (editorial board members). He has been selected as the Clarivate "Highly Cited Researcher" (*Agricultural Sciences*) from 2021 to 2023; the Stanford University "World Top 2% Scientists" (*Food Science*) from 2020 to 2024; and the Scilit "Top Cited Scholar" (*Food Science & Technology and Phytochemicals*) in 2023 and 2024.

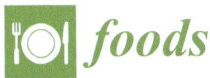

Article

DNA Barcoding Unveils Novel Discoveries in Authenticating High-Value Snow Lotus Seed Food Products

Gang Zhao [1,2], Lingyu Li [3], Xing Shen [1], Ruimin Zhong [2], Qingping Zhong [1] and Hongtao Lei [1,*]

1. Guangdong Provincial Key Laboratory of Food Quality and Safety, South China Agricultural University, Guangzhou 510642, China; gangzhao@scau.edu.cn (G.Z.); shenxing325@163.com (X.S.); zhongqp@scau.edu.cn (Q.Z.)
2. Guangdong Provincial Key Laboratory of Utilization and Conservation of Food and Medicinal Resources in Northern Region, Shaoguan University, Shaoguan 512005, China; zhongrm9898@163.com
3. College of Plant Protection, South China Agricultural University, Guangzhou 510642, China; lilingyu7788@163.com
* Correspondence: hongtao@scau.edu.cn; Tel.: +86-20-8528-3925; Fax: +86-20-8528-0270

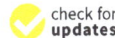

Citation: Zhao, G.; Li, L.; Shen, X.; Zhong, R.; Zhong, Q.; Lei, H. DNA Barcoding Unveils Novel Discoveries in Authenticating High-Value Snow Lotus Seed Food Products. *Foods* **2024**, *13*, 2580. https://doi.org/10.3390/foods13162580

Academic Editors: Mircea Oroian and Pedro Vicente Martínez-Culebras

Received: 4 July 2024
Revised: 10 August 2024
Accepted: 16 August 2024
Published: 18 August 2024

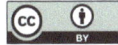

Copyright: © 2024 by the authors. Licensee MDPI, Basel, Switzerland. This article is an open access article distributed under the terms and conditions of the Creative Commons Attribution (CC BY) license (https://creativecommons.org/licenses/by/4.0/).

Abstract: Snow Lotus Seed (SLS), esteemed for its nutritional and market value, faces challenges of authentication due to the absence of appropriate testing standards and methods. This results in frequent adulteration of SLS sourced from *Gleditsia sinensis* (*G. sinensis*) with other plant seeds endosperm. Traditional chloroplast DNA barcoding methods are inadequate for species identification due to the absence of chloroplasts in *G. sinensis* seeds endosperm. In this study, the homology of 11 ITS genes among 6 common *Gleditsia* species was analyzed. Universal primers suitable for these species were designed and screened. A DNA barcoding method for distinguishing SLS species was developed using Sanger sequencing technology, leveraging existing GenBank and Barcode of Life Data System (BOLD) databases. Optimized sample pretreatment facilitated effective DNA extraction from phytopolysaccharide-rich SLS. Through testing of commercial SLS products, the species origin has been successfully identified. Additionally, a novel instance of food fraud was uncovered, where the *Caesalpinia spinosa* endosperm was used to counterfeit SLS for the first time. The study established that the developed DNA barcoding method is effective for authenticating SLS species. It is of great significance for combating food fraud related to SLS, ensuring food safety, and promoting the healthy development of the SLS industry.

Keywords: *Gleditsia sinensis*; DNA barcoding; species identification; food fraud; Snow Lotus Seed

1. Introduction

Snow Lotus Seed (SLS), known as "Zao Jiao Mi" in Chinese, is a product made from the dried mature fruits of the artificially cultivated *Gleditsia sinensis*, through the processes of pod removal, seed extraction, soaking, steaming, endosperm extraction, and drying [1]. After soaking in water, SLS becomes translucent and resembles the Tian Shan snow lotus, which is how it earned its name. It is primarily used in the preparation of sweet soups and desserts and is mainly produced in China's Guizhou and Yunnan provinces. The main component of SLS is oligosaccharides, and it is rich in plant dietary fiber and various minerals. With high energy and low fat, it is considered a healthy food choice and is well loved by many consumers [2]. Zhijin County in Guizhou Province is recognized as China's largest processing center for SLS, with an annual processing and sales volume exceeding 1000 tons, capturing over 90% of the market share. Its products are widely acclaimed and distributed globally. SLS has also become an important characteristic economic agricultural product for local farmers in Zhijin County to abolish poverty and become rich [3,4]. However, due to the limited annual production of SLS, its production and processing currently depend largely on manual labor, leading to low processing efficiency. This is a major reason for its relatively high market price. As a result, some unethical traders substitute the endosperm of other plant seeds for SLS processing and sales, seeking substantial profits from this practice. The shape and color of these plant seed endosperms closely resemble those of *Gleditsia sinensis*. After being processed into finished SLS products, consumers find it even more difficult to accurately identify the species' origin based solely on appearance. On one hand, this type of food fraud seriously undermines consumer interests and fosters the detrimental "Bad money drives out good money" phenomenon, hindering the healthy and sustainable development of the SLS industry [5]. On the other hand, commercially available SLS products derived from unidentified plant seeds may pose certain food safety risks. Currently, there have been no reported methods for authenticating the species of SLS products, making law enforcement against SLS food fraud increasingly challenging. Therefore, there is an urgent need to develop accurate methods for verifying its species authenticity.

In recent years, food adulteration detection technology has emerged as a prominent research focus within the global food industry. DNA-based molecular biology techniques have gained widespread recognition as highly accurate methods for species identification. Technologies such as PCR and its derivatives are extensively employed to verify the authenticity of plant-derived species like coffee and fruit juices [6,7]. Researchers have also utilized methods such as SRAP, SSR, transcriptome analysis, and genome sequencing for identifying plant varieties and distinguishing between male and female plants [8–11]. However, these approaches often suffer from issues such as instability, complex analyses, cumbersome procedures, or high costs. Real-time PCR, considered the gold standard for biological species identification, excels in targeted identification of specific species but faces challenges in identifying unknown species [12]. With the advancement and widespread adoption of Sanger sequencing technology, DNA barcoding has emerged as a powerful tool for taxonomic studies, especially for identifying unknown species [13]. Chloroplast DNA (cpDNA) is particularly suitable for species differentiation due to its matrilineal inheritance in most plants and slow evolutionary rate [14,15]. Several cpDNA genes such as *rbcL*, *matK*, *psbA-trnH*, and *ycf1b* have been identified as effective targets for DNA barcoding to accurately distinguish plant species [16–19]. Among these, the *rbcL* and *matK* genes are established targets for standard plant species barcodes recognized by the Barcode of Life Data System (BOLD) [20]. However, as the endosperm of SLS contains abundant plant polysaccharides, its DNA content is naturally low and lacks chloroplast DNA. Processing steps such as steaming and drying further exacerbate DNA fragmentation and loss. Moreover, many traditional universal DNA barcodes for plants amplify long target segments (600~1200 bp) [21,22], with most targeting chloroplast genes, thus they are not suitable for species identification of SLS raw materials and commercial products.

Hence, in order to address the challenge of lacking available methods for species identification of raw materials and commercial products of SLS, this study constructed a DNA barcoding method for identifying the species origin of SLS by analyzing the sequence information from the ITS region of nuclear genes in various common *Gleditsia* species (Figure 1). Through testing, this method has good amplification performance and differentiation ability for common *Gleditsia* species and can be used for species identification of raw materials and commercially available products of SLS. This study offers technical support for verifying the authenticity of SLS species, which is crucial for combating food fraud, safeguarding consumer interests, and promoting the green, healthy, and sustainable development of SLS and its associated industries.

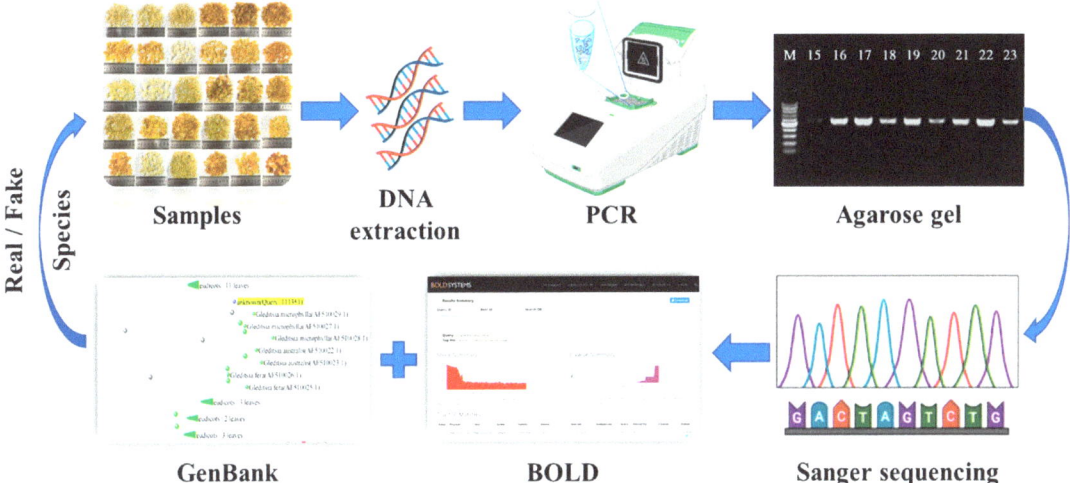

Figure 1. DNA barcoding assay for the authentication of commercially available SLS products.

2. Materials and Methods

2.1. Samples

The seeds of *Gleditsia sinensis*, *Gleditsia japonica*, and *Gleditsia microphylla* were obtained from Guangdong Provincial Key Laboratory of Food Quality and Safety. *Gleditsia delavayi* seeds were procured from the *Gleditsia delavayi* planting base (Meihui *Gleditsia delavayi* planting Base, Lianghe, China). *Gleditsia fera* seeds were collected from South China Agricultural University. After washing all seeds twice with sterilized water, they were soaked overnight in water at room temperature. Subsequently, the endosperm extracted by dissecting the seed coat with a surgical blade was dried at 60 °C in a DHG 9420(A) electric forced air-drying oven (Bluepard instruments Ltd., Shanghai, China) for 4 h [23]. Finally, the endosperm samples were stored at −20 °C. The 30 samples of commercially available SLS were procured from Yunnan (Samples 1~5), Guizhou (Samples 6~10), Shaanxi (Samples 10~15), Henan (Samples 15~20), Hebei (Samples 20~25), and Shandong (Samples 25~30) provinces (Figure 2).

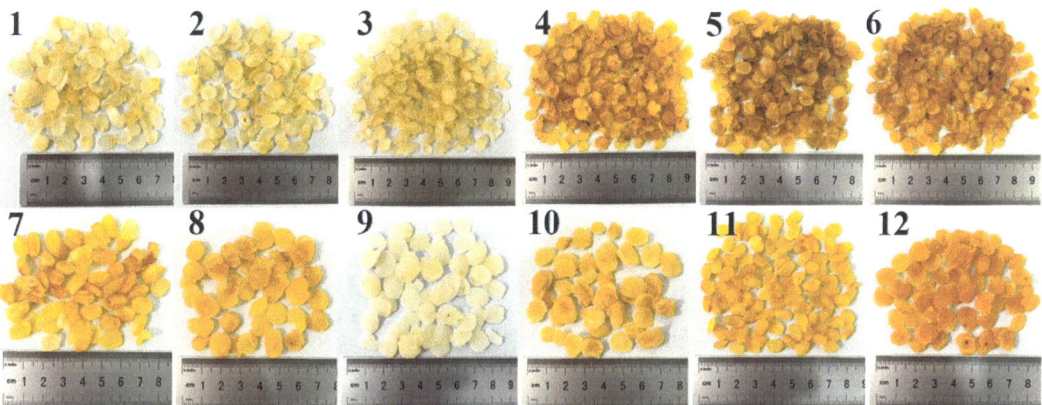

Figure 2. *Cont.*

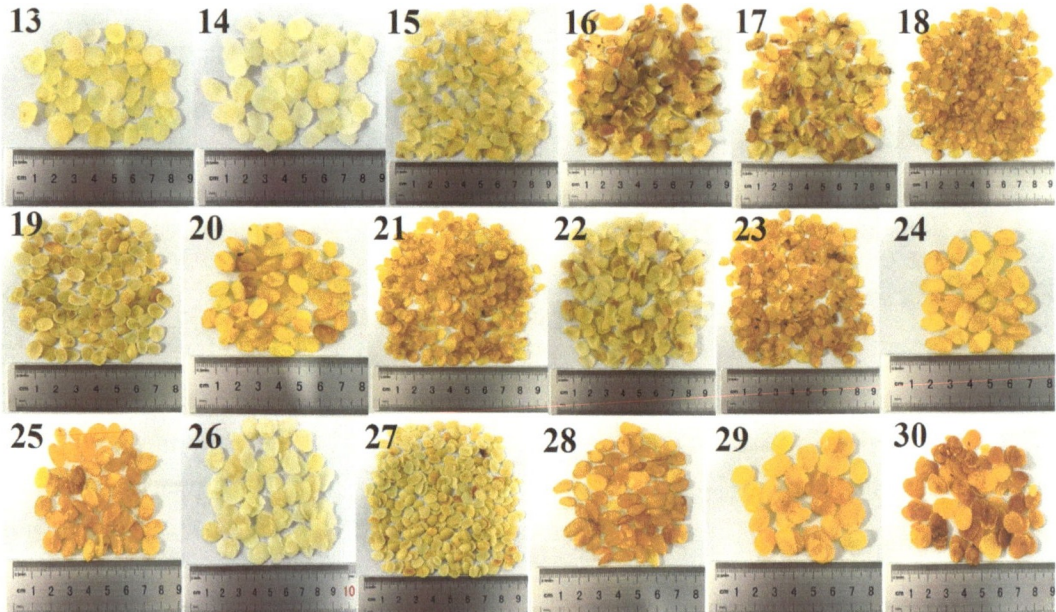

Figure 2. Thirty commercially available SLS products collected for this study.

2.2. DNA Extraction

The DNA was extracted from SLS samples using the DP360 Plant DNA Extraction Kit (Tiangen Biochemical Technology Ltd., Beijing, China), and the instructions were improved for use. Briefly, SLS samples were pulverized by a WFB-D1 wall-breaker (Westinghouse Electric Ltd., Ningbo, China) and passed through an 80-mesh sieve to remove large particles that were not completely pulverized. A 20 mg powder sample was mixed with 800 μL of lysis buffer and 20 μL of RNase A (10 mg/mL) in an EP tube at 65 °C for 10 min. Subsequently, 200 μL neutralization buffer was added to the tube and mixed thoroughly and place it on ice for 10 min. The sample was placed on ice for 10 min, and then the procedure was followed as described in the product manual until the sample DNA was obtained. Each sample was repeated 3 times and the DNA obtained was placed at −20 °C for storage.

2.3. Primer and PCR Amplification

A total of 11 ITS genes from *Gleditsia sinensis* (MH808446.1, AF510019.1), *Gleditsia japonica* (AF510012.1, AF510014.1, AF510010.1), and *Gleditsia microphylla* (AF510027.1), *Gleditsia triacanthos* (AF509977.1, AF509981.1, AF509974.1), *Gleditsia delavayi* (AF510009.1) and *Gleditsia fera* (AF510026.1) six *Gleditsia* species were downloaded from GeneBank database. Sequence homology analysis was performed using the "Clustal W Method" in MegAlign software version 7.1.0 (DNASTAR, Inc., Madison, WI, USA), and the conserved regions were selected for the design of generic DNA barcoding primers for *Gleditsia* (Figure 3). The four most common *Gleditsia* seed endosperm DNAs, *Gleditsia sinensis*, *Gleditsia japonica*, *Gleditsia microphylla*, and *Gleditsia delavayi*, were used for generalization testing of SLS DNA barcoding primers. Common plant DNA barcoding universal primers for ITS gene were also used for comparative suitability testing of SLS [24–26]. The PCR reaction was performed in 50 μL containing 41 μL of 1.1× T6 Super PCR Mix (Tsingke Biotech Ltd., Beijing, China), 2 μL of 10 μM each forward and reverse primer, and 5 μL of DNA template (10 ng/μL). The thermal cycling parameters were shown as follows: pre-denaturation at 98 °C for 2 min, followed by 39 cycles of 98 °C for 10 s, 56 °C for 15 s, and 72 °C for 15 s with a final extension at 72 °C for 5 min. Sterile ultrapure water as a template was used as a negative control to ensure that the PCR reaction was not contaminated. All primers (Table 1) were synthesized by GENEWIZ (GENEWIZ Biotechnology Ltd., Suzhou, China).

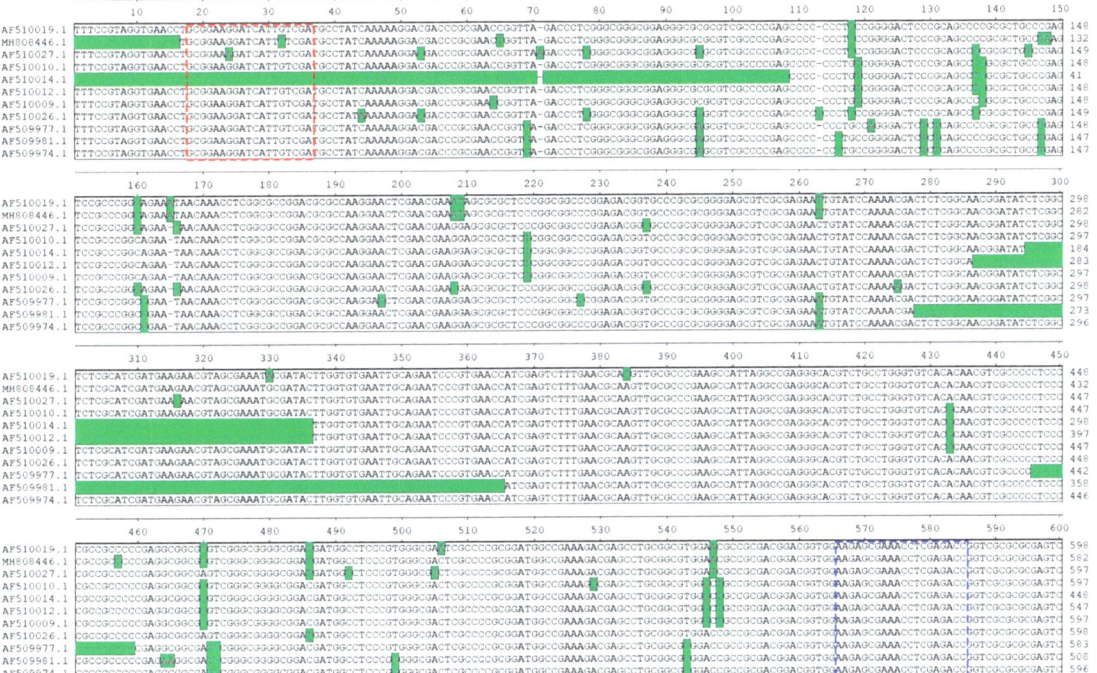

Figure 3. The homology analysis for 11 ITS genes from 6 *Gleditsia* species. The red and blue dashed boxes are the DNA barcoding forward and reverse primer design regions, respectively. Differential bases are labeled in green. The accession numbers of the ITS genes from top to bottom in the image belong to the following species: *Gleditsia sinensis*, *Gleditsia sinensis*, *Gleditsia microphylla*, *Gleditsia japonica*, *Gleditsia japonica*, *Gleditsia japonica*, *Gleditsia delavayi*, *Gleditsia fera*, *Gleditsia triacanthos*, *Gleditsia triacanthos*, *Gleditsia triacanthos*.

Table 1. Information of the oligonucleotides used in this work.

Primer	Oligonucleotide (5′-3′)	Amplicon (bp)	Reference
G-F	GCGGAAGGATCATTGTCGA	550	This study.
G-R	GGTCTCGAGGTTTCGCTCTT		
ITS-F	GGAAGTAAAAGTCGTAACAAGC	731	[25]
ITS-R	TCCTCCGCTTATTGATATGC		
ITS2-F	ATGCGATACTTGGTGTGAAT	450~550	[24]
ITS2-R	GACGCTTCTCCAGACTACAAT		

2.4. Sanger Sequencing

The above PCR amplification products and 100 bp DNA ladder (Tsingke Biotech Ltd., Beijing, China) were electrophoresed on a 2% agarose gel to determine the size of the bands. After confirming the successful amplification, the amplified products, together with the corresponding amplification primers, were submitted to GENEWIZ Biotechnology Ltd. for Sanger sequencing using the standard procedure of ABI 3730 DNA sequencing platform. To ensure the accuracy of the sequencing results, the PCR products were sequenced in both directions in this study. Sequencing results were returned by DNASTAR. Lasergene.v7 software (DNASTAR, Inc., Madison, WI, USA) for sequence splicing and manual sequence correction when necessary.

2.5. Phylogenetic Analysis

The acquired sequences were first subjected to homology analysis using the BLAST tool [27]. The phylogenetic analysis was conducted using the following BLAST tool workflow: the corrected sequence was inputted and searched against the nucleotide collection (nr/nt) within standard databases. The "Organism" field was specified as "plants", while other parameters were maintained at default settings. Sequence comparison was performed using the "Highly similar sequences (megablast)" algorithm in the Program Selection column. Subsequently, a Max Seq Difference of 0.75 was applied based on the BLAST results to construct a phylogenetic tree using the Neighbor Joining method [28].

This study also utilized the Barcode of Life Data System (BOLD) [29] to conduct secondary homology analysis on the acquired sample sequences, thereby reaffirming the origin of the analyzed specimens. Due to the limited gene targets, *rbcL* and *matK*, located exclusively in chloroplast DNA, the barcode database (Plant identification) within the BOLD System is insufficient for identifying SLS, which lacks chloroplast DNA. Consequently, corrected sequences from SLS samples were submitted to the "FUNGAL IDENTIFICATION [ITS]" database within the "IDENTIFICATION ENGINE" module for homology analysis.

3. Results and Discussion

3.1. DNA Barcoding Primers for SLS

The widely cited plant DNA barcoding universal primer pairs ITS-F/ITS-R and ITS2-F/ITS2-R were employed in this study to assess their amplification capability across five common varieties of SLS. Through multiple amplification tests, it was observed that both primer pairs exhibited limited universal amplification ability for SLS varieties sourced from the market (Figure 4A). Specifically, ITS-F/ITS-R showed better recognition and amplification performance for SLS DNA from *G. sinensis* and *G. fera*, but struggled with DNA from *G. microphylla*, *G. japonica*, and *G. delavayi*. Similarly, ITS2-F/ITS2-R effectively amplified SLS DNA from *G. microphylla* and *G. fera*, but encountered challenges in recognizing and amplifying DNA from *G. sinensis*, *G. japonica*, and *G. delavayi*. Upon analysis of this primer with *Gleditsia*, these two sets of reported universal primer pairs for plant DNA barcoding differed to some extent from the ITS gene sequences of *Gleditsia*, resulting in insufficient recognition and binding of different DNAs from *Gleditsia*, making it difficult to achieve universal amplification of SLS DNAs from common species sources. Thus, by reanalyzing the homology of 11 ITS genes of 6 *Gleditsia* species, this study designed and screened to obtain DNA barcoding universal amplification primers: G-F and G-R, suitable for common species of SLS in the market. Through testing, the G-F and G-R primers can better identify the DNA of five common *Gleditsia* species originating from SLS in the market, and all of them can obtain a single electrophoretic band amplicon of about 550 bp in size (Figure 4B), which can be used for Sanger sequencing and subsequent species analysis.

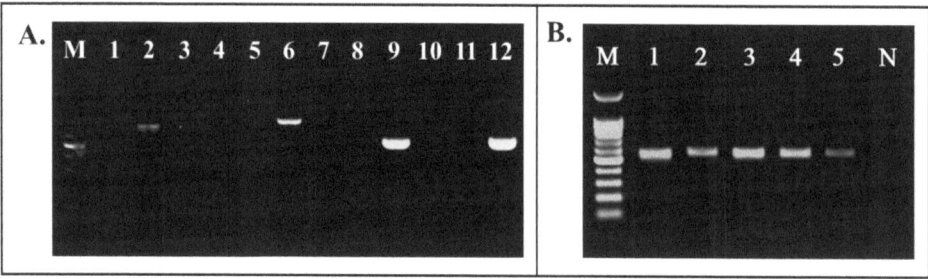

Figure 4. DNA barcoding primers were tested for amplification versatility against common *Gleditsia* species. (**A**) Amplification performance of primers ITS-F and ITS-R, and ITS2-F and ITS2-R on DNA

of different species of SLS. Numbers 1–6: ITS-F and ITS-R were used for amplification. Numbers 7–12: ITS2-F and ITS2-R were used for amplification. M: 100 bp DNA Ladder. Numbers 1–6 and 7–12: No template control, *Gleditsia sinensis*, *Gleditsia microphylla*, *Gleditsia japonica*, *Gleditsia delavayi*, and *Gleditsia fera*. (**B**) DNA from different species of SLS were tested for amplification versatility ability of primers G-F and G-R. M: 100 bp DNA Ladder. Numbers 1–4: DNA templates were obtained from *Gleditsia sinensis*, *Gleditsia microphylla*, *Gleditsia japonica*, and *Gleditsia delavayi*, respectively. Number 5: *Gleditsia fera*. N: No template control.

3.2. The Authenticity of Commercial SLS Products

After 30 commercial SLS products were sequenced by Sanger, the sequence results were verified by simultaneous comparison with both GenBank and BOLD databases, and the species with the highest homology and consistent results between the two databases were selected as the species to which the SLS products belonged. The results showed that 28 of the samples successfully obtained target amplicons and completed Sanger sequencing and subsequent analysis (Figure 5). Two samples (26 and 29) failed to yield PCR amplification despite multiple attempts at DNA extraction, primarily because successful DNA sample acquisition was never achieved for these samples. Additionally, alternative DNA extraction methods using Magnetic Particle Adsorption (CZ307, Biomed Biotech, Beijing, China) and CTAB precipitation [30] were also employed on samples 26 and 29, but these methods also yielded minimal results. After observing and sensory tasting of the two samples, it was found that both samples had noticeably larger shapes and sweeter tastes, indicating they were artificially manufactured SLS with added sucrose. Our analysis suggests that it is highly likely that the use of additives such as sucrose and edible gel during processing further prevented the already limited DNA in the samples from being released normally.

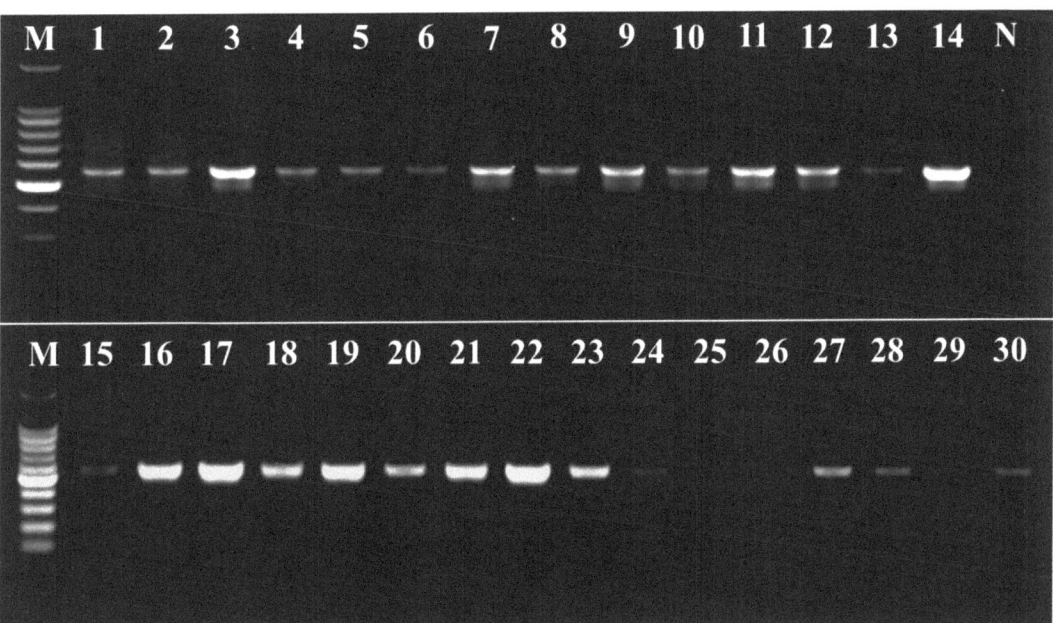

Figure 5. DNA barcoding universal primers for amplification assay of 30 commercial SLS products sold in the market. The amplicons of 30 SLS products using DNA barcoding primers G-F and G-R. Numbers 1–30: 30 commercial SLS products. M: 100 bp DNA Ladder. N: No template control.

Of the 28 successfully sequenced SLS products, only 8 samples were confirmed to be of true *G. sinensis* origin after comparison of the 2 databases, amounting to less than one-third

(26.6%) of the total samples (Table 2). Nearly two-thirds of the other number of products originated from *G. microphylla* (nine samples) and *G. japonica* (nine samples), which is a food fraud in the form of impersonation by a closely related species. Surprisingly, two samples (3 and 14) were found to not belong to any Gleditsia species based on the results of this sequencing analysis. The target sequences of these samples showed 100% homology with *Caesalpinia spinosa* in the BOLD database and with *Tara spinosa* in GenBank. Since *Tara spinosa* is a synonym of *Caesalpinia spinosa*, which belongs to the genus *Caesalpinia*, this represents food fraud involving species from a different genus. In conclusion, more than two-thirds of the 30 SLS products analyzed in this study were processed from seed endosperm of plants belonging to the same genus or different genera with *G. sinensis*. This widespread practice indicates prevalent food fraud involving SLS, highlighting the critical need to address the authenticity of SLS products.

Table 2. DNA barcode sequencing results of 30 SLS samples were compared with information from GenBank and BOLD databases.

Sample No.	GenBank				BOLD			Species Judgment [a]
	Species	Accession	Total Score	Similarity (%)	Species	Score	Similarity (%)	
1	Gleditsia sinensis	AF510020.1	1020	100	Gleditsia sinensis	548	99.64	R
2	Gleditsia sinensis	AF510020.1	1011	99.82	Gleditsia sinensis	543	99.63	R
3	Tara spinosa	OQ411711.1 OQ411709.1	872	100	Caesalpinia spinosa	472	100	F
4	Gleditsia microphylla	AF510027.1	667	100	Gleditsia microphylla	359	99.72	F
5	Gleditsia microphylla	AF510027.1	985	99.63	Gleditsia microphylla	533	98.9	F
6	Gleditsia microphylla	AF510027.1	662	100	Gleditsia microphylla	356	99.72	F
7	Gleditsia sinensis	AF510020.1	937	99.61	Gleditsia sinensis	504	99.41	R
8	Gleditsia japonica	MH710914.1	1002	99.82	Gleditsia japonica	539	100	F
9	Gleditsia japonica	MH710914.1	996	99.82	Gleditsia japonica	540	99.82	F
10	Gleditsia microphylla	AF510027.1	667	100	Gleditsia microphylla	359	99.72	F
11	Gleditsia japonica	MH710914.1	675	100	Gleditsia japonica	365	100	F
12	Gleditsia japonica	MH710914.1	680	100	Gleditsia japonica	368	100	F
13	Gleditsia microphylla	AF510027.1	665	99.73	Gleditsia microphylla	357	99.72	F
14	Tara spinosa	OQ411710.1	713	100	Caesalpinia spinosa	475	99.38	F
15	Gleditsia japonica	MH710914.1	1000	100	Gleditsia japonica	541	100	F
16	Gleditsia japonica	MH710914.1	1013	100	Gleditsia japonica	548	100	F
17	Gleditsia japonica	MH710914.1	1005	100	Gleditsia japonica	544	100	F
18	Gleditsia microphylla	AF510027.1	1005	99.64	Gleditsia microphylla	543	99.27	F

Table 2. Cont.

Sample No.	GenBank				BOLD			Species Judgment [a]
	Species	Accession	Total Score	Similarity (%)	Species	Score	Similarity (%)	
19	Gleditsia sinensis	AF510020.1	1024	100	Gleditsia sinensis	550	99.64	R
20	Gleditsia sinensis	AF510020.1	1013	100	Gleditsia sinensis	544	99.64	R
21	Gleditsia microphylla	AF510027.1	1000	99.82	Gleditsia microphylla	539	99.45	F
22	Gleditsia japonica	MH710914.1	1005	99.64	Gleditsia japonica	545	99.82	F
23	Gleditsia microphylla	AF510027.1	1005	99.82	Gleditsia microphylla	542	99.45	F
24	Gleditsia sinensi	AF510020.1	833	99.56	Gleditsia sinensis	449	99.12	R
25	Gleditsia sinensis	AF510020.1	992	100	Gleditsia sinensis	533	99.63	R
26	/	/	/	/	/	/	/	N
27	Gleditsia japonica	MH710914.1	1014	100	Gleditsia japonica	549	100	F
28	Gleditsia sinensis	AF510020.1	1003	100	Gleditsia sinensis	539	99.63	R
29	/	/	/	/	/	/	/	N
30	Gleditsia microphylla	AF510027.1	990	99.63	Gleditsia microphylla	535	99.26	F

[a] R: Real, the sample is sourced from *Gleditsia sinensis*. F: Fake, the sample is not sourced from *Gleditsia sinensis*. N: Sequencing was incomplete.

3.3. New Discovery for Authenticity Identification of SLS

After identifying the species origin of 30 commercial SLS products by the DNA barcoding method established in this study, only 26.6% of the samples were authentic SLS of *G. sinensis* origin, and the remaining samples were typically economically motivated adulteration (EMA) (Figure 6). Based on our field research at the SLS processing and distribution center in Guizhou, we believe there are currently three main instances of food fraud in the SLS products sold in the market: adulteration with closely related species belonging to the *Gleditsia* genus, misrepresentation of species such as *Caesalpinia spinosa* that do not belong to the *Gleditsia* genus, and the production of artificially enhanced SLS using sucrose and other additives for weight gain purposes.

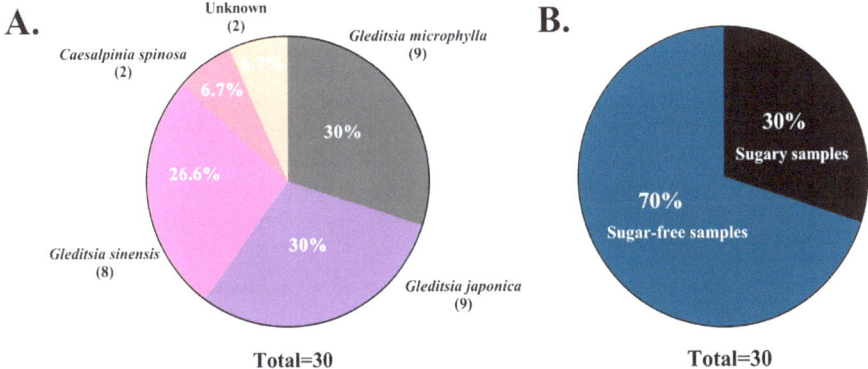

Figure 6. The authenticity of 30 commercial SLS products sold in the market. (**A**) Statistical results of species identification and classification of 30 commercially available SLS products. Two samples

(26 and 29) failed to identify the species, accounting for 6.7% of the total (Unknown). The remaining samples identified the species as *Gleditsia sinensis*, *Gleditsia microphylla*, *Gleditsia japonica*, and *Caesalpinia spinosa*, accounting for 26.6%, 30%, 30%, and 6.7% of the total tested samples, respectively. (**B**) Based on sensory tasting, 30% (9 out of 30) of the SLS products were found to be adulterated with added sugar for increased weight, while the remaining 70% (21 out of 30) were products without added sugar.

3.3.1. Adulteration of Closely Related Species of the Same Genus

Through our analysis of commercially available SLS products, we discovered that the endosperms from *Gleditsia microphylla* and *Gleditsia japonica* were frequently used to adulterate SLS, deceiving consumers into believing it was genuine *Gleditsia sinensis*. These adulterated samples, using closely related species to impersonate *G. sinensis*, accounted for 60% (*Gleditsia microphylla* 30% and *Gleditsia japonica* 30%) of the samples tested and represent a significant form of food fraud in the SLS market today (Figure 6A). *G. microphylla*, *G. japonica*, and *G. sinensis* are closely related species within the same genus, sharing similar genetic relationships and exhibiting very similar shapes and colors in their endosperms. This similarity makes it challenging to distinguish the origin of the species, whether in raw material form or as processed SLS products. Additionally, because the nursery costs for *G. microphylla* are significantly lower, only one-tenth of those for *G. sinensis* [31], and *G. japonica* seeds are smaller with less endosperm fullness, the prices of both *G. microphylla* and *G. japonica* seeds are lower compared to *G. sinensis* seeds. This has led to some growers and unscrupulous merchants selling seeds from *G. microphylla* and *G. japonica* disguised as *G. sinensis* seeds for the production of high-value SLS to make a profit. While the endosperms of *G. microphylla* and *G. japonica* also contain a considerable amount of plant polysaccharides and exhibit a translucent, gelatinous state when soaked in water, whether these endosperms can be safely consumed as food has not been definitively reported. Therefore, the practice of using closely related species from the genus *Gleditsia* to masquerade as *G. sinensis*-origin SLS not only infringes upon consumers' rights to accurate information but also poses potential food safety risks. Overall, this behavior highlights the need for stricter oversight and authentication measures in the SLS industry to ensure transparency and consumer safety.

3.3.2. Caesalpinia Spinosa: A Newly Identified Non-Gleditsia Species Involved in Adulterating SLS

In this study, 2 (sample 3 and 14) of the 30 commercial SLS products were identified as belonging to the *Caesalpinia spinosa* (*Tara spinosa*), accounting for 6.7% of the total samples (Figure 6A). It is distantly related to *G. sinensis* and belongs to a different genus in the *Fabaceae*. However, the *Caesalpinia spinosa* has pods with a similar appearance to the *G. sinensis*, and the seed endosperm is also rich in phytopolysaccharides, which are not directly distinguishable from SLS after processing. *Caesalpinia spinosa* is native to Peru and Ecuador in South America, and its seeds are the raw material for the production of the edible Tara gum [32,33]. Because of the large area under cultivation and the high yield and cheap price of the seeds of a single plant, there are unscrupulous merchants who use the endosperm of *Caesalpinia spinosa* seeds to process and pretend to be high-value SLS to obtain huge profits. Although the Tara gum produced from its seeds can be used as a food additive, it does not mean that the entire seed endosperm can be used directly as an edible part. Therefore, utilizing *Caesalpinia spinosa* seed endosperms in the production of SLS products still carries some undisclosed risks, greatly infringing upon consumers' right to knowledge and economic interests.

3.3.3. Artificially Manufactured Weighted SLS with Added Sucrose

Combined with the previous field research and the analysis of this commercially available samples of SLS, we also found food fraud in samples where sugar and other additives were mixed with low-grade or small SLS to increase the weight of the product for profit. In the blind SLS samples test, nine samples (sample 8, 9, 10, 12, 13, 14, 26, 29, 30) intentionally had sugar added to increase product weight, accounting for as much as 30%

of the total samples (Figure 6B). These sugared samples were all larger than the common SLS form, and the surface was not smooth, sticky to the touch, and sweet to the taste when licked directly. Two of these samples, moreover, were so likely to be due to, for example, excessive sugar adulteration, that the sample DNA could not be successfully extracted for subsequent analysis. In addition, the authors have made several field research trips to Maochang Town in Zhijin County, the largest SLS processing and distribution center in China. Through exchanges with local SLS manufacturing workers and wholesalers, it was indirectly confirmed that the use of white granulated sugar to adulterate SLS has become one of the most important means for some unscrupulous traders to obtain huge profits. As the price of sugar (~0.8 USD/kg) is much lower than the market price of SLS (60 USD/kg), the difference between the two is more than 60 times, and the use of sugar processing to obtain sugary SLS can be made to make SLS weigh 2–5 times than its original weight, leading to profit. This artificially weighted SLS, although it uses edible white sugar, is not only a consumer fraud, but a criminal offense against consumers expecting to stay in shape or for patient populations on low-sugar diets.

4. Conclusions

In this study, we developed a DNA barcoding method for the identification of species adulteration in raw materials for the production of high-value SLS and commercial products by designing ITS universal amplification primers. The method has good target identification and amplification performance for common *G. sinensis*, *G. microphylla*, *G. japonica*, *G. delavayi*, and *G. fera* species. By analyzing both GenBank and BOLD databases simultaneously, SLS from *G. microphylla* and *G. japonica* sources were accurately distinguished as *G. sinensis* sources. Moreover, the fraudulent use of the endosperm of the seed of a non-*Gleditsia* plant as SLS was also accurately identified. Through testing of commercial SLS products, this study found that more than 70% of the products were adulterated to varying degrees. Building on authors' previous field investigations, this study systematically reports, for the first time, three major kinds of food adulteration targeting high-value SLS products. The first new finding of food fraud in which the seed endosperm of *Caesalpinia spinosa*, a plant species of a different genera, was used for processing and was passed off as SLS. This study fills the gap in the authenticity identification method of high-value SLS species. It provides technical support to confirm the authenticity of raw material sources for SLS-processing enterprises, as well as for food regulatory-related agencies to combat SLS species fraud. It is also hoped that the establishment of the methodology in this study will draw the attention of the relevant food legislature to the establishment of relevant analytical and certification standards for high-value SLS so that healthier and safer SLS-related foods can be developed. This will promote the healthy and sustainable development of the SLS industry, and at the same time, it will also enable the consumers to obtain more protection for their health and economic interests.

Supplementary Materials: The following supporting information can be downloaded at: https://www.mdpi.com/article/10.3390/foods13162580/s1, The results (5′-3′) of Sanger sequencing for 30 Snow Lotus Seed products amplified using G-F/G-R primers.

Author Contributions: G.Z., Conceptualization, methodology, investigation, validation, data curation, writing—original draft, writing—review and editing, funding acquisition. L.L., writing—review and editing, visualization. X.S., conceptualization, supervision. R.Z., conceptualization. Q.Z., conceptualization. H.L., conceptualization, writing—review and editing, supervision, funding acquisition. All authors have read and agreed to the published version of the manuscript.

Funding: This work was supported by the China Postdoctoral Science Foundation (2023M731143), National Key Research and Development Program of China (2022YFD1601712), and the Guangdong Basic and Applied Basic Research Foundation (2023A1515110822).

Institutional Review Board Statement: Not applicable.

Informed Consent Statement: Not applicable.

Data Availability Statement: The original contributions presented in the study are included in the article and supplementary material, further inquiries can be directed to the corresponding author.

Conflicts of Interest: The authors declare no conflicts of interest.

References

1. *DBS52/061-2022*; Local Standard for Food Safety-Zaojiaomi. Guizhou health and Health Committee: Guiyang, China, 2022.
2. Liu, Y.; Shi, Z.J.; Peng, X.W.; Xu, J.Y.; Deng, J.; Zhao, P.; Zhang, X.; Kan, H. A polysaccharide from the seed of *Gleditsia japonica* var. delavayi: Extraction, purification, characterization and functional properties. *LWT Food Sci. Technol.* **2024**, *191*, 115660. [CrossRef]
3. Zhijin County, Guizhou: The Development of Zaojiaomi Industry to Help Rural Revitalization. Available online: https://www.gzzhijin.gov.cn/xwzx/jrzj/202111/t20211105_75135171.html (accessed on 21 June 2024).
4. Maochang, Zijin County: The Road to Industrial Breakthrough in the Largest Zaojiaomi Processing and Distribution Center of China. Available online: http://www.gzzhijin.gov.cn/xwzx/xzdt/202312/t20231220_83376396.html (accessed on 21 June 2024).
5. Kendall, H.; Clark, B.; Rhymer, C.; Kuznesof, S.; Hajslova, J.; Tomaniova, M.; Brereton, P.; Frewer, L. A systematic review of consumer perceptions of food fraud and authenticity: A European perspective. *Trends Food Sci. Technol.* **2019**, *94*, 79–90. [CrossRef]
6. Liang, Y.L.; Ding, Y.J.; Liu, X.; Zhou, P.F.; Ding, M.X.; Yin, J.J.; Song, Q.H. A duplex PCR–RFLP–CE for simultaneous detection of mandarin and grapefruit in orange juice. *Eur. Food Res. Technol.* **2021**, *247*, 1–7. [CrossRef]
7. Uncu, A.T.; Uncu, A.O. Plastid trnH-psbA intergenic spacer serves as a PCR-based marker to detect common grain adulterants of coffee (*Coffea arabica* L.). *Food Control* **2018**, *91*, 32–39. [CrossRef]
8. Shamustakimova, A.O.; Mavlyutov, Y.M.; Klimenko, I.A. Application of SRAP Markers for DNA Identification of Russian Alfalfa Cultivars. *Russ. J. Genet.* **2021**, *57*, 540–547. [CrossRef]
9. Li, J.J.; Ye, C.L. Genome-wide analysis of microsatellite and sex-linked marker identification in *Gleditsia sinensis*. *BMC Plant Biol.* **2020**, *20*, 338. [CrossRef] [PubMed]
10. Tan, W.; Gao, H.; Jiang, W.L.; Zhang, H.Y.; Yu, X.L.; Liu, E.W.; Tian, X.X. The complete chloroplast genome of *Gleditsia sinensis* and *Gleditsia japonica*: Genome organization, comparative analysis, and development of taxon specific DNA mini-barcodes. *Sci. Rep.* **2020**, *10*, 16309. [CrossRef] [PubMed]
11. Wu, Y.; Zhang, R.; Staton, M.; Schlarbaum, S.E.; Coggeshall, M.V.; Severson, J.R.; Carlson, J.E.; Zembower, N.; Liang, H.; Xu, Y.; et al. Development of genic and genomic microsatellites in *Gleditsia triacanthos* L. (Fabaceae) using illumine sequencing. *Ann. For. Res.* **2017**, *60*, 343–350.
12. Kang, T.S. Basic principles for developing real-time PCR methods used in food analysis: A review. *Trends Food Sci. Technol.* **2019**, *91*, 574–585. [CrossRef]
13. Mishra, P.; Kumar, A.; Nagireddy, A.; Mani, D.N.; Shukla, A.K.; Tiwari, R.; Sundaresan, V. DNA barcoding: An efficient tool to overcome authentication challenges in the herbal market. *Plant Biotechnol. J.* **2016**, *14*, 8–21. [CrossRef]
14. Al-Qurainy, F.; Khan, S.; Tarroum, M.; Al-Hemaid, F.M.; Ali, M.A. Molecular authentication of the medicinal herb *Ruta graveolens* (Rutaceae) and an adulterant using nuclear and chloroplast DNA markers. *Genet. Mol. Res.* **2011**, *10*, 2806–2816. [CrossRef] [PubMed]
15. Letsiou, S.; Madesis, P.; Vasdekis, E.; Montemurro, C.; Grigoriou, M.E.; Skavdis, G.; Moussis, V.; Koutelidakis, A.E.; Tzakos, A.G. DNA barcoding as a plant identification method. *Appl. Sci.* **2024**, *14*, 1415. [CrossRef]
16. Thongkhao, K.; Tungphatthong, C.; Phadungcharoen, T.; Sukrong, S. The use of plant DNA barcoding coupled with HRM analysis to differentiate edible vegetables from poisonous plants for food safety. *Food Control* **2020**, *109*, 106896. [CrossRef]
17. Wang, J.L.; Yan, Z.F.; Zhong, P.; Shen, Z.B.; Yang, G.F.; Ma, L.C. Screening of universal DNA barcodes for identifying grass species of Gramineae. *Front. Plant Sci.* **2022**, *13*, 998863. [CrossRef] [PubMed]
18. Yang, X.; Yu, X.L.; Zhang, X.Y.; Guo, H.; Xing, Z.M.; Xu, L.W.; Wang, J.; Shen, Y.Y.; Yu, J.; Lv, P.F.; et al. Development of Mini-Barcode Based on Chloroplast Genome and Its Application in Metabarcoding Molecular Identification of Chinese Medicinal Material Radix Paeoniae Rubra (Chishao). *Front. Plant Sci.* **2022**, *13*, 819822. [CrossRef] [PubMed]
19. Zhang, D.Q.; Jiang, B. Species identification in complex groups of medicinal plants based on DNA barcoding: A case study on *Astragalus* spp. (Fabaceae) from southwest China. *Conserv. Genet. Resour.* **2020**, *12*, 469–478. [CrossRef]
20. Hollingsworth, P.M.; Forrest, L.L.; Spouge, J.L.; Hajibabaei, M.; Ratnasingham, S.; van der Bank, M.; Chase, M.W.; Cowan, R.S.; Erickson, D.L.; Fazekas, A.J.; et al. A DNA barcode for land plants. *Proc. Natl. Acad. Sci. USA* **2009**, *106*, 12794–12797.
21. Jamdade, R.; Upadhyay, M.; Shaer, K.A.; Harthi, E.A.; Sallani, M.A.; Jasmi, M.A.; Ketbi, A.A. Evaluation of Arabian Vascular Plant Barcodes (rbcL and matK): Precision of Unsupervised and Supervised Learning Methods towards Accurate Identification. *Plants* **2021**, *10*, 2741. [CrossRef] [PubMed]
22. Li, W.T.; Yang, S.H.; Ni, L.H.; Zhao, Z.L.; Xu, H.X. Determination of the Genomic DNA Degradation Rate of the Chinese Herb *Gentianae crassicaulis* Radix During Processing and Storage. *Pharmacogn. Mag.* **2023**, *19*, 520–529. [CrossRef]
23. *T/GZSX 064-2020*; Technical Regulations for Production and Processing of Zaojiaomi. Guizhou Food Industry Association: Guiyang, China, 2020.
24. Chen, S.L.; Yao, H.; Han, J.P.; Liu, C.; Song, J.Y.; Shi, L.C.; Zhu, Y.J.; Ma, X.Y.; Gao, T.; Pang, X.H.; et al. Validation of the ITS2 region as a novel DNA barcode for identifying medicinal plant species. *PLoS ONE* **2010**, *5*, e8613. [CrossRef]

25. Gu, W.; Song, J.Y.; Cao, Y.; Sun, Q.W.; Yao, H.; Wu, Q.N.; Chao, J.G.; Zhou, J.J.; Xue, W.D.; Duan, J.A. Application of the ITS2 Region for Barcoding Medicinal Plants of Selaginellaceae in Pteridophyta. *PLoS ONE* **2013**, *8*, e67818. [CrossRef] [PubMed]
26. Qian, Z.H.; Munywoki, J.M.; Wang, Q.F.; Malombe, I.; Li, Z.Z.; Chen, J.M. Molecular Identification of African Nymphaea Species (Water Lily) Based on ITS, trnT-trnF and rpl16. *Plants* **2022**, *11*, 2431. [CrossRef] [PubMed]
27. Basic Local Alignment Search Tool. Available online: https://blast.ncbi.nlm.nih.gov/Blast.cgi (accessed on 8 August 2024).
28. Saitou, N.; Nei, M. The Neighbor-joining Method: A New Method for Reconstructing Phylogenetic Trees. *Mol. Biol. Evol.* **1987**, *4*, 406–425. [PubMed]
29. Barcode of Life Data System. Available online: http://www.boldsystems.org/index.php/ (accessed on 8 August 2024).
30. Healey, A.; Furtado, A.; Cooper, T.; Henry, R.J. Protocol: A simple method for extracting next-generation sequencing quality genomic DNA from recalcitrant plant species. *Plant Methods* **2014**, *10*, 21. [CrossRef]
31. He, S.L. Key Technologies for High-Yield and Efficient Cultivation of *Gleditsia sinensis* for Obtaining the Thorn. Available online: http://www.lczmcn.com/sf_B3AEB904EC204D76A19FFF2918415309_264_luoyanglinzhan.html (accessed on 21 June 2024).
32. Fierro, O.; Siano, F.; Bianco, M.; Vasca, E.; Picariello, G. Comprehensive molecular level characterization of protein- and polyphenol-rich tara (*Caesalpinia spinosa*) seed germ flour suggests novel hypothesis about possible accidental hazards. *Food Res. Int.* **2024**, *181*, 114119. [CrossRef] [PubMed]
33. Raj, V.; Chun, K.; Lee, S. State-of-the-art advancement in tara gum polysaccharide (*Caesalpinia spinosa*) modifications and their potential applications for drug delivery and the food industry. *Carbohydr. Polym.* **2024**, *323*, 121440. [CrossRef] [PubMed]

Disclaimer/Publisher's Note: The statements, opinions and data contained in all publications are solely those of the individual author(s) and contributor(s) and not of MDPI and/or the editor(s). MDPI and/or the editor(s) disclaim responsibility for any injury to people or property resulting from any ideas, methods, instructions or products referred to in the content.

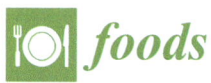 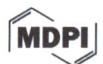

Article

Laser-Induced Breakdown Spectroscopy–Visible and Near-Infrared Spectroscopy Fusion Based on Deep Learning Network for Identification of Adulterated Polygonati Rhizoma

Feng Chen [1], Mengsheng Zhang [1], Weihua Huang [1], Harse Sattar [2,*] and Lianbo Guo [1,*]

1 Wuhan National Laboratory for Optoelectronics (WNLO), Huazhong University of Science and Technology (HUST), Wuhan 430074, China
2 School of Integrated Circuits, Huazhong University of Science and Technology (HUST), Wuhan 430074, China
* Correspondence: harissattar@hust.edu.cn (H.S.); lbguo@hust.edu.cn (L.G.)

Abstract: The geographical origin of foods greatly influences their quality and price, leading to adulteration between high-priced and low-priced regions in the market. The rapid detection of such adulteration is crucial for food safety and fair competition. To detect the adulteration of Polygonati Rhizoma from different regions, we proposed LIBS-VNIR fusion based on the deep learning network (LVDLNet), which combines laser-induced breakdown spectroscopy (LIBS) containing element information with visible and near-infrared spectroscopy (VNIR) containing molecular information. The LVDLNet model achieved accuracy of 98.75%, macro-F measure of 98.50%, macro-precision of 98.78%, and macro-recall of 98.75%. The model, which increased these metrics from about 87% for LIBS and about 93% for VNIR to more than 98%, significantly improved the identification ability. Furthermore, tests on different adulterated source samples confirmed the model's robustness, with all metrics improving from about 87% for LIBS and 86% for VNIR to above 96%. Compared to conventional machine learning algorithms, LVDLNet also demonstrated its superior performance. The results indicated that the LVDLNet model can effectively integrate element information and molecular information to identify the adulterated Polygonati Rhizoma. This work shows that the scheme is a potent tool for food identification applications.

Keywords: LIBS; VNIR; Polygonati Rhizoma; deep learning; adulteration

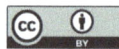

1. Introduction

Polygonati Rhizoma (PR), which is called Huangjing in China, is the rhizome of a liliaceous plant from the genus *Polygonatum* Mill and has been used in traditional food and medicine in China for centuries [1]. PR contains a range of essential compounds such as sugars, lipids, proteins, carotenoids, vitamins, amino acids, and trace elements, which can resist hidden hunger and makes it a potential high-quality crop [2,3]. Rich in compounds like polysaccharides and flavonoids, it offers numerous health benefits, including anti-aging, anti-diabetic, anti-fatigue, and anti-cancer effects [4–7]. PR has traditionally been used in clinical practices to treat age-related diseases, diabetes, lung diseases, fatigue, feebleness, and indigestion in China, India, Pakistan, Iran, and Japan [4,8]. The wide range of medicinal benefits and the increasing demand for PR in various therapeutic applications underscore the importance of ensuring its authenticity and quality. PR is cultivated in various geographical regions, with China being the main producer. However, the geographical origin of PR affects the quality, drug effect, and price [9,10]. Products certified as protected geographical indications (PGIs) are more popular with consumers and have higher prices. Consequently, unscrupulous traders often mislabel the origins or adulterate PGI products with inferior products or products from other regions to increase profits, causing both healthy and wealthy losses to consumers [9]. In the market, consumers are concerned about whether the product is pure, adulterated, or pure counterfeit. Therefore, the accurate identification of adulterated PR from different geographical origins is essential to protect consumer health and maintain fair trade practices.

Current identification methods for the geographical origin of foods and medicinal materials primarily include manual identification, chromatography, mass spectrometry, and DNA molecular identification [11–15]. However, manual identification requires extensive professional knowledge and is unsuitable for processing products (dry whole root, slice, powder). Chromatography, mass spectrometry, and DNA molecular identification are time-consuming, expensive, environmentally unfriendly, and complicated to operate [15–17]. Also, the adulteration of powder samples from different geographical origins has created challenges in these technologies. Therefore, there is an urgent need for a real-time, rapid, direct, efficient, and high-precision method to identify adulterated foods or medicinal materials from different regions.

Currently, some researchers use laser-induced breakdown spectroscopy (LIBS) and near-infrared spectroscopy (NIR) LIBS to identify geographical origin and adulterated foods or medicinal materials products, due to their advantages such as fast and in situ analysis [18–21]. For instance, Nie et al. employed visible and near-infrared spectroscopy (VNIR) for the quantitative analysis of the adulteration of *Sophora flavescens* powder or corn flour in Notoginseng powder, yielding a predictive R-squared value within the range of 0.86 to 0.94 [22]. Zhao et al. demonstrated the utility of LIBS in analyzing Chinese yam adulterated with cassava and the rhizome of winged yam, with R-squared values reaching 0.9570 [23]. Akin et al. employed LIBS in the analysis of corn and sorghum flour mixtures, achieving a good R-squared result of 0.965 [24]. Some researchers have also fused LIBS and VNIR to achieve better identification results [25]. For example, Zhao et al. used the fusion of LIBS and hyperspectral imaging (400–1000 nm) data to improve ginseng samples' geographical origin identification accuracy from 96.9% and 94.75% to 98.8% [26]. Collectively, these studies described above verified the potential of LIBS and NIR techniques in the identification of adulterated samples, especially the fusion of LIBS and VNIR, which has a better effect. Combining the elemental and molecular information obtained from these two techniques makes it possible to achieve a more comprehensive and accurate identification of adulterated materials. The subtle chemical and morphological changes between these materials of the same species but with different geographical origins pose a significant challenge for adulteration identification, and single-modal analysis makes it difficult to achieve a high level of identification accuracy. However, there is no report on the identification of adulterated PR from different geographical origins. For food quality identification, the research on the fusion method of LIBS and VNIR at the atomic and molecular levels is rarely studied.

Since foods or herbal medicines are rich in elemental and molecular information, based on the complementary advantages of LIBS in elemental analysis and VNIR in molecular analysis, together, they can provide a comprehensive assessment of the authenticity of PR. Therefore, the purpose of this study is to propose a deep learning model that effectively combines LIBS and VNIR to improve the accuracy of adulteration identification. We proposed an LIBS-VNIR fusion based on a deep learning network (LVDLNet) to detect adulteration in PR sourced from different regions in this study. The model was explained and verified from different aspects. Finally, the study confirmed that the fusion of LIBS and VNIR was feasible and effective in identifying adulterated PR. This work provides a powerful solution for the efficient, accurate, precise, and robust detection of adulteration, which is expected to enhance the integrity and safety of the food supply chain.

2. Samples and Experimental System
2.1. Sample Preparation

The highest quality PR, produced in Jiuhua Mountain and its surrounding areas in Qingyang County, southern Anhui, is certified as a PGI in China [6,27]. In this experiment, PR from Qingyang County was adulterated with cheaper PR from Dandong City, Liaoning Province. To ensure the authenticity of the samples, our staff personally collected the PR from their respective regions of origin. After the collection, the samples were cleansed with deionized water to eliminate surface dust and debris. Subsequently, they were sliced to a thickness of approximately 2 mm. These slices were then dried to constant weight at a controlled temperature of 60 °C within an electric blast drying oven (101-0B, Shaoxing Shangcheng Instrument Manufacturing Co., Ltd., Shaoxing, China). The dried samples were subsequently crushed and ground to a fine powder, passing through an 80-mesh sieve to ensure uniformity.

In actual market conditions, there are instances where cheaper Polygonati Rhizoma (PR) is used to completely impersonate more expensive PR from famous origins. There are also situations where the cheaper PR is mixed into the more expensive PR for sale, and a small amount of adulteration is insignificant for counterfeiters. To simulate the market adulteration practices, PR from Dandong City was systematically blended with PR from Qingyang County in incremental proportions ranging from 0% to 100% in steps of 20% (w/w). The adulterated samples contained 0, 20, 40, 60, 80, and 100% (w/w) adulterated levels. Specifically, the adulteration percentages refer to the weight percentage of PR from Dandong City in the mixture. For instance, a 0% level indicates pure PR from Qingyang County, while a 100% level signifies a mixture composed entirely of PR from Dandong City. Intermediate levels at 20%, 40%, 60%, and 80% represent the respective proportions of the Dandong City PR in the blend. The resulting mixtures were then compacted into pellets, each weighing two grams, using an electric tablet press exerting a substantial pressure of 24 tons over one minute. The pressed pellets, characterized by a thickness of approximately 3 mm and a diameter of 20 mm, were employed for our subsequent analyses. Two replicate samples were made for each concentration gradient to eliminate individual differences in samples. A total of 12 pressed pellets were prepared for measurement without further treatment. To evaluate the robustness of our proposed model, we also prepared another batch of samples by blending PR from Baise City in Guangxi Province with authentic PR from Qingyang County, adhering to the stringent criteria outlined in our previous methodology.

2.2. Setup and Measurement

The schematic diagram of the experimental setup used in this work is shown in Figure 1. This experimental setup mainly consisted of two parts: one was the VNIR acquisition setup, and the other was the LIBS acquisition setup. The VNIR spectra of the samples were collected first. All VNIR spectra were collected using a VNIR spectrometer (QE65pro, spectral ranges: 350–1100 nm; Ocean Optics, Inc., Dunedin, USA) equipped with a Halogen lamp light source (Avalight-HAL-Mini, Avantes B.V., Apeldoom, Netherlands). The samples were placed on an X-Y-Z motion platform (DZY110TA-3Z, Beijing Jiangyun Juli Technology Co., Ltd., Beijing, China) to enable spectral collection at different positions. For the spectral collection process, a precision optical fiber probe was positioned perpendicularly above each sample, thereby enabling the acquisition of the diffuse reflectance spectra. The integration time for each scan was 10 milliseconds, and each spectrum was obtained by averaging ten consecutive scans at each spatial point. In total, 100 distinct spectra per pellet sample were collected at 100 different spatial points. Consequently, for each proportion (adulteration level) of the adulterated samples, we amassed 200 spectra, culminating in a comprehensive dataset comprising 1200 VNIR spectra for six adulteration levels. Each VNIR spectrum had a dimension of 1×997.

After the VNIR acquisition, the samples were moved to the LIBS acquisition setup through the displacement platform. For the LIBS acquisition setup, a Q-switched Nd: YAG laser (Beamtech Optronics, Nimma-400; pulse duration: 8 ns; flattened Gaussian beam; Beamtech Optronics Co., Ltd., Beijing, China) operating at 532 nm, 1 Hz, and 130 mJ was used as the ablation source. The laser beam was reflected by a 45° mirror and focused by a quartz lens (focal length: 150 mm) onto the sample surface to generate plasmas. The plasma emission was collected by a collector and transmitted by fiber to a six-channel spectrometer (AvaSpec-ULS4096CL-EVO; spectral ranges: 196–874 nm; minimum gate width: 9 μs; Avantes B.V., Apeldoom, Netherlands). The gate delay and width were set to 2 μs, and

9 µs, respectively. A digital delay generator (LDG 3.0, Wuhan NRD Laser Engineering Co., Ltd., Wuhan, China) synchronized the laser and spectrograph. The experiment was conducted in the air atmosphere. For each pellet sample, 400 spectra were obtained and then averaged to 100 spectra to improve the stability of spectral intensity. Thus, 200 spectra for each proportion and 1200 spectra in total were obtained. Each LIBS spectrum had a dimension of 1 × 24,564.

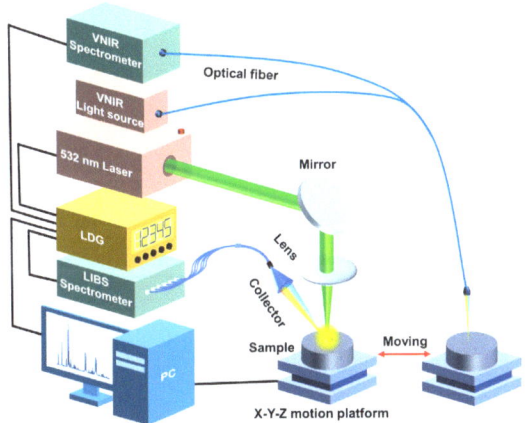

Figure 1. A schematic diagram of the experimental setup.

3. Method

3.1. The Framework of LVDLNet

To realize the identification of adulteration, we propose the LVDLNet framework shown in Figure 2. The proposed LVDLNet includes three main parts: DL-LIBS, which extracts element information; DL-VNIR, which extracts molecular information; and the information fusion part.

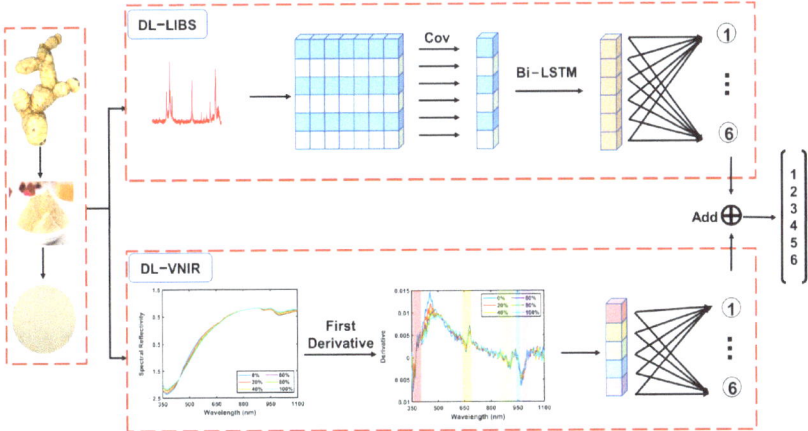

Figure 2. The framework of the proposed LVDLNet. (DL-LIBS: LIBS data processing based on deep learning; DL-VNIR: VNIR data processing based on deep learning; Cov: convolution; Bi-LSTM: bidirectional long short-term memory; Add: Add function; A box of a certain color corresponds to boxes or region of the same color; Numbers 1 to 6 represent the classification results of different adulteration levels).

3.2. Element Information Extraction by DL-LIBS

The LIBS spectrum can provide element information. The LIBS spectrum lines of PR from two different origins are shown in Figure 3. It can be seen that the LIBS spectral lines of PR from different origins are similar and contain the same elements, with variations primarily in intensity. Distinguishing the origin based solely on individual elemental spectral lines poses challenges, particularly when PR from different sources is mixed. Hence, employing chemometrics becomes essential for discerning these differences.

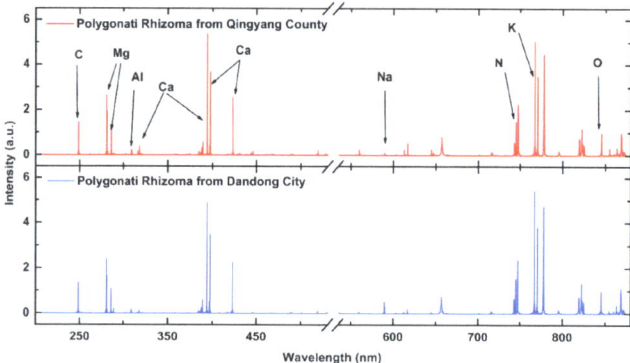

Figure 3. The LIBS spectra of Polygonati Rhizoma from Qingyang County and Dandong City.

The characteristic dimension of LIBS full spectrum is 24,564, which contains much invalid information. To reduce background and noise interference, researchers usually select the spectral peak of the element spectral line for analysis [28,29]. Only a few researchers selected the spectral interval (the interval of spectral line profile), which contains the characteristics of spectral wing and the Full Width at Half Maximum (FWHM) [30]. Selecting only the spectral peak will lead the loss of some effective information. Therefore, the selection of a spectral line profile interval is considered in this study. Specifically, for the analysis of PR, we have identified 18 elemental spectral lines with robust signal quality. These lines, with varying numbers of data points across their waveform intervals, are detailed in Table 1. It is observed that each spectral line is characterized by a unique distribution of points, with an average of approximately 14 points. Figure 4 illustrates the waveform intervals for two typical elemental lines: (a) Si I 288.17 nm, which comprises 7 points; and (b) Ca II 396.79 nm, which includes 22 points. Notably, the central 14 points of Ca II 396.79 nm can contain almost the entire waveform of the spectral line, exceeding the FWHM while retaining the critical information for analysis.

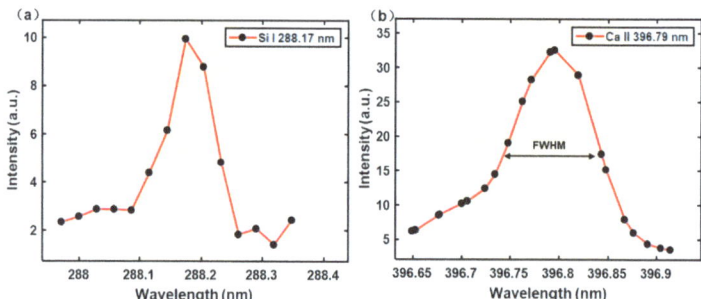

Figure 4. The interval of two typical elemental lines: (**a**) Si I 288.17 nm and (**b**) Ca II 396.79 nm. (The yellow area represents the coverage of the selected element spectral line waveform interval; FWHM: Full Width at Half Maximum).

Table 1. The LIBS elements' spectral interval and number of points.

Elements	Wavelength (nm)	Interval (nm)	Points	Operation	Points after Operation
C	247.86	247.72–248.04	11	Zero Padding	14
Mg	280.28	280.16–280.46	11	Zero Padding	14
Mg	285.23	285.08–285.37	11	Zero Padding	14
Si	288.17	288.09–288.26	7	Zero Padding	14
Al	309.29	309.23–309.36	10	Zero Padding	14
Ca	315.89	315.79–315.98	14	Retention	14
Ca	317.93	317.83–318.08	18	Interception	14
Ca	393.34	393.12–393.51	17	Interception	14
Ca	396.79	396.65–396.94	22	Interception	14
Ca	422.64	422.49–422.75	11	Zero Padding	14
Na	588.99	588.90–589.11	14	Retention	14
Na	589.59	589.52–598.71	14	Retention	14
N	742.53	742.30–742.75	9	Zero Padding	14
N	744.35	744.07–744.79	14	Retention	14
N	746.89	746.66–747.38	14	Retention	14
K	766.55	766.23–766.92	14	Retention	14
K	769.89	769.62–770.31	14	Retention	14
O	844.64	844.38–844.96	14	Retention	14

To extract elemental information from the LIBS spectrum effectively, we introduce a deep learning model, as illustrated in Figure 5, termed DL-LIBS. This model initiates the extraction process by performing a convolution operation on the elemental spectral interval to capture the waveform information inherent to each line. To simplify this operation, we standardized the size of the convolution kernel to ensure that it encompassed the complete waveform of each spectral line. Given that 14 data points can contain almost the entire waveform of the vast majority of spectral lines, we set 14 as the convolution kernel size. This selection ensured that the kernel width was sufficient to cover the spectral line's FWHM, thereby providing a robust basis for the convolution operation.

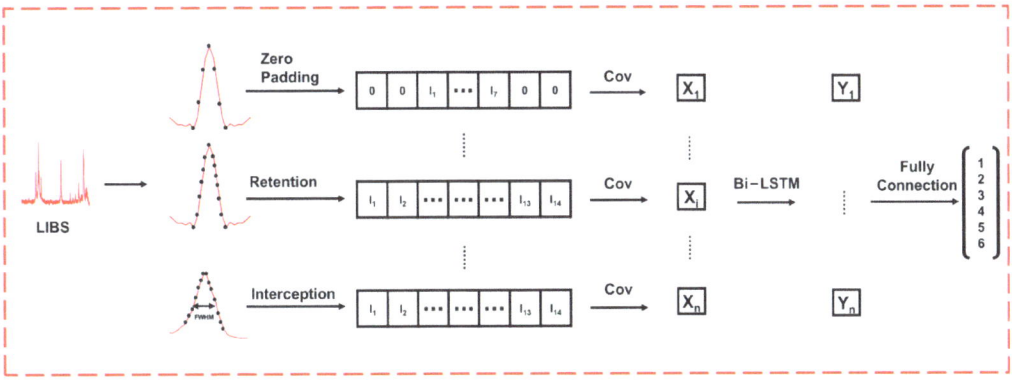

Figure 5. The framework of DL-LIBS. (LIBS: Laser-induced breakdown spectroscopy).

To standardize the data to a consistent set of 14 points, we employed a triad of strategies tailored to varying spectral profiles: (a) Zero Padding: When the spectral interval comprised fewer than 14 data points, we increased the interval with zero values at both sides, thereby expanding the point total to 14; (b) Retention: For intervals that naturally aligned with the 14-point criterion, we maintained the existing data points without alteration; (c) Interception: When the spectral interval exceeded 14 points, we selectively extracted a central subset of 14 points, while ensuring that this selection spanned beyond the FWHM to preserve the most representative segment of the spectral line. The treatment of each spectral line interval is also shown in Table 1. These standardization strategies allow for a uniform input into the subsequent stages of the model. After the convolution operation, the 18 result values obtained from the 18 spectral lines were fed into the bidirectional long short-term memory (Bi-LSTM) network. The network can identify the nonlinear relationship between spectral lines, improving the accuracy of element information extraction. Next, the extracted LIBS element information was input into the fully connected layer to achieve preliminary classification.

3.3. Molecular Information Extraction by DL-VNIR

Given the challenges in distinguishing mixed adulterated PR using elemental information alone, this study introduces the utilization of VNIR molecular information to augment the identification analysis. The VNIR spectra of PR with different adulteration concentrations are shown in Figure 6. The VNIR spectra of PR elucidate the presence of multiple absorption bands, with the band situated at approximately 670 nm corresponding to the characteristic chlorophyll absorption band [31]. Additionally, the band observed near 920 nm is associated with the second overtone of the O-H stretching vibration, while the band at 970 nm corresponds to the second overtone of another O-H stretching mode [32]. It can be seen that the VNIR spectra with different adulteration degrees have higher similarity and slightly different intensities.

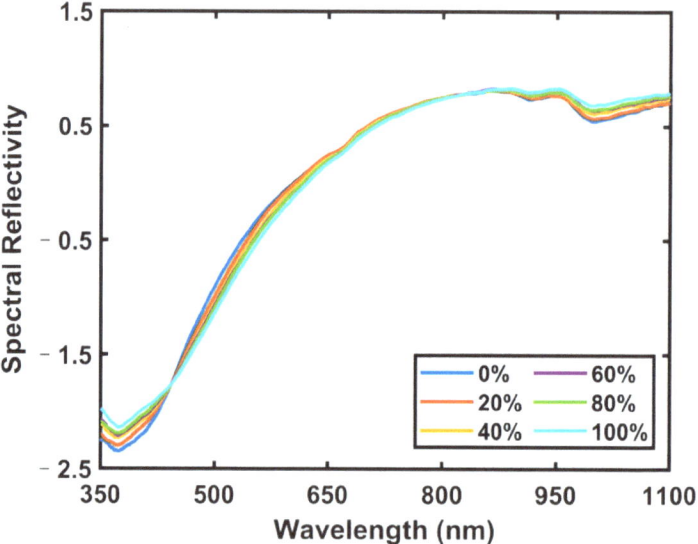

Figure 6. The VNIR spectra of Polygonati Rhizoma with different adulteration concentrations.

To extract effective molecular information from the VNIR spectra, we present the framework for the DL-VNIR model in Figure 7. The complexity of near-infrared spectra, characterized by significant overlap and discontinuity, poses a challenge to the direct extraction of component-related information and the subsequent provision of spectral analysis. Unlike discrete points, near-infrared spectra are often manifested as broad bands, a consequence of the myriad vibrational and rotational modes through which molecules interact with light, leading to an extensive array of absorption features. Conventional approaches to feature selection in near-infrared spectroscopy, such as peak and trough detection, have focused on isolated points within these spectral features, often overlooking the information contained within the complete waveform [33,34]. Unlike these traditional methods, our strategy involved an initial selection of the waveband data encompassing both peaks and troughs. The selected intervals of VNIR are shown in Table 2. This selection process targeted five specific wavebands, each representing a significant peak or trough. By employing this refined approach, we effectively condensed the original VNIR data dimensionality from 1044 to 375, retaining valid information while reducing the complexity of the dataset.

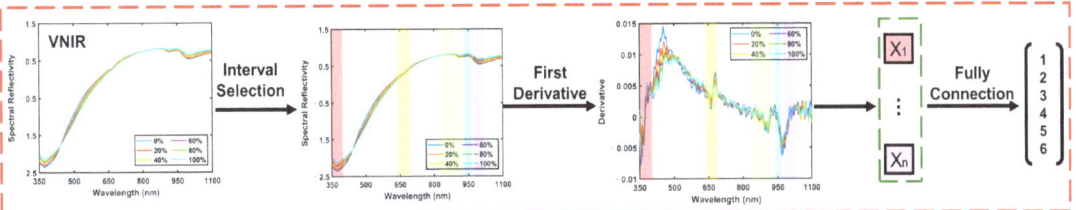

Figure 7. The framework of DL-VNIR. (VNIR: visible and near-infrared spectroscopy; Different colored areas represent different intervals of selection. Boxes of different colors correspond to intervals of the same color).

Table 2. The selected intervals of VNIR.

Interval (nm)	Points
350.00–400.02	63
639.88–690.76	67
830.92–930.41	136
940.65–960.35	27
966.90–1026.31	82

Subsequently, we computed the first derivative of the selected intervals, capitalizing on each waveform's unique degree of change characteristic. We could quantify the absorption variation rate across specific wavelength ranges by utilizing the spectrum slope. This approach effectively mitigated the interference from noise and baseline fluctuations, thereby enhancing the sensitivity of the analysis to subtle changes in sample concentration, composition, or structural attributes [31]. Such optimization is instrumental in elevating the precision of VNIR spectral analysis. The calculated waveform slopes were fed into a fully connected layer. Ultimately, this facilitated the extraction of molecular information and enabled VNIR to preliminary classify the samples.

3.4. Information Fusion

In this study, we harnessed the complementary strengths of LIBS and VNIR to perform an analysis of the samples. LIBS provides an in-depth elemental fingerprint, while VNIR offers a detailed molecular profile. Integrating these two modalities is essential for thoroughly understanding the sample characteristics. In the information fusion part, we adopted the Add function to amalgamate LIBS and VNIR data, which is an effective approach in dual-mode data fusion. By combining the data of LIBS and VNIR, this method maintains the integrity and unique attributes of element and molecular information and avoids the possibility of excessive information mixing. The flexibility of the Add function makes it suitable for processing input data of different dimensions and effectively avoids the loss of information [35]. After the operation of the Add function, the Add feature vector was sent to the classification layer to obtain the final results. This final step was crucial as it translated the integrated information into a definitive classification outcome.

3.5. Implementation Details

Both LIBS and VNIR obtained 1200 spectra. The dataset was randomly divided into a training set, validation set, and test set according to the ratio of 7:1:2. Thus, the dataset had 840 pairs for training, 120 for validating, and 240 for testing. The training set was used to train the model to establish a prediction model. The validation set was a set of samples left separately during the model training process, which was used to evaluate the performance of the model during the training process and to adjust the parameters and select the model. During the training process, by evaluating the performance of the model on the validation set, the overfitting or underfitting of the model could be found in time, and the hyperparameters of the model could be adjusted according to the results of the validation set. The test set was used to evaluate the final performance and generalization ability of the model. It was a dataset used to simulate the performance of the model in real scenes. All the results presented in this study are test set results. To avoid overfitting, we used data enhancement technology in the training set. Specifically, by adding white noise to the spectral data, and then combining the original spectral data with the spectrum after adding noise, the data expansion of the training set sample was realized. In addition, in the model design, batch normalization and a Dropout layer were added to reduce the risk of overfitting of the model.

In this work, the macro-average evaluation criteria was used to evaluate the model performance. The accuracy (Acc), macro-precision (Mac_P), macro-recall (Mac_R), and macro-F measure (Mac_F) were applied as evaluation metrics [36]. Acc is the ratio of the number of correctly classified samples to the total number of samples. Mac_P is the arithmetic mean of the precision of each category, where the precision is the proportion of the actual positive samples in the predicted positive samples. Mac_R is the arithmetic mean of the recall of each category, where the recall is the proportion of the actual positive sample and the predicted positive sample. Mac_F is the weighted harmonic average of precision and recall, providing a single score that balances both the precision and recall of the model. These metrics offer a comprehensive assessment of the model's predictive capabilities and are essential for understanding the reliability of our results. The data processing was carried out on PyTorch 2.0 with a PC of INTEL i7 12700KF CPU (Intel Corporation, Santa Clara, USA), 32G DDR4 RAM (Kingston Technology Corporation, Fountain Valley, USA), and an NVIDIA RTX 3060 GPU (NVIDIA Corporation, Santa Clara, USA)). The size of the GPU was 12 G. The epoch and the batch size were set to 500 and 32, respectively. The learning rate was all set to 0.0005.

4. Results and Discussion

4.1. Visualization Analysis with t-SNE

To observe the clustering effect of different adulterated samples, the full spectral data were visually analyzed with t-SNE. Figure 8 shows the visualization result of t-SNE. It can be seen from the figure that there is a particular clustering effect for different adulterated samples, indicating the feasibility of classification using both LIBS and VNIR data.

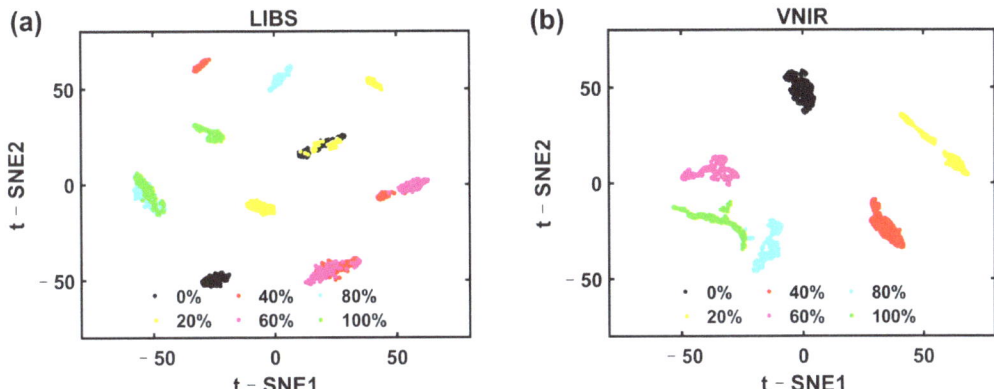

Figure 8. The visualization results with t-SNE based on (**a**) LIBS and (**b**) VNIR.

4.2. Comparison with Different Baseline Models

In LVDLNet, we used DL-LIBS to extract element information and make a preliminary classification, and DL-VNIR was used to extract molecular information and make a preliminary classification. Then, the two kinds of information were fused to realize the final classification. Table 3 shows the results of a single modality and dual modalities. The four evaluation metrics of DL-LIBS and DL-VNIR were less than 88%, and 94%, respectively. However, the LVDLNet model achieved good results. The *Acc*, *Mac_F*, *Mac_P*, and *Mac_R* of the LVDLNet model were 98.75%, 98.50%, 98.78%, and 98.75%, respectively. The four indicators of the LVDLNet model all exceeded 98%, demonstrating its ability to effectively synthesize LIBS and VNIR data for the enhanced classification accuracy of adulterated PR. Additionally, the confusion matrices for the baseline models are depicted in Figure 9, which facilitates a clear comparison of the classification proficiency between the LVDLNet model and the individual DL-LIBS and DL-VNIR models. For example, in the case of a 0% adulteration level, seven spectral lines from the LIBS data were mistakenly identified as corresponding to a 60% adulteration level, while three spectral lines from the VNIR data suffered the same error. The predictive accuracy for all these lines was successfully rectified upon implementing the fusion process. This further shows that the fusion of LIBS element information and VNIR molecular information can improve classification accuracy.

Table 3. Comparison results of baseline models.

Models	Acc	Mac_F	Mac_P	Mac_R
DL-LIBS	0.8708	0.8710	0.8780	0.8708
DL-VNIR	0.9375	0.9373	0.9378	0.9375
LVDLNet	0.9875	0.9850	0.9878	0.9875

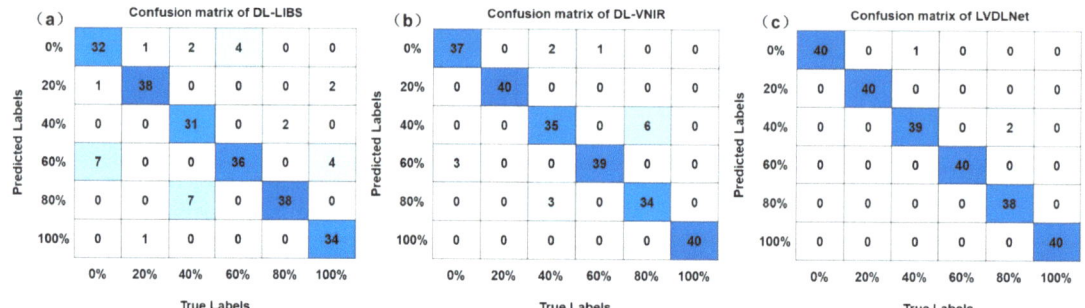

Figure 9. The confusion matrix of baseline modes: (**a**) DL-LIBS, (**b**) DL-VNIR, (**c**) LVDLNet.

4.3. Effectiveness of Interval Selection

To verify the effectiveness of the selected intervals in this work, the classification effects of different feature inputs were compared. In the comparison, the LIBS spectral peak and intervals were selected as the feature inputs, and the VNIR intervals and full spectra were chosen as the feature inputs. In addition to the DL-LIBS and DL-VNIR models, Principal Component Analysis (PCA) and Support Vector Machine (SVM) were used for verification. PCA and SVM are commonly used in spectral analysis for feature extraction and pattern recognition algorithms, respectively.

The results are shown in Table 4. For DL-LIBS, when the LIBS peak was used as the input, the result was poor, and the four evaluation metrics were about 50%. However, when the LIBS interval was used as the input, the metrics increased to over 87%. For DL-VNIR, the VNIR full-spectra analysis showed slightly higher results than the selected intervals. However, the difference in this result was considered negligible when considering that the intervals with fewer features achieved a classification accuracy similar to full spectra. When using the PCA-SVM model, the spectral interval could also produce better results for LIBS and VNIR data. The above results verify the effectiveness of the selected intervals for the information extraction of LIBS and VNIR in this work. Compared to the LIBS peaks, the LIBS intervals contain more spectral information. Compared to the VNIR full spectra, the selected VNIR intervals essentially contain the information of the full spectrum.

Table 4. Comparison of results under different feature inputs.

Models	Input	Acc	Mac_F	Mac_P	Mac_R
DL-LIBS	LIBS Peaks	0.5042	0.4909	0.4783	0.5042
	LIBS Intervals	0.8708	0.8710	0.8780	0.8708
DL-VNIR	VNIR Intervals	0.9375	0.9373	0.9378	0.9375
	VNIR Full Spectra	0.9458	0.9452	0.9450	0.9458
PCA-SVM	LIBS Peaks	0.7875	0.7871	0.7873	0.7875
	LIBS Intervals	0.8250	0.8236	0.8233	0.8250
	VNIR Intervals	0.9000	0.9006	0.9014	0.9000
	VNIR Full Spectra	0.8958	0.8928	0.8969	0.8958

4.4. Comparison with Conventional Machine Learning

To evaluate the performance of the model, the result of the deep learning model proposed in this work was compared with the results of conventional machine learning models.

The analysis encompassed four distinct conventional machine learning classifiers: Linear Discriminant Analysis (LDA), K-Nearest Neighbors (KNN), SVM, and Extreme Learning Machine (ELM). Similarly, PCA was first used for the feature extraction of selected LIBS and VNIR intervals. After feature extraction, the features were input into the classification model for classification. The classification results for the LIBS and VNIR datasets are presented in Table 5.

Table 5. Comparison results of conventional machine learning and deep learning.

Models	Acc		Mac_F		Mac_P		Mac_R	
	LIBS	VNIR	LIBS	VNIR	LIBS	VNIR	LIBS	VNIR
PCA-LDA	0.6083	0.8750	0.6016	0.8732	0.5976	0.8723	0.6083	0.8750
PCA-KNN	0.7625	0.8708	0.7626	0.8708	0.7643	0.8723	0.7625	0.8708
PCA-SVM	0.8250	0.9000	0.8236	0.9006	0.8233	0.9014	0.8250	0.9000
PCA-ELM	0.7333	0.8792	0.7342	0.8757	0.7406	0.8827	0.7333	0.8792
DL-LIBS	0.8708	-	0.8710	-	0.8780	-	0.8708	-
DL-VNIR	-	0.9375	-	0.9373	-	0.9378	-	0.9378
LVDLNet	0.9875		0.9850		0.9878		0.9875	

Among the four conventional machine learning models, PCA-SVM achieved the best results for both LIBS and VNIR data. However, the deep learning model proposed in this work attained better results. For LIBS data, DL-LIBS improved the results of PCA-SVM from about 82% to more than 87%. For VNIR data, DL-VNIR improved the results of PCA-SVM from about 90% to more than 93%. Moreover, by the fusion of LIBS and VNIR, the LVDLNet model improved the indicators to more than 98%. This demonstrates the superiority of the proposed deep learning model over conventional machine learning technology. Deep learning models can better capture nonlinear relationships in data and adapt to complex and variable data than conventional machine learning.

4.5. Universal Verification

To establish the broad applicability of our model, additional verification was conducted using adulterated samples which blended PR from Baise City in Guangxi Province with the authentic PR from Qingyang County. The results are shown in Table 6. As shown in the table, the results of LVDLNet were also better than the single-modality results of DL-LIBS and DL-VNIR. The Acc, Mac_F, Mac_P, and Mac_R of the LVDLNet model were 96.25%, 96.25%, 96.30%, and 96.25%, respectively. LVDLNet raised the evaluation indexes from 87% of DL-LIBS and 86% of DL-VNIR to over 96%. This verifies that the models proposed in this study can effectively identify adulterated PR between different geographical origins, proving the effectiveness and robustness of the proposed models.

Table 6. Results of universal verification.

Models	Acc	Mac_F	Mac_P	Mac_R
DL-LIBS	0.8792	0.8776	0.8777	0.8792
DL-VNIR	0.8625	0.8563	0.8607	0.8625
LVDLNet	0.9625	0.9625	0.9630	0.9625

5. Conclusions

Food adulteration identification is essential for protecting consumers' interests, but no universal method has been widely adopted, especially in industrial scenarios. This study presented a novel deep learning framework, LIBS-VNIR fusion based on a deep learning network (LVDLNet), for identifying adulterated Polygonati Rhizoma (PR). In the LVDLNet model, an interval point standardization strategy in LIBS and a refined peak and trough focus in VNIR data processing improved signal clarity and extraction efficiency. By integrating LIBS elemental information with VNIR molecular information, we enhanced the accuracy of authentication. The LVDLNet model achieved good results, with the accuracy (*Acc*), macro-F measure (*Mac_F*), macro-precision (*Mac_P*), and macro-recall (*Mac_R*) being 98.75%, 98.50%, 98.78%, and 98.75%, respectively. It significantly enhanced the classification evaluation metrics, increasing them from approximately 87% for LIBS and 93% for VNIR to over 98%. Additionally, tests on various adulterated source samples further confirmed the efficacy of the LVDLNet model, with all four classification metrics improved from about 87% for LIBS and 86% for VNIR to above 96%. In addition, this work confirmed the classification effect of the proposed method from different feature inputs and conventional machine learning models. All in all, this study presented a pioneering deep learning framework that synergizes LIBS and VNIR to effectively detect adulterated PR, offering a novel perspective and methodology for identifying food adulteration. Future work can apply this deep learning framework to a wider range of samples, including more different origins and different types of foods, which may be affected by adulteration.

Author Contributions: Conceptualization, L.G. and H.S.; methodology, F.C.; software, W.H.; validation, M.Z., W.H. and F.C.; formal analysis, F.C. and M.Z.; investigation, F.C.; resources, L.G.; data curation, F.C. and M.Z.; writing—original draft preparation, F.C.; writing—review and editing, F.C., M.Z., H.S. and L.G.; visualization, M.Z. and W.H.; supervision, L.G. and H.S.; project administration, L.G. and H.S.; funding acquisition, L.G. All authors have read and agreed to the published version of the manuscript.

Funding: This research was financially supported by the National Natural Science Foundation of China (No. 62075069).

Institutional Review Board Statement: Not applicable.

Informed Consent Statement: Not applicable.

Data Availability Statement: The original contributions presented in the study are included in the article, further inquiries can be directed to the corresponding authors.

Conflicts of Interest: The authors declare no conflicts of interest.

References

1. Song, Y.; Guo, T.; Liu, S.; Gao, Y.; Wang, Y. Identification of *Polygonati rhizoma* in Three Species and from Different Producing Areas of Each Species Using HS-GC-IMS. *LWT* **2022**, *172*, 114142. [CrossRef]
2. Zhao, L.; Xu, C.; Zhou, W.; Li, Y.; Xie, Y.; Hu, H.; Wang, Z. *Polygonati rhizoma* with the Homology of Medicine and Food: A Review of Ethnopharmacology, Botany, Phytochemistry, Pharmacology and Applications. *J. Ethnopharmacol.* **2023**, *309*, 116296. [CrossRef]
3. Pan, M.; Wu, Y.; Sun, C.; Ma, H.; Ye, X.; Li, X. *Polygonati rhizoma*: A Review on the Extraction, Purification, Structural Characterization, Biosynthesis of the Main Secondary Metabolites and Anti-Aging Effects. *J. Ethnopharmacol.* **2024**, *327*, 118002. [CrossRef] [PubMed]
4. Zhao, P.; Zhao, C.; Li, X.; Gao, Q.; Huang, L.; Xiao, P.; Gao, W. The Genus Polygonatum: A Review of Ethnopharmacology, Phytochemistry and Pharmacology. *J. Ethnopharmacol.* **2018**, *214*, 274–291. [CrossRef]
5. He, Y.; Chen, Z.; Nie, X.; Wang, D.; Zhang, Q.; Peng, T.; Zhang, C.; Wu, D.; Zhang, J. Recent Advances in Polysaccharides from Edible and Medicinal *Polygonati rhizoma*: From Bench to Market. *Int. J. Biol. Macromol.* **2022**, *195*, 102–116. [CrossRef]
6. Du, L.; Nong, M.-N.; Zhao, J.-M.; Peng, X.-M.; Zong, S.-H.; Zeng, G.-F. *Polygonatum sibiricum* Polysaccharide Inhibits Osteoporosis by Promoting Osteoblast Formation and Blocking Osteoclastogenesis through Wnt/β-Catenin Signalling Pathway. *Sci. Rep.* **2016**, *6*, 32261. [CrossRef]
7. Liu, T.; Xu, B. Polygonatum cyrtonema *Hua* (Huangjing). In *Dietary Chinese Herbs: Chemistry, Pharmacology and Clinical Evidence*; Liu, Y., Wang, Z., Zhang, J., Eds.; Springer: Vienna, Austria, 2015; pp. 213–218.
8. Lamardi, S.N.S.; Ghambariyn, S.; Ardekani, M.R.S.; Amin, G. Major Phytosterol from *Polygonatum orientale* Desf. Rhizome. *J. Pharm. Health Sci.* **2017**, *5*, 43–49.
9. Fu, H.; Wei, L.; Chen, H.; Yang, X.; Kang, L.; Hao, Q.; Zhou, L.; Zhan, Z.; Liu, Z.; Yang, J.; et al. Combining Stable C, N, O, H, Sr Isotope and Multi-Element with Chemometrics for Identifying the Geographical Origins and Farming Patterns of Huangjing Herb. *J. Food Compos. Anal.* **2021**, *102*, 103972. [CrossRef]
10. Cheng, H.; Liu, J.; Xu, J.; Shi, S.; Yu, N.; Peng, D.; Xing, L.; Wu, Z. Study on Suitable Areas of *Polygonatum cyrtonema* Hua in Anhui Province. *Chin. J. Inf. Tradit. Chin. Med.* **2021**, *28*, 6–10.

11. Martín-Torres, S.; Jiménez-Carvelo, A.M.; González-Casado, A.; Cuadros-Rodríguez, L. Authentication of the Geographical Origin and the Botanical Variety of Avocados Using Liquid Chromatography Fingerprinting and Deep Learning Methods. *Chemom. Intell. Lab. Syst.* **2020**, *199*, 103960. [CrossRef]
12. Wang, F.; Zhao, H.; Yu, C.; Tang, J.; Wu, W.; Yang, Q. Determination of the Geographical Origin of Maize (*Zea mays* L.)) Using Mineral Element Fingerprints. *J. Sci. Food Agric.* **2020**, *100*, 1294–1300. [CrossRef] [PubMed]
13. Esteki, M.; Farajmand, B.; Amanifar, S.; Barkhordari, R.; Ahadiyan, Z.; Dashtaki, E.; Mohammadlou, M.; Vander Heyden, Y. Classification and Authentication of Iranian Walnuts According to Their Geographical Origin Based on Gas Chromatographic Fatty Acid Fingerprint Analysis Using Pattern Recognition Methods. *Chemom. Intell. Lab. Syst.* **2017**, *171*, 251–258. [CrossRef]
14. Muñoz-Falcón, J.E.; Prohens, J.; Vilanova, S.; Ribas, F.; Castro, A.; Nuez, F. Distinguishing a Protected Geographical Indication Vegetable (Almagro Eggplant) from Closely Related Varieties with Selected Morphological Traits and Molecular Markers. *J. Sci. Food Agric.* **2009**, *89*, 320–328. [CrossRef]
15. Jiao, J.; Jia, X.; Liu, P.; Zhang, Q.; Liu, F.; Ma, C.; Xi, P.; Liang, Z. Species Identification of *Polygonati rhizoma* in China by Both Morphological and Molecular Marker Methods. *Comptes Rendus Biol.* **2018**, *341*, 102–110. [CrossRef]
16. Kakouri, E.; Revelou, P.-K.; Kanakis, C.; Daferera, D.; Pappas, C.S.; Tarantilis, P.A. Authentication of the Botanical and Geographical Origin and Detection of Adulteration of Olive Oil Using Gas Chromatography, Infrared and Raman Spectroscopy Techniques: A Review. *Foods* **2021**, *10*, 1565. [CrossRef] [PubMed]
17. Epova, E.N.; Bérail, S.; Séby, F.; Vacchina, V.; Bareille, G.; Médina, B.; Sarthou, L.; Donard, O.F.X. Strontium Elemental and Isotopic Signatures of Bordeaux Wines for Authenticity and Geographical Origin Assessment. *Food Chem.* **2019**, *294*, 35–45. [CrossRef]
18. Senesi, G.S.; Cabral, J.; Menegatti, C.R.; Marangoni, B.; Nicolodelli, G. Recent Advances and Future Trends in LIBS Applications to Agricultural Materials and Their Food Derivatives: An Overview of Developments in the Last Decade (2010–2019). Part II. Crop Plants and Their Food Derivatives. *TrAC Trends Anal. Chem.* **2019**, *118*, 453–469. [CrossRef]
19. Fernandes Andrade, D.; Pereira-Filho, E.R.; Amarasiriwardena, D. Current Trends in Laser-Induced Breakdown Spectroscopy: A Tutorial Review. *Appl. Spectrosc. Rev.* **2021**, *56*, 98–114. [CrossRef]
20. Zhang, C.; Su, J. Application of near Infrared Spectroscopy to the Analysis and Fast Quality Assessment of Traditional Chinese Medicinal Products. *Acta Pharm. Sin. B* **2014**, *4*, 182–192. [CrossRef]
21. Eum, C.; Jang, D.; Kim, J.; Choi, S.; Cha, K.; Chung, H. Improving the Accuracy of Spectroscopic Identification of Geographical Origins of Agricultural Samples through Cooperative Combination of Near-Infrared and Laser-Induced Breakdown Spectroscopy. *Spectrochim. Acta Part B At. Spectrosc.* **2018**, *149*, 281–287. [CrossRef]
22. Nie, P.; Wu, D.; Sun, D.-W.; Cao, F.; Bao, Y.; He, Y. Potential of Visible and Near Infrared Spectroscopy and Pattern Recognition for Rapid Quantification of Notoginseng Powder with Adulterants. *Sensors* **2013**, *13*, 13820–13834. [CrossRef] [PubMed]
23. Zhao, Z.; Wang, Q.; Xu, X.; Chen, F.; Teng, G.; Wei, K.; Chen, G.; Cai, Y.; Guo, L. Accurate Identification and Quantification of Chinese Yam Powder Adulteration Using Laser-Induced Breakdown Spectroscopy. *Foods* **2022**, *11*, 1216. [CrossRef] [PubMed]
24. Akın, P.A.; Sezer, B.; Bean, S.R.; Peiris, K.; Tilley, M.; Apaydın, H.; Boyacı, İ.H. Analysis of Corn and Sorghum Flour Mixtures Using Laser-induced Breakdown Spectroscopy. *J. Sci. Food Agric.* **2021**, *101*, 1076–1084. [CrossRef] [PubMed]
25. Xu, Z.; Li, X.; Cheng, W.; Zhao, G.; Tang, L.; Yang, Y.; Wu, Y.; Zhang, P.; Wang, Q. Rapid and Accurate Determination Methods Based on Data Fusion of Laser-Induced Breakdown Spectra and near-Infrared Spectra for Main Elemental Contents in Compound Fertilizers. *Talanta* **2024**, *266*, 125004. [CrossRef]
26. Zhao, S.; Song, W.; Hou, Z.; Wang, Z. Classification of Ginseng According to Plant Species, Geographical Origin, and Age Using Laser-Induced Breakdown Spectroscopy and Hyperspectral Imaging. *J. Anal. At. Spectrom.* **2021**, *36*, 1704–1711. [CrossRef]
27. Liu, H.; Cheng, H.; Xu, J.; Hu, J.; Zhao, C.; Xing, L.; Wang, M.; Wu, Z.; Peng, D.; Yu, N.; et al. Genetic Diversity and Population Structure of *Polygonatum cyrtonema* Hua in China Using SSR Markers. *PLoS ONE* **2023**, *18*, e0290605. [CrossRef] [PubMed]
28. Ferreira, D.S.; Pereira, F.M.V.; Olivieri, A.C.; Pereira-Filho, E.R. Electronic Waste Analysis Using Laser-Induced Breakdown Spectroscopy (LIBS) and X-Ray Fluorescence (XRF): Critical Evaluation of Data Fusion for the Determination of Al, Cu and Fe. *Anal. Chim. Acta* **2024**, *1303*, 342522. [CrossRef]
29. Naseri, A.; Khalilzadeh, J.; Reza Darbani, S.M.; Akbari, M.R.; Eslamimajd, A. Laser-Induced Breakdown Spectroscopy Combined with Multivariate Linear Discriminant Analysis for Discriminating Different Growth Phases of Bacteria. *J. Anal. At. Spectrom.* **2024**, *39*, 1131–1141. [CrossRef]
30. Gong, A.; Guo, L.; Yu, Y.; Xia, Y.; Deng, X.; Hu, Z. Spectrum-Image Dual-Modality Fusion Empowered Accurate and Efficient Classification System for Traditional Chinese Medicine. *Inf. Fusion* **2024**, *101*, 101981. [CrossRef]
31. Zahir, S.A.D.M.; Omar, A.F.; Jamlos, M.F.; Azmi, M.A.M.; Muncan, J. A Review of Visible and Near-Infrared (Vis-NIR) Spectroscopy Application in Plant Stress Detection. *Sens. Actuators A Phys.* **2022**, *338*, 113468. [CrossRef]
32. Pissard, A.; Marques, E.J.N.; Dardenne, P.; Lateur, M.; Pasquini, C.; Pimentel, M.F.; Fernández Pierna, J.A.; Baeten, V. Evaluation of a Handheld Ultra-Compact NIR Spectrometer for Rapid and Non-Destructive Determination of Apple Fruit Quality. *Postharvest Biol. Technol.* **2021**, *172*, 111375. [CrossRef]
33. Yun, Y.-H.; Li, H.-D.; Deng, B.-C.; Cao, D.-S. An Overview of Variable Selection Methods in Multivariate Analysis of Near-Infrared Spectra. *TrAC Trends Anal. Chem.* **2019**, *113*, 102–115. [CrossRef]
34. Mehmood, T.; Liland, K.H.; Snipen, L.; Sæbø, S. A Review of Variable Selection Methods in Partial Least Squares Regression. *Chemom. Intell. Lab. Syst.* **2012**, *118*, 62–69. [CrossRef]

35. Zhang, D.; Nayak, R.; Bashar, M.A. Exploring Fusion Strategies in Deep Learning Models for Multi-Modal Classification. In *Data Mining. AusDM 2021. Communications in Computer and Information Science*; Xu, Y., Wang, R., Lord, A., Boo, Y.L., Nayak, R., Zhao, Y., Williams, G., Eds.; Springer: Singapore, 2021; pp. 102–117.
36. Zhou, Z.-H. Model Selection and Evaluation. In *Machine Learning*; Zhou, Z.-H., Ed.; Springer: Singapore, 2021; pp. 25–55.

Disclaimer/Publisher's Note: The statements, opinions and data contained in all publications are solely those of the individual author(s) and contributor(s) and not of MDPI and/or the editor(s). MDPI and/or the editor(s) disclaim responsibility for any injury to people or property resulting from any ideas, methods, instructions or products referred to in the content.

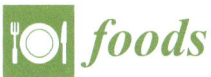

Article

Exploring the Influence of Soil Types on the Mineral Profile of Honey: Implications for Geographical Origin Prediction

Simona Schmidlová [1], Zdeňka Javůrková [1], Bohuslava Tremlová [1], Józef Hernik [2], Barbara Prus [2], Slavomír Marcinčák [3], Dana Marcinčáková [4], Pavel Štarha [5], Helena Čížková [6], Vojtěch Kružík [6], Zsanett Bodor [7], Csilla Benedek [7], Dalibor Titěra [8], Jana Boržíková [9] and Matej Pospiech [1],*

1. Department of Plant Origin Food Sciences, Faculty of Veterinary Hygiene and Ecology, University of Veterinary Sciences Brno, 612 42 Brno, Czech Republic; s.ljasovska@gmail.com (S.S.); javurkovaz@vfu.cz (Z.J.); tremlovab@vfu.cz (B.T.)
2. Department of Land Management and Landscape Architecture, Faculty of Environmental Engineering and Land Surveying, University of Agriculture in Krakow, 31-120 Krakow, Poland; jozef.hernik@urk.edu.pl (J.H.); barbara.prus@urk.edu.pl (B.P.)
3. Department of Food Hygiene, Technology and Safety, University of Veterinary Medicine and Pharmacy in Košice, 041 81 Košice, Slovakia; slavomir.marcincak@uvlf.sk
4. Department of Pharmacology and Toxicology, University of Veterinary Medicine and Pharmacy in Košice, 041 81 Košice, Slovakia; dana.marcincakova@uvlf.sk
5. Department of Computer Graphics and Geometry, Faculty of Mechanical Engineering, Brno University of Technology, 616 69 Brno, Czech Republic; starha@fme.vutbr.cz
6. Department of Food Preservation, Faculty of Food and Biochemical Technology, University of Chemistry and Technology, 160 00 Prague, Czech Republic; helena.cizkova@vscht.cz (H.Č.); vojtech.kruzik@vscht.cz (V.K.)
7. Department of Dietetics and Nutritional Science, Faculty of Health Sciences, Semmelweis University, 1088 Budapest, Hungary; zsanett.bodor93@gmail.com (Z.B.); benedek.csilla.se.etk@gmail.com (C.B.)
8. Bee Research Institute, Maslovice-Dol 94, 252 66 Libcice nad Vltavou, Czech Republic; titera@beedol.cz
9. State Veterinary and Food Institute Dolný Kubín, Veterinary and Food Institute Košice, Hlinková 1, 043 65 Košice, Slovakia; borzikova@svu-ke.sk
* Correspondence: mpospiech@vfu.cz

Abstract: Honey contains a wide range of inorganic substances. Their content can be influenced, i.e., by the type of soil on which the bee pasture is located. As part of this study, the mineral profile of 32 samples of honey from hobby beekeepers from the Czech Republic was evaluated and then compared with soil types in the vicinity of the beehive location. Pearson's correlation coefficient was used to express the relationship between mineral substances and soil type. There was a high correlation between antroposol and Zn (R = 0.98), Pb (R = 0.96), then between ranker and Mn (0.95), then regosol and Al (R = 0.97) ($p < 0.05$). A high negative correlation was found between regosol and Mg (R = −0.97), Cr (R = −0.98) and between redzinas and Al (R = −0.97) ($p < 0.05$). Both positive and negative high correlations were confirmed for phaeozem. The CART method subsequently proved that the characteristic elements for individual soil types are B, Ca, Mg, Ni, and Mn. The soil types of cambisol, fluvisol, gleysol, anthrosol, and kastanozem had the closest relationship with the elements mentioned, and it can therefore be assumed that their occurrence indicates the presence of these soil types within the range of beehive location.

Keywords: traces elements; Czech beekeepers; sustainability; GIS

1. Introduction

Honey is very variable in its composition. In addition to basic substances such as sugars and water, honey also contains a diverse array of mineral components, including essential minerals and potentially toxic elements. The composition of honey is strongly influenced by natural and anthropogenic influences. Although mineral substances and potentially toxic elements subgroups are less significant components of honey by volume, they play a vital role in evaluating its quality [1,2].

It is essential that honey is free of potential contaminating substances. It is estimated that the honey bee forages on plants growing in an area from 7 to 28 km^2, depending on their need for food and its availability [3]. Honey bees collect pollen as a source of amino acids, fats, minerals, proteins, starch, sterols and vitamins. A diverse selection of floral sources is required for a bee to get all her nutritional needs [4]. Honey bees interact with a variety of matrices that can be measured for contaminant accumulation, such as freshly collected pollen, honey, stored pollen, and beeswax. Honey composition is the result of many processes, is useful for gathering information about the environment, and can be a suitable bioindicator of environmental pollution [5,6].

The idea of using bees and honey in the field of the environment goes back to J. Svoboda (1961) and E. Crane (1984), who believed that bees could provide valuable data on the environmental impact the authors proved that potentially toxic elements such as Cd, Pb and metalloid As in bees and bee products correspond as indicators of environmental pollution [7,8]. In research from 1962, J. Svoboda's team recorded an increase in the content of the radionuclide strontium 90 in the environment through the monitoring of bees—most likely as a result of nuclear testing. In the following years, bees were increasingly used to monitor environmental pollution by potentially toxic elements in geological and urban surveys [9,10]. As Leita et al. (1996) [11] suggested, a network of hives located next to polluted areas can provide data for monitoring heavy metal emissions from specific sources. Ruschioni et al. (2013) [12] also show that trends in metal contamination correlate with weather patterns and anthropogenic activities in the region where samples were obtained. Honey has nutritional, medicinal, and prophylactic properties, which are contributed to by its chemical components. The concentration of mineral compounds ranges from 0.1% to 1.0%. In comparison with nectar honeys, honeydew honeys are higher in minerals, resulting in higher electrolytic conductivity [13]. Also, the mineral content influences the color and taste of honeys. The higher the quantity of metals and the darker the color is, the stronger the taste they will have [14]. The mineral profile is dominated by potassium, followed by calcium, magnesium, sodium, sulfur, and phosphorus. Trace elements include iron, copper, zinc, and manganese [15,16]. The main mineral substances come mainly from soil and nectar-bearing plants but can also come from anthropogenic sources [17,18].

There are relations between the mineral profile of honey and a soil type [19,20]. According to the international soil classification system, soils are divided into different groups, especially by particle size, texture classes, and mineral composition [21,22].

The Czech Republic has a very diverse spectrum of soil types. The mountains are dominated by coniferous forests, under which podzol soils are formed. In the lowlands, which are a very warm region, chernozems are found. The occurrence of different types of soils is also influenced by altitude, slope, and biota. For example, alluvial soils, for the formation of which sufficient water is essential, are most often found near watercourses [23]. The Czech Geological Survey provides a detailed map of soil types, of which it is possible to evaluate the connection with the location of bee colonies. The mutual relationship between soil type and mineral substances in honey can be used to predict the geographical origin of honey. The aim of this study was to verify the influence of soil types according to the international classification on the mineral profile of honey depending on the total area of the soil type in the beehive location. A partial goal was to verify the correlation dependence of the mineral composition of honey and soil type and to describe the mineral profile depending on the soil type.

2. Materials and Methods

In this study, 32 multifloral honey samples were collected and harvested between 2019 and 2020 in the Czech Republic, Moravia. The honeys were collected from hobby beekeepers and harvested at the University of Veterinary Sciences with the same equipment to eliminate the impact of different harvesters. The pollen profile and locality are summarized in Table S1 and Figure S1. The quantitative melissopalynology analysis was performed with semiautomated acquisition according to the previous study [24].

The World Reference Base for Soil Resources (WRB) classification system [22] was used. The area of WRB for the beehive location was processed by QGIS 3.28 (QGIS Development Team, 2023); soil data were taken from the national geoportal https://geoportal.gov.cz/ (accessed on 1st April 2024) [25], where the soils are classified according to new soil systems [26].

In the collected data, 16 soil types were observed with different area sizes. The area and frequency of each soil type are detailed in Table 1. In general, hive locations were represented by more than one soil type, and the same soil type was observed in different hive locations. The evaluated area of soil type was represented by approximate bee flying distances of 3 km. In total, the 28.27 km^2 for each hive location were evaluated. Honey samples were collected in situ by the research team directly from the hives. The GPS coordinates, land use data, and botanical profiles of the surrounding area were documented in a detailed questionnaire. The GPS coordinates of each hive served as the central point for a 3 km radius buffer zone. Within this defined buffer zone, soil-type data were extracted and analyzed.

Table 1. Soil type frequency and area.

Categories	Frequencies	Lands Area (km^2)	%
Anthrosol	8	24.147	2.669
Cambisol	26	427.149	47.218
Chernozem	7	92.438	10.218
Fluvisol	26	95.405	10.546
Gleysol	21	36.620	4.048
Kastanozem	14	66.888	7.394
Luvisol	13	52.301	5.781
Pararendzina	6	20.171	2.230
Pelozem	6	31.849	3.521
Phaeozem	2	8.905	0.984
Podzol	2	10.307	1.139
Pseudogley	15	20.158	2.228
Ranker	5	1.242	0.137
Regosol	7	11.010	1.217
Rendzinas	4	2.663	0.294
Water Bodies	8	3.388	0.375

The mineral content was determined by Inductively Coupled Plasma Mass Spectrometry ICP-MS 7900 (Agilent, Santa Clara, CA, USA) according to the STN EN 15763 [27], UNI EN 13805 [28], and UNI EN 13804 [29] in honey samples. The B, Na, Mg, Al, K, Ca, Cr, Mn, Fe, Ni, Cu, Zn, As, and Pb content were determined in each sample. The methods, including qualitative parameters, are described in Document S1.

The data were statistically evaluated by Xlstat 2024.2.0 (Adinsoft, Denver, CO, USA). The data follow normal distribution according to the Shapiro–Wilk test. For comparison of mineral content, ANOVA (post-hoc, Tukey HSD) and Pearson correlation coefficient were used. Due to the variation in soil types across different locations, statistical analyses were conducted using weighted correction methods. This approach adjusts for differences in sample size, ensuring that each observation contributes appropriately to the analysis. Weighted corrections were applied to ANOVA, Pearson correlation, and Classification and Regression Trees CART analyses. CART, based on a machine learning algorithm, was used to distinguish soil type based on mineral profile. The location of the hive positions was visualized in Excel 356 (Microsoft, Redmond, WA, USA).

3. Results and Discussion

The average mineral profile of Czech honey and its comparison with other European countries is shown in Table 2. The influence of the habitat of bees on the quality of their honey has been investigated in many studies [17]. Habitats influence the characteristic properties of honey, not only from the point of view of sensory uniqueness or the content of biologically active substances but also from the point of view of the mineral profile of the substances contained. The mineral composition of honey has been used in several studies, both for the characterization of bee honey [30–34] as well as a tool for proof of honey adulteration [33,35–38]. The mineral composition of honey is related to bee pasture [39] and is therefore significantly influenced by botanical taxa in the vicinity of the site [40] but also by geographic location and soil composition [41].

The measured values point to differences in the mineral composition of honey, which are related to both its botanical and geographical origin. However, it is clear from the comparison that K (1365.2 mg/kg) is the most represented element, followed by Ca (148.8 mg/kg), Na (36.9 mg/kg), and Mg (35.1 mg/kg). The greatest representation of K agrees with the results of other authors [33,35,39,41]. The representation of Ca and Na may differ depending on the country where the honey comes from when Italy (Latium region) and Turkey (Antolia) had a greater representation of Na [41,42]. In other studies, Ca was more represented, see Table 2, the same finding was confirmed in the Czech Republic (Moravia). All of the major mineral elements did not exceed the tolerable upper intake level (UI) for the adults, which are for Ca, Mg and Zn Fe, 2500, 250, and 25 mg/kg, respectively. For K, Mn, Mn, and Fe, there is not evidence in the EU for tolerable upper intake levels [43–45]. Considering the consumption of 1.7 kg [46] in the EU, honey is not a risk food, even in terms of potentially toxic elements.

Table 2. Comparison of the average mineral profile of honeys from different geographical areas.

	Present Study (Moravia Region) ($n = 32$)	Italy [a] (Siena) ($n = 50$)	Italy [b] (Latium Region) ($n = 84$)	Spain [c] ($n = 40$)	Spain [d] (Galicia) ($n = 22$)	Spain [e] ($n = $**)	Turkey [f] (Anatolia) ($n = 30$)	Ireland [g] ($n = 50$)	Portugal (Castelo Branco) [h] ($n = 16$)	Poland [i] ($n = 30$)	Hungary [j] ($n = 34$)
K (mg/kg)	1365.2	1195	472	1124	1345	1778	296	566	701.87	1585.6	610.2
Ca (mg/kg)	148.8	257	47.7	169	**	113	51	111	28.36	35.52	92.3
Na (mg/kg)	36.9	96.6	96	76	115	279	118	98	31.04	29	**
Mg (mg/kg)	35.1	56.7	37	39	77	136	33	31	74.00	**	17.6
Zn (mg/kg)	3.5	1.82	3.1	3.9	2.0	5.65	2.7	5	1.23	2.6	3.7
Mn (mg/kg)	2.3	1.54	3.0	3.4	5.2	**	1.0	4	2.78	2.72	2.1
Fe (mg/kg)	0.7	3.07	4.5	**	3.7	9.19	6.6	8	0.97	3.8	1.4
B (mg/kg)	11.1	**	**	5.43	**	**	**	**	**	5.17	**

** Not provided, [a] [41]; [b] [34]; [c] [35]; [d] [47]; [e] [29]; [f] [42]; [g] [48]; [h] [49]; [i] [50]; [j] [51].

As already mentioned, there can be more reasons for the different representations of mineral substances. Our study has shown that one of the factors influencing the mineral composition, specifically the content of K, Mg, and Mn, is the type of soil on which the colonies are located. Mineral representation in plants depends on the type of soil and the density of the root system, the amount of precipitation, and the mineral composition of the subsoil [52]. The average values of mineral substances in honey with respect to the soil types of the observed beehive location are indicated in Table 3. The most K was found in honey with a majority of podzol; on the contrary, the lowest amount was found in honeys from phaeozem, chernozem, and pseoudogley ($p < 0.05$). Higher K values in some types of soils can be explained by the fertilization of these soils [53]. Podzol soils also yielded higher amounts of Mg in honey ($p < 0.05$). High amounts of Ca were found in the honeys around the gleysols and rankers, but no statistically significant difference was found between the Ca content in the soils.

Table 3. Comparison of the major mineral substance profiles of soil types in honey (mg/kg).

Soil	Al	B	Ca	K	Mg	Mn	Na	Zn
Gleysol	392.2 [a]	9.7 [a]	196.9 [a]	1604.9 [abcd]	34.1 [ab]	1.8 [a]	41.7 [ab]	3.8 [a]
Cambisol	513.1 [a]	10.3 [a]	167.7 [a]	1463.3 [abcd]	34.7 [ab]	2.8 [a]	35.6 [b]	4.1 [a]
Luvisol	431.8 [a]	10.6 [a]	163.9 [a]	1559.6 [abcd]	32.3 [ab]	1.9 [a]	42.8 [ab]	3.7 [a]
Anthrosol	20.6 [a]	14.7 [a]	161.3 [a]	1427.8 [abcd]	35.9± [ab]	1.1 [a]	36.4 [b]	6.3 [a]
Podzol	11 [a]	14.1 [a]	174.7 [a]	2099 [a]	45.7 [a]	2.8 [a]	32.7 [b]	2.9 [a]
Pelozem	25.3 [a]	14.7 [a]	163.9 [a]	1844.6 [abc]	43.7 [ab]	2.5 [a]	32.4 [b]	2.9 [a]
Rendzinas	49.6 [a]	9.6 [a]	152.5 [a]	1884.6 [ab]	33.4 [ab]	4.1 [a]	31.8 [b]	5.3 [a]
Fluvisol	318.1 [a]	10.7 [a]	129.5 [a]	1398.6 [abcd]	33.9 [ab]	2.5 [a]	35.5 [b]	2.9 [a]
Ranker	144.6 [a]	11 [a]	189.2 [a]	1272.6 [abcd]	38.3 [ab]	1.5 [a]	33.2 [b]	2.8 [a]
Kastanozem	553.4 [a]	11.2 [a]	127.6 [a]	963.7 [abcd]	29.2 [ab]	1.7 [a]	35.5 [b]	3.6 [a]
Chernozem	318.2 [a]	11.7 [a]	125.3 [a]	665.1 [cd]	28.6 [ab]	0.5 [a]	45.1 [ab]	3.4 [a]
Pseudogley	54.5 [a]	15.1 [a]	119.2 [a]	666.6 [cd]	29 [ab]	1.4 [a]	32.6 [b]	3.1 [a]
Pararendzina	13.1 [a]	13.7 [a]	115.3 [a]	878.7 [bcd]	32.7 [ab]	1.7 [a]	25.1 [b]	3.6 [a]
Regosol	71.9 [a]	15.7 [a]	133.5 [a]	985.6 [abcd]	30.2 [ab]	1.2 [a]	28.4 [b]	2.7 [a]
Phaeozem	31.9 [a]	9.7 [a]	96.1 [a]	477.7 [d]	26.3 [ab]	0.3 [a]	64 [a]	1.7 [a]
Water Bodies	36.6 [a]	10.7 [a]	109.7 [a]	916.6 [abcd]	24.5 [b]	1.8 [a]	26.5 [b]	2.3 [a]

Different letters mean significant differences between raw ($p < 0.05$).

For B, Al, Ca, Cr, Mn, Fe, Ni, Cu, Zn, As, and Pb, statistical differences in the content of mineral substances in honey and the types of soil were not confirmed. This finding is due to the large variability of the measured values, while differences in the mineral composition of individual soil types were observed (Tables 3 and 4), especially for B, Al, Mn, and Zn ($p > 0.05$).

Table 4. Comparison of the minor mineral substances profiles of soil types in honey (mg/kg).

Soil	As	Cr	Cu	Fe	Ni	Pb
Gleysol	0.008	0.151	0.302	0.787	0.211	0.090
Cambisol	0.006	0.131	0.342	0.717	0.224	0.100
Luvisol	0.007	0.141	0.299	0.796	0.200	0.095
Anthrosol	0.008	0.151	0.370	0.749	0.173	0.086
Podzol	0.009	0.130	0.387	0.576	0.261	0.059
Pelozem	0.009	0.121	0.361	0.562	0.249	0.060
Rendzinas	0.008	0.130	0.366	0.591	0.184	0.072
Fluvisol	0.007	0.111	0.322	0.662	0.165	0.082
Ranker	0.005	0.128	0.425	0.621	0.144	0.066
Kastanozem	0.008	0.109	0.264	0.863	0.148	0.067
Chernozem	0.006	0.113	0.307	0.698	0.126	0.074
Pseudogley	0.005	0.132	0.183	0.562	0.211	0.048
Pararendzina	0.005	0.119	0.223	0.606	0.201	0.070
Regosol	0.006	0.092	0.249	0.502	0.165	0.052
Phaeozem	0.007	0.120	0.256	0.543	0.107	0.055
Water Bodies	0.006	0.100	0.172	0.481	0.127	0.043

Note: As, Cr, Cu, Fe, Ni, and Pb were no significant differences between raw ($p < 0.05$).

The minor mineral substances such as As, Cr, Cu, Fe, Ni, and Pb are summarized in Table 4. Potentially toxic elements such as Pb and metalloid As can contaminate honey due to environmental pollution and Al. Higher concentration in Al in comparison with Pb and As was also confirmed in the Hungarian study, but the total amount of Al was lower than was detected in our study [51]. In our study, statistical differences between soil types and Pb and As were not determined. Cu, Fe, Ni, and Zn are essential nutrients for organisms, including bees and plants. Statistical differences with soil type have not been confirmed (Table 4). Low concentrations of minor mineral substances in honey were also confirmed in other studies [51,54].

In order to better express the relationship between mineral substances and soil types, the Pearson correlation coefficient was further used. The correlation between soil type and mineral substances is shown in Table 5. There was a high correlation between antroposol area and Zn (R = 0.98), Pb (R = 0.96), then between ranker area and Mn (0.95), then regosol area and Al (R = 0.97) ($p < 0.05$). A high negative correlation was between regosol area and Mg (R = -0.97), Cr (R = -0.98) and between the redzinas area and Al (R = -0.97) ($p < 0.05$).

A positive and negative high correlation was also confirmed for phaeozem, but this result is compromised by an error, which is due to the small representation of this soil in the analyzed localities, both in terms of total representation (1%) and frequency (number of occurrences: 2) (Table 5). At the same time, the frequency corresponded to two beehive locations where the phaeozem represented 20% and 10% of the given locality. Further research is still needed to define a conclusion for this type of soil so that it is included in more locations in a wider representation.

The relationship between mineral composition and plants has been confirmed in various studies, mostly focusing on plant mass, leaves, seeds, and roots [55–58]. Several studies [59,60] confirmed the effect of soil type on the nectar production of the nectar-bearing plant called mānuka (*Leptospermum scoparium*). Ca, Mn, and Fe contained in soil types had a positive effect on production. The amount of Ca also affects the number of flowers on plants [61,62]. The influence of soil type on the growth of other honey plants (*Salix caprea* and *Prunus padus*) was confirmed by [61]. On another honey plant, *Allium ursinum*, the influence of soil mineral composition on nectar production was also confirmed, where the influence of phosphorus was confirmed. The influence of humus, K, Fe, and Mn on the number of flowers was confirmed, while Mn also had an influence on the total nectar content. From the above, we expected that the effect on the mineral substances in honey is manifested due to higher nectar-producing capacity and the number of flowers on soils with a suitable mineral composition and a layer of humus. In our study, statistical differences between the type of soil and the content of Ca, Fe, and Mn in honey were not confirmed (Table 3), but the correlation dependence with the type of soil was confirmed (Table 5).

Therefore, methods of higher statistics were applied to verify the relationship between soil type and mineral composition, which allows for the comparison of several variable parameters. Classification and Regression Trees (CART) were utilized. CART is a machine learning algorithm that recursively splits the dataset based on features to predict a target variable (response). It constructs a decision tree suitable for classification, where the target variable represents categories or classes. In regression, the target variable represents a continuous variable. The CART reaches the best correct classification rate in comparison with not supervised (PCA) and supervised (LDA and QDA) classification for mineral substances [36] and for other honey parameters [63].

Table 5. Correlation between the area of soil type and mineral content in honey in the observed localities.

	B	Na	Mg	Al	K	Ca	Cr	Mn	Fe	Ni	Cu	Zn	As	Pb	No. of Locality
Anthrosol	**0.712**	0.240	−0.144	0.045	0.344	0.742	0.595	−0.227	0.824	−0.054	0.812	0.982	0.375	0.956	8
Cambisol	−0.013	0.037	−0.034	0.041	0.087	0.243	0.191	0.018	0.031	0.290	0.001	0.263	0.087	−0.027	26
Chernozem	0.134	−0.530	−0.176	−0.263	−0.457	−0.063	−0.486	−0.370	−0.371	−0.437	−0.291	−0.349	−0.717	−0.357	7
Fluvisol	0.329	−0.140	−0.129	−0.139	−0.251	−0.513	−0.387	−0.192	−0.181	−0.337	−0.287	−0.356	0.026	−0.139	26
Gleysol	−0.674	0.519	−0.343	−0.163	0.344	0.296	0.574	−0.457	0.237	−0.372	−0.383	−0.166	0.489	−0.172	21
Kastanozem	−0.510	0.001	−0.594	−0.169	−0.339	−0.479	−0.215	−0.077	−0.199	−0.452	−0.444	−0.301	0.140	−0.375	14
Luvisol	−0.187	0.103	−0.037	−0.319	0.405	0.753	0.573	−0.489	−0.148	−0.035	−0.328	0.159	0.267	−0.266	13
Pararendzina	0.585	−0.333	0.180	−0.636	−0.822	−0.635	0.007	−0.517	0.293	0.196	−0.569	−0.294	−0.669	−0.081	6
Pelozem	−0.210	−0.158	−0.057	−0.306	0.218	0.285	0.259	0.138	0.027	−0.062	0.050	−0.239	0.026	−0.285	6
Phaeozem	**−0.978**	**0.978**	**−0.978**	**−0.978**	**0.978**	**−0.978**	**−0.978**	**−0.978**	**−0.978**	**−0.978**	**0.978**	**−0.978**	**0.978**	**0.978**	2
Podzol	0.000	0.000	0.000	0.000	0.000	0.000	0.000	0.000	0.000	0.000	0.000	0.000	0.000	0.000	2
Pseudogley	0.458	−0.440	−0.503	−0.448	−0.530	−0.374	−0.238	−0.534	0.047	−0.539	−0.583	−0.520	−0.178	−0.761	15
Ranker	−0.247	0.235	0.687	−0.559	0.709	0.818	0.713	**0.954**	0.288	0.169	0.598	−0.386	0.450	−0.235	5
Regosol	**0.629**	**−0.741**	**−0.971**	**0.973**	**−0.946**	**−0.943**	**−0.982**	−0.723	−0.886	**−0.930**	**−0.906**	−0.638	−0.568	−0.588	7
Rendzinas	0.165	0.290	0.796	**−0.970**	0.809	0.485	0.704	0.139	0.304	0.471	0.629	0.375	**0.929**	0.387	4
Water Bodies	−0.107	−0.233	−0.932	−0.046	−0.366	−0.431	−0.085	−0.484	−0.182	−0.698	−0.684	−0.242	0.512	−0.560	8

Value in bold means significant correlation ($p < 0.05$); dark grey means positive correlation higher than 95%; light grey higher than 90%; dark blue negative means correlation higher than 95%; and light blue higher than 90%.

According to the CART, the B, Ca, Mg, Ni, and Mn in honey samples are characteristic of all soil types in our study. The soil types of cambisol, fluvisol, gleysol, anthrosol, and kastanozem were most closely related to the above-mentioned mineral substances found in honey and can, therefore, be assumed to have a major influence on the mineral content of honey (Table 6). An overall summary of the classification is provided in Figure S2. Cambisol and fuvisol are the most common soils in the Czech Republic. While cambisols are represented both in hilly areas and uplands and in mountains; fuvisols, on the other hand, were formed mainly in lowlands, especially along larger rivers [64]. In the Czech Republic, 58% of agricultural land is of the cambisol type [65]. These soils are poor in minerals; thus, in order to achieve adequate production, crops grown on them must be regularly fertilized, which affects their mineral profile [66]. According to CART, therefore, honeys with a large proportion of cambisol were mainly represented by a low content of B, Ca, and Mg, with the exception of the Ni content in honey, which increased with a larger area of cambisol in the vicinity of bee colonies.

Table 6. Regression classification rules for mineral substances.

Nodes	Soil (Prediction)	Rules
Node 1	Cambisol	All cases
Node 2	Cambisol	If B ≤ 14.59 then Soil = Cambisol in 62.9% of cases
Node 3	Cambisol	If B (14.59; 15.87] then Soil = Cambisol in 8.8% of cases
Node 4	Cambisol	If B (15.87; 16.49] then Soil = Cambisol in 10% of cases
Node 5	Gleysol	If B (16.49; 17.05] then Soil = Gleysol in 11.8% of cases
Node 6	Fluvisol	If B > 17.05 then Soil = Fluvisol in 6.5% of cases
Node 7	Fluvisol	If B ≤ 14.59 and Ca ≤ 162.10 then Soil = Fluvisol in 41.8% of cases
Node 8	Cambisol	If B ≤ 14.59 and Ca (162.10; 179.20] then Soil = Cambisol in 5.3% of cases
Node 9	Cambisol	If B ≤ 14.59 and Ca (179.20; 189.20] then Soil = Cambisol in 5.3% of cases
Node 10	Anthrosol	If B ≤ 14.59 and Ca (189.20; 215.30] then Soil = Anthrosol in 2.4% of cases
Node 11	Cambisol	If B ≤ 14.59 and Ca > 215.30 then Soil = Cambisol in 8.2% of cases
Node 12	Cambisol	If B (14.59; 15.87] and Mg ≤ 30.22 then Soil = Cambisol in 4.1% of cases
Node 13	Anthrosol	If B (14.59; 15.87] and Mg > 30.22 then Soil = Anthrosol in 4.7% of cases
Node 14	Cambisol	If B (15.87; 16.49] and Ca ≤ 109.60 then Soil = Cambisol in 8.2% of cases
Node 15	Cambisol	If B (15.87; 16.49] and Ca > 109.60 then Soil = Cambisol in 1.8% of cases
Node 16	Kastanozem	If B (16.49; 17.05] and Ni ≤ 0.13 then Soil = Kastanozem in 5.9% of cases
Node 17	Cambisol	If B (16.49; 17.05] and Ni (0.13; 0.27] then Soil = Cambisol in 4.1% of cases
Node 18	Cambisol	If B (16.49; 17.05] and Ni > 0.27 then Soil = Cambisol in 1.8% of cases
Node 19	Anthrosol	If B > 17.05 and Mg ≤ 34.69 then Soil = Anthrosol in 4.7% of cases
Node 20	Fluvisol	If B > 17.05 and Mg > 34.69 then Soil = Fluvisol in 1.8% of cases
Node 21	Fluvisol	If B ≤ 14.59 and Ca ≤ 162.10 and Mg ≤ 31.49 then Soil = Fluvisol in 29.4% of cases
Node 22	Cambisol	If B ≤ 14.59 and Ca ≤ 162.10 and Mg (31.49; 37.11] then Soil = Cambisol in 4.1% of cases
Node 23	Cambisol	If B ≤ 14.59 and Ca ≤ 162.10 and Mg (37.11; 42.41] then Soil = Cambisol in 4.1% of cases
Node 24	Anthrosol	If B ≤ 14.59 and Ca ≤ 162.10 and Mg > 42.41 then Soil = Anthrosol in 4.1% of cases
Node 25	Cambisol	If B ≤ 14.59 and Ca (179.20; 189.20] and Mg ≤ 37.65 then Soil = Cambisol in 2.9% of cases
Node 26	Cambisol	If B ≤ 14.59 and Ca (179.20; 189.20] and Mg > 37.65 then Soil = Cambisol in 2.4% of cases
Node 27	Cambisol	If B ≤ 14.59 and Ca > 215.30 and Mn ≤ 2 then Soil = Cambisol in 7.1% of cases
Node 28	Cambisol	If B ≤ 14.59 and Ca > 215.30 and Mn > 2 then Soil = Cambisol in 1.2% of cases

The presence of fluvisol in the vicinity of the beehive location was manifested by a low content of B, Ca, and Mg in honey (29.4% of cases) or a low content of B and Ca (41.8% of cases) but in some cases, the presence of this type of soil led to a high content of B (6.5% of cases). These differences are explained by the type of soil, where fluvisol represents river sediments that can be affected by anthropogenic activity [67]. This fact is also indicated by the high content of Pb (Table 3), although in the discrimination according to CART, Pb was not significant, which is caused by the variability of this factor. Another type of soil that has been confirmed to have an effect on the mineral composition of honey is anthrosol. This type of soil is significantly transformed by human activity, mostly with originally less fertile soil [68], which, within the CART discrimination, was manifested by a higher representation of Ca and Mg. A high content of Ca and Mg is typical for anthrosol, while their higher content is due to both anthropogenic activity and sandy or sandstone subsoil [68,69]. Another type of soil influencing the mineral profile of honey, according to CART, was kastanozem. This type of soil is typical for pastures, steppes, meadows, and anthropogenic analogs [70]. Kastanozem was manifested by a high content of B and a low content of Ni. These soils are characterized by available Ca, Mg, and Na cations. In our study, only a higher Na content (Table 3) was confirmed in honey in relation to the amount of kastanozem in the location of the bee colonies. The content of B and Ni can be affected by anthropogenic activity (fertilization), but there is not enough information in the scientific literature about its content and availability for plants. Pollution as the reason for their higher content cannot be assumed because other metals such as Pb, As, Cu, and Zn have not been confirmed in honey.

4. Conclusions

The mineral profile of honey can be influenced, among mechanisms, by the type of soil on which the beehive is located and which occurs within its flying range. In this study, positive high correlations were confirmed with certain soil types and specific elements, namely phaeozem with Na and K, as well as ranker with Mn, regosol with Al, and anthrosol with Zn and Pb, while a negative correlation between phaeozem with B, Mg, Al, Ca, Cr, Mn, Fe, Ni, Zn, regosol with Mg, Cr, and rendzinas with Al ($p < 0.05$). The higher statistics methods subsequently proved that some elements are characteristic of the given soil type. Using CART analysis, the linear regression dependence between Ca, B, Mg, and Mn and the cambisol, anthrosol, fluvisol, and kastanozem soils was confirmed. The mutual relationship between soil type and mineral substances in honey can be used to predict the geographical origin of honey. When working with national map data, soil profiles can be used to predict the mineral profile of honey using minerals such as B, Ca, Mg, Ni, and Mn and subsequently authenticate its geographical origin.

Supplementary Materials: The following supporting information can be downloaded at: https://www.mdpi.com/article/10.3390/foods13132006/s1, Table S1: Pollen profile of analyzed samples; Figure S1: Location of analyzed samples, Figure S2: CART Classification tree of soil types; Document S1: ICP-MS 7900 methods.

Author Contributions: Conceptualization, M.P. and B.P.; methodology, D.T., J.H. and Z.B.; validation, H.Č., P.Š., D.M., J.B. and V.K.; formal analysis, S.S., V.K. and S.M.; resources, C.B., Z.J., S.M., J.H. and D.T.; data curation, M.P.; writing—original draft preparation, S.S. and M.P.; writing—review and editing, D.T., H.Č. and D.M.; visualization, Z.J.; supervision, B.T.; project administration, M.P.; funding acquisition, M.P. All authors have read and agreed to the published version of the manuscript.

Funding: The project is financed by the governments of the Czech Republic, Hungary, Poland, and Slovakia through Visegrad Grants from the International Visegrad Fund No. 22220064. The mission of the fund is to advance ideas for sustainable regional cooperation in Central Europe.

Institutional Review Board Statement: Not applicable.

Informed Consent Statement: Not applicable.

Data Availability Statement: The original contributions presented in the study are included in the article and Supplementary Materials; further inquiries can be directed to the corresponding author.

Conflicts of Interest: The authors declare no conflicts of interest. The funders had no role in the design of the study; in the collection, analyses, or interpretation of data; in the writing of the manuscript, and in the decision to publish the results.

References

1. Bogdanov, S.; Haldimann, M.; Luginbühl, W.; Gallmann, P. Minerals in Honey: Environmental, Geographical and Botanical Aspects. *J. Apic. Res.* **2007**, *46*, 269–275. [CrossRef]
2. Alvarez-Suarez, J.M.; Tulipani, S.; Romandini, S.; Bertoli, E.; Battino, M. Contribution of Honey in Nutrition and Human Health: A Review. *Med. J. Nutr. Metab.* **2010**, *3*, 15–23. [CrossRef]

3. van der Steen, J.J.M. The Foraging Honey Bee. *Br. Bee J.* **2015**, *2015*, 43–46.
4. Pound, M.J.; Vinkenoog, R.; Hornby, S.; Benn, J.; Goldberg, S.; Keating, B.; Woollard, F. Determining If Honey Bees (*Apis mellifera*) Collect Pollen from Anemophilous Plants in the UK. *Palynology* **2022**, *47*, 2154867. [CrossRef]
5. Cunningham, M.M.; Tran, L.; McKee, C.G.; Ortega Polo, R.; Newman, T.; Lansing, L.; Griffiths, J.S.; Bilodeau, G.J.; Rott, M.; Marta Guarna, M. Honey Bees as Biomonitors of Environmental Contaminants, Pathogens, and Climate Change. *Ecol. Indic.* **2022**, *134*, 108457. [CrossRef]
6. Bratu, I.; Georgescu, C. Chemical Contamination of Bee Honey—Identifying Sensor of the Environment Pollution. *J. Cent. Eur. Agric.* **2005**, *6*, 95–98.
7. Crane, E. Bees, Honey and Pollen as Indicators of Metals in the Environment. *Bee World* **1984**, *61*, 47–49. [CrossRef]
8. Svoboda, J. *Poisoning of Bees by Industrial Arsenic Emissions*; Ceská Akademie Zemědelskych Věd: Prague, Czechia, 1961; pp. 1499–1506.
9. Celli, G.; Maccagnani, B. Honey Bees as Bioindicators of Environmental Pollution. *Bull. Insectology* **2003**, *56*, 137–139.
10. Svoboda, J. Teneur En Strontium 90 Dans Les Abeilles et Dans Leurs Produits. *Bull. Apic.* **1962**, *5*, 101–103.
11. Leita, L.; Muhlbachova, G.; Cesco, S.; Barbattini, R.; Mondini, C. Investigation of the Use of Honey Bees and Honey Bee Products to Assess Heavy Metals Contamination. *Environ. Monit. Assess.* **1996**, *43*, 1–9. [CrossRef]
12. Ruschioni, S.; Riolo, P.; Minuz, R.L.; Stefano, M.; Cannella, M.; Porrini, C.; Isidoro, N. Biomonitoring with Honeybees of Heavy Metals and Pesticides in Nature Reserves of the Marche Region (Italy). *Biol. Trace Elem. Res.* **2013**, *154*, 226–233. [CrossRef] [PubMed]
13. Persano Oddo, L.; Piro, R. Main European Unifloral Honeys: Descriptive Sheets. *Apidologie* **2004**, *35*, S38–S81. [CrossRef]
14. González-Miret, M.L.; Terrab, A.; Hernanz, D.; Fernández-Recamales, M.Á.; Heredia, F.J. Multivariate Correlation between Color and Mineral Composition of Honeys and by Their Botanical Origin. *J. Agric. Food Chem.* **2005**, *53*, 2574–2580. [CrossRef] [PubMed]
15. Lachman, J.; Kolihová, D.; Miholová, D.; Košata, J.; Titěra, D.; Kult, K. Analysis of Minority Honey Components: Possible Use for the Evaluation of Honey Quality. *Food Chem.* **2007**, *101*, 973–979. [CrossRef]
16. Anklam, E. A Review of the Analytical Methods to Determine the Geographical and Botanical Origin of Honey. *Food Chem.* **1998**, *63*, 549–562. [CrossRef]
17. Porrini, C.; Sabatini, A.G.; Girotti, S.; Ghini, S.; Medrzycki, P.; Grillenzoni, F.; Bortolotti, L.; Gattavecchia, E.; Celli, G. Honey bees and bee products as monitors of the environmental contamination. *Apiacta* **2003**, *38*, 63–70.
18. Solayman, M.; Islam, M.A.; Paul, S.; Ali, Y.; Khalil, M.I.; Alam, N.; Gan, S.H. Physicochemical Properties, Minerals, Trace Elements, and Heavy Metals in Honey of Different Origins: A Comprehensive Review. *Compr. Rev. Food Sci. Food Saf.* **2016**, *15*, 219–233. [CrossRef]
19. González-Porto, A.V.; Martín Arroyo, T.; Bartolomé Esteban, C. How Soil Type (Gypsum or Limestone) Influences the Properties and Composition of Thyme Honey. *Springerplus* **2016**, *5*, 1663. [CrossRef] [PubMed]
20. Sakač, M.B.; Jovanov, P.T.; Marić, A.Z.; Pezo, L.L.; Kevrešan, Ž.S.; Novaković, A.R.; Nedeljković, N.M. Physicochemical Properties and Mineral Content of Honey Samples from Vojvodina (Republic of Serbia). *Food Chem.* **2019**, *276*, 15–21. [CrossRef]
21. Helfenstein, J.; Jegminat, J.; Mclaren, T.I.; Frossard, E. Soil Solution Phosphorus Turnover: Derivation, Interpretation, and Insights from a Global Compilation of Isotope Exchange Kinetic Studies. *Biogeosciences* **2018**, *15*, 105–114. [CrossRef]
22. IUSS Working Group WRB. *World Reference Base for Soil Resources 2014, Update 2015*; Food and Agriculture Organization of the United Nations: Rome, Italy, 2015; Volume 106, ISBN 9789251083697.
23. Hajková, M.; Svobodová, J. *Geography; Thematic Atlas Czech Republic; Cartographic Skills*; Masaryk Univerzity: Brno, Czech Republic, 2017.
24. Pospiech, M.; Javůrková, Z.; Hrabec, P.; Štarha, P.; Ljasovská, S.; Bednář, J.; Tremlová, B. Identification of Pollen Taxa by Different Microscopy Techniques. *PLoS ONE* **2021**, *16*, e0256808. [CrossRef]
25. CENIA Národní Geoportál INSPIRE. Available online: https://geoportal.gov.cz/web/guest/map?openNode=Stanovi%C5%A1t%C4%9B+a+biotopy&keywordList=inspire (accessed on 23 March 2024).
26. Nachtergaele, F.O.; Spaargaren, O.; Deckers, J.A.; Ahrens, B. New Developments in Soil Classification: World Reference Base for Soil Resources. *Geoderma* **2000**, *96*, 345–357. [CrossRef]
27. STN EN 15763; Foodstuffs—Determination of Trace Elements—Determination of Arsenic, Cadmium, Mercury, and Lead in Foodstuffs by Inductively Coupled Plasma Mass Spectrometry (ICP-MS) after Pressure Digestion. European Committee For Standardization: Brussels, Belgium, 2010.
28. UNI EN 13805; Foodstuffs—Determination of Trace Elements—Pressure Digestion. British Standards Institution: London, UK, 2014.
29. UNI EN 13804; Foodstuffs—Determination of Trace Elements—Performance Criteria, General Considerations, and Sample Preparation. European Committee For Standardization: Brussels, Belgium, 2013.
30. Silva, L.R.; Videira, R.; Monteiro, A.P.; Valentão, P.; Andrade, P.B. Honey from Luso Region (Portugal): Physicochemical Characteristics and Mineral Contents. *Microchem. J.* **2009**, *93*, 73–77. [CrossRef]
31. Alves, A.; Ramos, A.; Gonçalves, M.M.; Bernardo, M.; Mendes, B. Antioxidant Activity, Quality Parameters and Mineral Content of Portuguese Monofloral Honeys. *J. Food Compos. Anal.* **2013**, *30*, 130–138. [CrossRef]
32. Terrab, A.; Recamales, A.F.; Hernanz, D.; Heredia, F.J. Characterisation of Spanish Thyme Honeys by Their Physicochemical Characteristics and Mineral Contents. *Food Chem.* **2004**, *88*, 537–542. [CrossRef]

33. Kek, S.P.; Chin, N.L.; Tan, S.W.; Yusof, Y.A.; Chua, L.S. Classification of Honey from Its Bee Origin via Chemical Profiles and Mineral Content. *Food Anal. Methods* **2017**, *10*, 19–30. [CrossRef]
34. Conti, M.E. Lazio Region (Central Italy) Honeys: A Survey of Mineral Content and Typical Quality Parameters. *Food Control* **2000**, *11*, 459–463. [CrossRef]
35. Fernández-Torres, R.; Luis Pérez-Bernal, J.; Bello-López, A.; Callejón-Mochón, M.; Carlos Jiménez-Sánchez, J.; Guiraúm-Pérez, A. Mineral Content and Botanical Origin of Spanish Honeys. *Talanta* **2005**, *65*, 686–691. [CrossRef]
36. Pasquini, B.; Goodarzi, M.; Orlandini, S.; Beretta, G.; Furlanetto, S.; Dejaegher, B. Geographical Characterisation of Honeys According to Their Mineral Content and Antioxidant Activity Using a Chemometric Approach. *Int. J. Food Sci. Technol.* **2014**, *49*, 1351–1359. [CrossRef]
37. Taha, E.K.A. Chemical Composition and Amounts of Mineral Elements in Honeybee-Collected Pollen in Relation to Botanical Origin. *J. Apic. Sci.* **2015**, *59*, 75–81. [CrossRef]
38. Louppis, A.P.; Karabagias, I.K.; Kontakos, S.; Kontominas, M.G.; Papastephanou, C.; Konstantinos Karabagias, I.; Kontakos, S.; Kontominas, M.G.; Papastephanou, C. Botanical Discrimination of Greek Unifloral Honeys Based on Mineral Content in Combination with Physicochemical Parameter Analysis, Using a Validated Chemometric Approach. *Microchem. J.* **2017**, *135*, 180–189. [CrossRef]
39. Rashed, M.N.; Soltan, M.E. Major and Trace Elements in Different Types of Egyptian Mono-Floral and Non-Floral Bee Honeys. *J. Food Compos. Anal.* **2004**, *17*, 725–735. [CrossRef]
40. Di Bella, G.; Lo Turco, V.; Potortì, A.G.; Bua, G.D.; Fede, M.R.; Dugo, G. Geographical Discrimination of Italian Honey by Multi-Element Analysis with a Chemometric Approach. *J. Food Compos. Anal.* **2015**, *44*, 25–35. [CrossRef]
41. Pisani, A.; Protano, G.; Riccobono, F. Minor and Trace Elements in Different Honey Types Produced in Siena County (Italy). *Food Chem.* **2008**, *107*, 1553–1560. [CrossRef]
42. Yilmaz, H.; Yavuz, Ö. Content of Some Trace Metals in Honey from South-Eastern Anatolia. *Food Chem.* **1999**, *65*, 475–476. [CrossRef]
43. European Food Safety Authority (EFSA). Opinion of the Scientific Panel on Dietetic Products, Nutrition and Allergies [NDA] Related to the Tolerable Upper Intake Level of Sodium. *EFSA J.* **2005**, *3*, 209. [CrossRef]
44. Allen, L.H.; Carriquiry, A.L.; Murphy, S.P. Perspective: Proposed Harmonized Nutrient Reference Values for Populations. *Adv. Nutr.* **2020**, *11*, 469–483. [CrossRef]
45. Godswill, A.G.; Somtochukwu, I.V.; Ikechukwu, A.O.; Kate, E.C. Health Benefits of Micronutrients (Vitamins and Minerals) and Their Associated Deficiency Diseases: A Systematic Review. *Int. J. Food Sci.* **2020**, *3*, 1–32. [CrossRef]
46. Vida-Aliz, V.; Ferenczi, F. Trends in Honey Consumption and Purchasing Habits in the European Union. *Appl. Stud. Agribus. Commer.* **2023**, *17*. [CrossRef]
47. Latorre, M.J.; Peña, R.; Pita, C.; Botana, A.; García, S.; Herrero, C. Chemometric Classification of Honeys According to Their Type. II. Metal Content Data. *Food Chem.* **1999**, *66*, 263–268. [CrossRef]
48. Downey, G.; Hussey, K.; Daniel Kelly, J.; Walshe, T.F.; Martin, P.G. Preliminary Contribution to the Characterisation of Artisanal Honey Produced on the Island of Ireland by Palynological and Physico-Chemical Data. *Food Chem.* **2005**, *91*, 347–354. [CrossRef]
49. Silva, L.R.; Sousa, A.; Taveira, M. Characterization of Portuguese Honey from Castelo Branco Region According to Their Pollen Spectrum, Physicochemical Characteristics and Mineral Contents. *J. Food Sci. Technol.* **2017**, *54*, 2551–2561. [CrossRef] [PubMed]
50. Madejczyk, M.; Baralkiewicz, D. Characterization of Polish Rape and Honeydew Honey According to Their Mineral Contents Using ICP-MS and F-AAS/AES. *Anal. Chim. Acta* **2008**, *617*, 11–17. [CrossRef] [PubMed]
51. Czipa, N.; Andrási, D.; Kovács, B. Determination of Essential and Toxic Elements in Hungarian Honeys. *Food Chem.* **2014**, *175*, 536–542. [CrossRef] [PubMed]
52. Christophe, C.; Gil, K.; Laurent, S.-A.; Paul-Olivier, R.; Marie-Pierre, T. Relationship between Soil Nutritive Resources and the Growth and Mineral Nutrition of a Beech (*Fagus sylvatica*) Stand along a Soil Sequence. *Catena* **2017**, *155*, 156–169. [CrossRef]
53. Wyszkowski, M.; Brodowska, M.S. Content of Trace Elements in Soil Fertilized with Potassium and Nitrogen. *Agriculture* **2020**, *10*, 398. [CrossRef]
54. Mititelu, M.; Udeanu, D.I.; Docea, A.O.; Tsatsakis, A.; Calina, D.; Arsene, A.L.; Nedelescu, M.; Neacsu, S.M.; Velescu, B.Ș.; Ghica, M. New Method for Risk Assessment in Environmental Health: The Paradigm of Heavy Metals in Honey. *Environ. Res.* **2023**, *236*, 115194. [CrossRef]
55. Joy, E.J.M.; Broadley, M.R.; Young, S.D.; Black, C.R.; Chilimba, A.D.C.; Ander, E.L.; Barlow, T.S.; Watts, M.J. Soil Type Influences Crop Mineral Composition in Malawi. *Sci. Total Environ.* **2015**, *505*, 587–595. [CrossRef] [PubMed]
56. Jordan-Meille, L.; Holland, J.E.; McGrath, S.P.; Glendining, M.J.; Thomas, C.L.; Haefele, S.M. The Grain Mineral Composition of Barley, Oat and Wheat on Soils with PH and Soil Phosphorus Gradients. *Eur. J. Agron.* **2021**, *126*, 126281. [CrossRef]
57. Pongrac, P.; McNicol, J.W.; Lilly, A.; Thompson, J.A.; Wright, G.; Hillier, S.; White, P.J. Mineral Element Composition of Cabbage as Affected by Soil Type and Phosphorus and Zinc Fertilisation. *Plant Soil* **2019**, *434*, 151–165. [CrossRef]
58. Kaiser, M.; Ellerbrock, R.H.; Wulf, M.; Dultz, S.; Hierath, C.; Sommer, M. The Influence of Mineral Characteristics on Organic Matter Content, Composition, and Stability of Topsoils under Long-Term Arable and Forest Land Use. *J. Geophys. Res. Biogeosci* **2012**, *117*, 2018. [CrossRef]
59. Nickless, E.M.; Anderson, C.W.N.; Hamilton, G.; Stephens, J.M.; Wargent, J. Soil Influences on Plant Growth, Floral Density and Nectar Yield in Three Cultivars of Mānuka (*Leptospermum scoparium*). *N. Z. J. Bot.* **2017**, *55*, 100–117. [CrossRef]

60. Meister, A.; Gutierrez-Gines, M.J.; Maxfield, A.; Gaw, S.; Dickinson, N.; Horswell, J.; Robinson, B. Chemical Elements and the Quality of Mānuka (*Leptospermum scoparium*) Honey. *Foods* **2021**, *10*, 1670. [CrossRef]
61. Wielgolaski, F.E. Phenological Modifications in Plants by Various Edaphic Factors. *Int. J. Biometeorol.* **2001**, *45*, 196–202. [CrossRef] [PubMed]
62. Cardoso, F.C.G.; Marques, R.; Botosso, P.C.; Marques, M.C.M. Stem Growth and Phenology of Two Tropical Trees in Contrasting Soil Conditions. *Plant Soil* **2012**, *354*, 269–281. [CrossRef]
63. Popek, S.; Halagarda, M.; Kursa, K. A New Model to Identify Botanical Origin of Polish Honeys Based on the Physicochemical Parameters and Chemometric Analysis. *LWT* **2017**, *77*, 482–487. [CrossRef]
64. Tomášek, M. *Atlas Půd České Republiky (Soil Atlas of the Czech Republic)*; Český Geologický Ústav: Prague, Czech Republic, 1995; Volume 1.
65. Růžek, L.; Růžková, M.; Voříšek, K.; Kubát, J.; Friedlová, M.; Mikanová, O. Chemical and Microbiological Characterization of Cambisols, Luvisols and Stagnosols. *Plant Soil Environ.* **2009**, *55*, 231–237. [CrossRef]
66. Hejcman, M.; Kunzová, E. Sustainability of Winter Wheat Production on Sandy-Loamy Cambisol in the Czech Republic: Results from a Long-Term Fertilizer and Crop Rotation Experiment. *Field Crops Res.* **2010**, *115*, 191–199. [CrossRef]
67. Gaberšek, M.; Gosar, M. Geochemistry of Urban Soil in the Industrial Town of Maribor, Slovenia. *J. Geochem. Explor.* **2018**, *187*, 141–154. [CrossRef]
68. Vasilchenko, A.V.; Vasilchenko, A.S. Plaggic Anthrosol in Modern Research: Genesis, Properties and Carbon Sequestration Potential. *Catena* **2024**, *234*, 107626. [CrossRef]
69. Krupski, M.; Kabala, C.; Sady, A.; Gliński, R.; Wojcieszak, J. Double-and Triple-Depth Digging and Anthrosol Formation in a Medieval and Modern-Era City (Wrocław, SW Poland). Geoarchaeological Research on Past Horticultural Practices. *Catena* **2017**, *153*, 9–20. [CrossRef]
70. Sorokin, A.S.; Abrosimov, K.N.; Lebedeva, M.P.; Kust, G.S. Composition and Structure of Aggregates from Compacted Soil Horizons in the Southern Steppe Zone of European Russia. *Eurasian Soil Sci.* **2016**, *49*, 355–367. [CrossRef]

Disclaimer/Publisher's Note: The statements, opinions and data contained in all publications are solely those of the individual author(s) and contributor(s) and not of MDPI and/or the editor(s). MDPI and/or the editor(s) disclaim responsibility for any injury to people or property resulting from any ideas, methods, instructions or products referred to in the content.

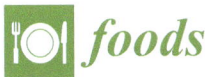

Article

Effects of Geographical Origin and Tree Age on the Stable Isotopes and Multi-Elements of Pu-erh Tea

Ming-Ming Chen [1,2,†], Qiu-Hong Liao [1,†], Li-Li Qian [2], Hai-Dan Zou [1], Yan-Long Li [1], Yan Song [1], Yu Xia [1], Yi Liu [1], Hong-Yan Liu [1,*] and Ze-Long Liu [3,*]

[1] Institute of Urban Agriculture, Chinese Academy of Agricultural Sciences, Chengdu National Agricultural Science & Technology Center, Chengdu 610213, China; chenmingming515@163.com (M.-M.C.); liaoqiuhong@caas.cn (Q.-H.L.); zellazou@foxmail.com (H.-D.Z.); a99008191@163.com (Y.-L.L.); seany_lib@163.com (Y.S.); xiayu03@caas.cn (Y.X.); liuyi03@caas.cn (Y.L.)
[2] College of Food Science, Heilongjiang Bayi Agricultural University, Daqing 163319, China; qianlili286@163.com
[3] China Food Flavor and Nutrition Health Innovation Center, Beijing Technology and Business University, Beijing 102488, China
* Correspondence: liuhongyan01@caas.cn (H.-Y.L.); liuzelong@btbu.edu.cn (Z.-L.L.)
[†] These authors contributed equally to this work.

Abstract: Pu-erh tea is a famous tea worldwide, and identification of the geographical origin of Pu-erh tea can not only protect manufacture's interests, but also boost consumers' confidence. However, tree age may also influence the fingerprints of Pu-erh tea. In order to study the effects of the geographical origin and tree age on the interactions of stable isotopes and multi-elements of Pu-erh tea, 53 Pu-erh tea leaves with three different age stages from three different areas in Yunnan were collected in 2023. The $\delta^{13}C$, $\delta^{15}N$ values and 25 elements were determined and analyzed. The results showed that $\delta^{13}C$, $\delta^{15}N$, Mg, Mn, Fe, Cu, Zn, Rb, Sr, Y, La, Pr, Nd, Sm, Eu, Gd, Tb, Dy, Ho, Er, Tm, Yb, and Lu had significant differences among different geographical origins ($p < 0.05$). Mn content was significantly influenced by region and tree age interaction. Based on multi-way analysis of variance, principal component analysis and step-wised discriminant analysis, 24 parameters were found to be closely related to the geographical origin rather than tree age, and the geographical origin of Pu-erh tea can be 100.0% discriminated in cross-validation with six parameters ($\delta^{13}C$, $\delta^{15}N$, Mn, Mg, La, and Tb). The study could provide references for the establishment of a database for the traceability of Pu-erh tea, and even the identification of tea sample regions with different tree ages.

Keywords: geographical origin; pu-erh tea; tree ages; mineral elements; stable isotope

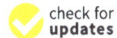

Citation: Chen, M.-M.; Liao, Q.-H.; Qian, L.-L.; Zou, H.-D.; Li, Y.-L.; Song, Y.; Xia, Y.; Liu, Y.; Liu, H.-Y.; Liu, Z.-L. Effects of Geographical Origin and Tree Age on the Stable Isotopes and Multi-Elements of Pu-erh Tea. *Foods* 2024, *13*, 473. https://doi.org/10.3390/foods13030473

Received: 15 December 2023
Revised: 24 January 2024
Accepted: 26 January 2024
Published: 2 February 2024

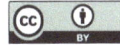

Copyright: © 2024 by the authors. Licensee MDPI, Basel, Switzerland. This article is an open access article distributed under the terms and conditions of the Creative Commons Attribution (CC BY) license (https://creativecommons.org/licenses/by/4.0/).

1. Introduction

Pu-erh tea, made by large-leaf tea species (*Camellia sinensis var.assamica*), is one of the top ten famous teas in China and is a geographical landmark product of Yunnan [1]. Pu-erh tea is made from Yunnan large-leaf sun-blue maocha. Under the protection of geographical indications, the tea is made by special processing technology, including primary processing (picking, fixing, rolling, and sun-drying) and the blending and pressing of Pu-erh raw tea, the mentation and finishing of Pu-erh ripe tea, as well as the post processing [2]. Exceptionally, plenty of nutrients such as protein, amino acids, carbohydrates, tea polyphenols, and tea pigments have been reported in Pu-erh tea [3]. Pu-erh has multiple health benefits such as anti-cancer [4], antioxidant [5], anti-hypertensive [6], and hypolipidemic properties [7–9]. In recent years, the demand for Pu-erh tea has increased rapidly, and consumers have increasingly higher requirements for the quality of Pu-erh tea. The government and enterprises are committed to promoting the development of Pu-erh tea production in the direction of intensification, continuity, technology and digitization.

At present, Pu-erh tea has been listed as a geographical indication product. However, due to its high quality and price, especially raw Pu-erh tea, there are frequently phenomena of substandard quality and fake origin in the market. As a result, there is an urgent need to establish a stable and reliable traceability technology of raw Pu-erh tea's origin, and to obtain a fresh and authentic identification model by sampling from the original place of origin. Currently, the common traceability methods applied to tea, herbs and spices include chromatographic, spectroscopic and electrochemical methods such as high-performance liquid chromatography [10], gas chromatography mass spectrometry [11], near-infrared spectroscopy [12,13], electronic nose and electronic tongue [14]. In addition, mineral elements [15–17] and stable isotopic ratios [18] were also effective fingerprints for geographical traceability. Liu et al. detected four stable isotopes (C, N, H, and O) and 20 elements in green tea samples from different provinces of China, and the correct discrimination rate of green tea samples from different origins was 92.30% [19]. Ni et al. examined the ability to discriminate the geographic origin of green tea by determining the multi-element content and stable isotope signature of flat green tea samples from different origins, combined with the decision tree (DT) method. Under the validation of cross-validation and the "blind" dataset, the prediction accuracy was more than 70.00%, and the discrimination accuracy of green tea from different origins was 90.00% [20].

Among them, the multi-element and stable isotopic ratios were closely related with local geological background (soil [21], water [22], etc.) and environment (temperature [23], precipitation [24], etc.), which proved to be effective tools for geographical traceability. As for the geographical traceability of Pu-erh tea, Zhang et al. analyzed 41 elements in 98 Pu-erh tea samples in Yunnan Province. The results showed that the average concentrations of Fe and Pb in tea samples from Pu-erh were significantly higher than those in other production areas, Mn and Cr were generally higher in Xishuangbanna production area, while Ba and rare earth elements showed higher concentrations in Lancang Pu-erh tea samples. As a result, the geographical origins of Pu-erh tea could be distinguished based on the concentrations of 12 elements combined with chemometric analysis [25]. Li et al. conducted an exploration of the content of eight microelements in raw Pu-erh tea to assess the safety risk related to the storage year [26]. The above literature indicates that researchers mostly focus on mineral element and isotope analysis of tea leaves from different regions, and it is feasible to identify the origin of Pu-erh tea by mass-spectrometric techniques. However, the mineral element and isotopic ratios of tea leaves are not only related to the origin (soil, water, climate) [27,28], but the above parameters may also be influenced by factors such as variety and age of the tree [29,30]. However, there are few reports on the influence of tree age on the fingerprint analysis of fresh Pu 'er leaves from different geographical origin. Therefore, we will focus on the of different origin, tree age and other factors as a new research idea in this paper.

In this study, the stable isotopic ratios and mineral elemental contents in fresh leaves of Pu-erh tea from different regions and tree ages were collected. The C and N stable isotopes and the elemental contents in tea leaves were analyzed. The indicators mainly influenced by the region and less affected by tree age were screened to establish the robust discriminative model. Based on the above results, the study could lay the theoretical research foundation for the systematic research and database construction work on the origin traceability technology of Pu-erh tea.

2. Materials and Methods
2.1. Sample Cultivation and Collection

The main production areas (Jinggu County and Ning'er County in Yunnan Pu'er tea City, and Bangdong Township in Lincang City) were selected within the limited area of Geographical Indication Product Pu-erh tea [31]. Two tea gardens were selected in each county. About 200 g of young 'bud' leaves (one bud and two leaf) from large-leaf tea species was sampled from tea trees at each sampling site from 26 to 29 March in 2023. Furthermore, specific information including the geographical location information (longitude, latitude, and altitude information) and tree age of Pu-erh tea trees was also recorded. The detailed information is shown in Table 1.

Table 1. The sample numbers, location, and tree age of tea geographical origins.

Region	Number of Samples	N Latitude (deg)	E Longitude (deg)	Altitude (m)	Tree Age (Year)
Jinggu	24	23.7227	100.6877	1842–1901	20~100 (12), 100~200 (6), >200 (6)
Bangdong	14	23.9374–23.9397	100.3532–100.3562	1633–1739	20~100 (8), 100~200 (3), >200 (3)
Ning'er	15	23.2548	101.0822	1614	20~100 (5), 100~200 (5), >200 (5)

2.2. Sample Pretreatment

The leaves were cleaned before drying so as to remove dust and dirt. All tea samples were put into a dryer at 40 °C to obtain a constant weight. Subsequently, the dried samples were finely ground into a uniform powder using a plant crusher. The resulting powder was then passed through a 100-mesh sieve to achieve a homogeneous particle size. All samples were uniformly stored at 4 °C for further analysis.

2.3. Multi-Element Analysis

The digestion process for each sample closely followed the methodology outlined in our prior research [1]. Approximately 0.25 g of the homogenized sample was subjected to a 2-h treatment with 6 mL of concentrated HNO_3 in Teflon digestion vessels. Subsequently, 2 mL of BV-III grade H_2O_2 was added to each vessel and allowed to react for 30 min. After the release of nitrogen oxides, the digestion vessels were introduced into a microwave digestion instrument (CEM MARS Xpress, Charlotte, NC, USA) and heated gradually to 180 °C for 40 min.

The ICP-MS operational parameters were as follows: radio frequency power at 1280 W, atomizing chamber temperature at 2 °C. The cooling gas, carrier gas, and auxiliary gas were set at flow rates of 1.47 L min^{-1}, 1 L min^{-1}, and 1 L min^{-1}, respectively. To ensure accuracy, the CRM of tea flour (GBW10016) underwent digestion and determination using the same procedure. All sample determinations were performed in triplicate, with a re-measurement undertaken if the relative standard deviation of internal standard concentration exceeded 5%. Element concentration data were corrected based on dry matter after being adjusted for water content measured before digestion. The quality control (LOD, LOQ, recovery, etc.) of the instrument for the mineral element determination is shown in Table S1.

2.4. Stable Carbon and Nitrogen Isotope Analysis

Dry tea samples (0.5–0.6 mg) were carefully weighed into 6.0 mm × 4.0 mm tin capsules and introduced into an elemental analyzer (vario PYRO cube, Elementar Company, Langenselbold, Germany) equipped with an autosampler. Carbon and nitrogen elements within the samples were combusted at 1020 °C, converting them into CO_2 and NOx gases. Subsequently, the NOx was reduced to N_2 through a copper wire at 600 °C before entering an isotope ratio mass spectrometer (IsoPrime100, Isoprime Company, Stockport, UK) via a Conflo III dilutor.

The final stable isotope ratios are expressed as δ notation relative to international standard (Vienna Pee Dee Belimnite (VPDB) for carbon, atmospheric nitrogen (AIR) for nitrogen), according to the following equation:

$$\delta\ (‰) = (R_{sample}/R_{standard} - 1) \times 1000,$$

where δ (‰) represents the $\delta^{13}C$ and $\delta^{15}N$ values, and R is the ratio of $^{13}C/^{12}C$ or $^{15}N/^{14}N$.

For scale normalization and quality assurance, tea samples were analyzed together with reference materials including USGS40 (L-glutamic acid; $\delta^{13}C_{VPDB} = -26.389‰$, $\delta^{15}N_{air} = -4.5‰$) and urea ($\delta^{13}C_{VPDB} = -43.26‰$, $\delta^{15}N_{air} = -0.56‰$) for $\delta^{13}C$ and $\delta^{15}N$ values. Each sample was analyzed three times. The instrumental precision for stable isotope ratio measurements based on the reference materials was $\leq 0.2‰$ for $\delta^{13}C$ values, $\leq 0.2‰$ for $\delta^{15}N$ values, $\leq 3‰$ values, respectively.

2.5. Statistical Analysis

The statistical analyses of the data, including one-way analysis of variance (one-way ANOVA), multiway analysis of variance (multiway ANOVA), principal component analysis (PCA) and linear discriminant analysis (LDA), were carried out with SPSS for Windows version 22.0 (SPSS Inc., Chicago, IL, USA).

One-way ANOVA was applied to elements to test whether the differences in average elemental values are related to considered geographical origins. With post-hoc analysis conducted using either Dunnett's or Tukey's test for multiple comparisons according to the result of Bartlett's test for equal variances. Multiway ANOVA was applied was to quantify the contributions of geographical origin, tree age and their interactions (three factors) to the total variance in element levels. A factor with a larger ratio of relative variance indicates the greater influence relative to the other factors.

Principal component analysis (PCA) is used to transform a set of correlated variables into a set of uncorrelated principal components (PCs) that explain the greatest possible amount of variation in the data, and to provide a comprehensive data visualization [32]. Upon applying PCA to the analytical data for three geographical origins, tea samples could be preliminarily clustered (the first four PCs). In addition, we used Fisher's linear discrimination analysis (LDA) to assess the effectiveness of the elements for the identification of tea origin traceability. Linear discriminant analysis (LDA) is a supervised procedure that maximizes the variances between categories and minimizes the variances within categories by creating new variables (discriminant functions). The reliability of the discriminant model was also verified by the cross-validation method (leave-one-out method).

3. Results

3.1. Comparison of Isotopic Ratios and Mineral Contents from Different Regions

The mean values and standard deviations of mineral element contents in Pu-erh tea samples from different regions are shown in Table 2. The mineral elements (Mg, Mn, Fe, Cu, Zn, Rb, Sr, Y, La, Pr, Nd, Sm, Eu, Gd, Tb, Dy, Ho, Er, Tm, Yb and Lu) and isotopes ($\delta^{15}N$ and $\delta^{13}C$) had significant differences among different geographical origins ($p < 0.05$). The mineral elements (Mg, Mn, Fe, Cu, Rb, Sr, La, Pr, Nd, Sm, Eu, Gd, Tb, Dy, Ho, Er, Tm, Yb and Lu) and isotopes ($\delta^{15}N$ and $\delta^{13}C$) had significant differences between the two geographical origins of Jinggu and Bangdong ($p < 0.01$). The mineral elements (Mn, Y, Gd, Tb, Dy, Ho, Er, Tm, Yb and Lu) had significant differences between the two geographical origins of Jinggu and Ning'er ($p < 0.01$). The mineral elements (Mg, Mn, Rb, Sr, Y, La, Pr, Nd, Sm, Eu, Gd, Tb, Dy, Ho, Er, Tm, Yb and Lu) and isotopes ($\delta^{15}N$ and $\delta^{13}C$) had significant differences between the two geographical origins of Bangdong and Ning'er ($p < 0.01$). Specifically, the highest elemental content of K was found in Ning'er tea samples, and the Fe, Sr, Tb contents and $\delta^{15}N$ were significantly higher in Pu-erh tea samples from Jinggu than in other regions, the elemental contents of Mg, K and Ca were higher in Pu-erh tea samples from Bangdong, while the $\delta^{13}C$ value and the elemental contents of Mg, Mn, Y, Sm, Eu, Gd, Dy, Ho, Er, Tm, Yb, and Lu were significantly higher in Pu-erh tea samples from Ning'er than in other regions. Box plots of stable isotope ratios and mineral contents in Pu-erh tea in different regions are shown in Figure 1.

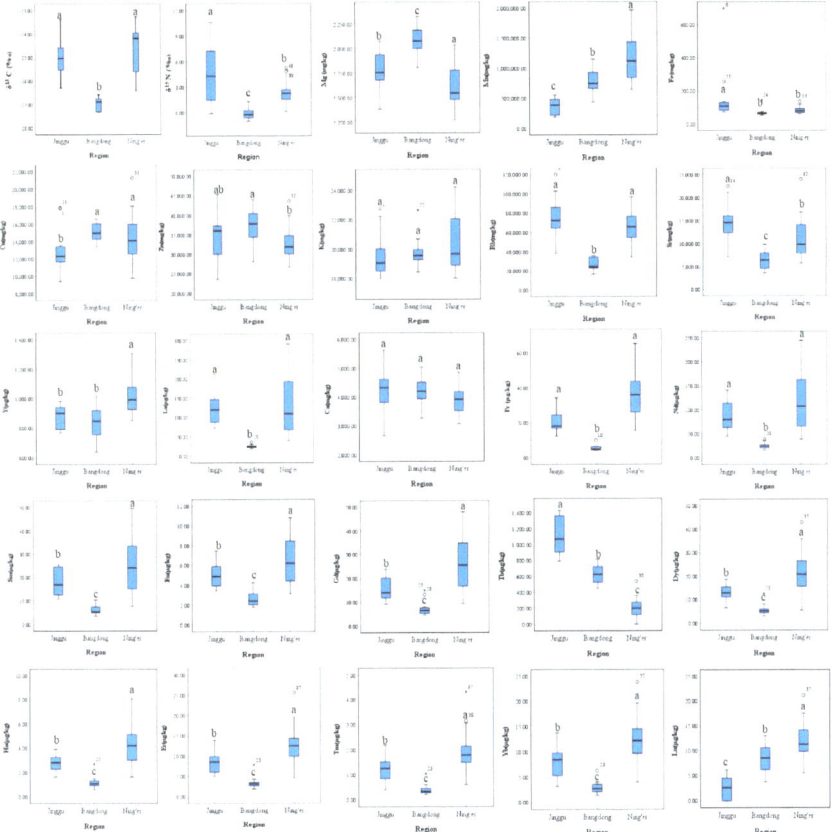

Figure 1. Box plots of stable isotope ratio and mineral content in Pu-erh tea in different regions. a–c in the same row indicated that there are significant differences among regions at $p < 0.05$ level. Note: ○ indicates outliers, and the number in the upper right corner represents the number of in-dividuals that are outliers; * denotes outliers, the number in the upper right corner represents the number of individuals that are outliers.

Table 2. Stable isotope ratios and mineral contents in Pu-erh tea from different regions.

Element	Jinggu	Bangdong	Ning'er
$\delta^{13}C$ (‰) *	−25.16 ± 0.83 [a]	−26.77 ± 0.61 [b]	−24.82 ± 1.16 [a]
$\delta^{15}N$ (‰) **	4.06 ± 3.35 [a]	−0.11 ± 0.66 [c]	2.39 ± 1.30 [b]
Mg (mg/kg) **	1776.176 ± 184.688 [b]	2077.253 ± 152.236 [c]	1601.886 ± 201.680 [a]
K (mg/kg)	19,617.81 ± 1591.58 [a]	19,701.25 ± 1035.70 [a]	20,368.84 ± 1833.42 [a]
Ca (mg/kg)	4193.70 ± 820.56 [a]	4184.00 ± 486.66 [a]	3864.72 ± 469.04 [a]
Mn (mg/kg) **	376 ± 139 [c]	790 ± 219 [b]	1159 ± 359 [a]
Fe (mg/kg) *	155 ± 164 [a]	70 ± 22 [b]	84 ± 20 [b]
Cu (mg/kg) *	12.7 ± 2.5 [b]	15.2 ± 1.1 [a]	14.3 ± 2.5 [a]
Zn (mg/kg) *	34.7 ± 5.9 [ab]	37.3 ± 4.8 [a]	32.9 ± 4.2 [b]
Rb (mg/kg) *	75 ± 21 [a]	28 ± 6 [b]	65 ± 17 [a]
Sr (mg/kg) **	14 ± 5 [a]	7 ± 2 [c]	11 ± 4 [b]
Y (μg/kg) *	876.96 ± 79.77 [b]	843.16 ± 120.60 [b]	1020.33 ± 125.51 [a]
La (μg/kg) *	119.86 ± 38.80 [a]	25.08 ± 4.42 [b]	123.80 ± 68.58 [a]
Pr (μg/kg) *	24 ± 8 [a]	6 ± 2 [b]	29 ± 14 [a]
Nd (μg/kg) *	88.38 ± 30.35 [a]	24.53 ± 6.16 [b]	115.51 ± 54.43 [a]

Table 2. *Cont.*

Element	Jinggu	Bangdong	Ning'er
Sm (µg/kg) **	18 ± 6 [b]	6 ± 2 [c]	25 ± 12 [a]
Eu (µg/kg) **	5.0 ± 1.2 [b]	2.7 ± 0.8 [c]	6.5 ± 2.3 [a]
Gd (µg/kg) **	16 ± 5 [b]	7 ± 3 [c]	26 ± 11 [a]
Tb (µg/kg) **	1122.8 ± 238.5 [a]	630.6 ± 124.7 [b]	219.6 ± 110.1 [c]
Dy (µg/kg) **	13 ± 4 [b]	6 ± 2 [c]	21 ± 9 [a]
Ho (µg/kg) **	2.7 ± 0.7 [b]	1.2 ± 0.5 [c]	4.3 ± 1.6 [a]
Er (µg/kg) **	9 ± 3 [b]	3 ± 1 [c]	13 ± 5 [a]
Tm (µg/kg) **	1.2 ± 0.5 [b]	0.4 ± 0.2 [c]	1.9 ± 0.8 [a]
Yb (µg/kg) **	8 ± 3 [b]	3 ± 1 [c]	13 ± 5 [a]
Lu (µg/kg) **	3.6 ± 1.8 [c]	8.5 ± 2.9 [b]	11.8 ± 3.9 [a]

Data are shown as the mean ± standard deviation. [a–c] in the same row indicated that there are significant differences among regions at $p < 0.05$ level. * means significant difference ($p < 0.05$), ** means highly significant difference ($p < 0.01$).

The mean values and standard deviations of mineral element contents in deep soil (30–60 cm) from different regions are shown in Table 3. The mineral elements (Mg, K, Ca, Mn, Fe, Cu, Zn, Rb, Sr, Y, La, Pr, Nd, Sm, Eu, Gd, Tb, Dy, Ho, Er, Tm, Yb and Lu) had significant differences among different geographical origins ($p < 0.05$). The mineral elements (Mg, K, Mn, Zn, Rb, Y, Pr, Nd, Sm, Eu, Gd, Tb, Dy, Ho and Er) had significant differences between Jinggu and Bangdong ($p < 0.01$). The mineral elements (Mg, K, Mn, Fe, Cu, Zn, Rb, Sr, Y, Eu, Tb, Dy, Ho, Er, Tm, Yb and Lu) had significant differences between Jinggu and Ning'er ($p < 0.01$). The mineral elements (Mg, Fe, Cu, Zn, Rb and Sr) had significant differences between Bangdong and Ning'er ($p < 0.01$). In summary, the trends of the elements (Mn, Rb, Tb and Dy) in the soil in the three geographic regions were consistent with those in Pu-erh tea.

Table 3. Mineral contents in deep soil (30–60 cm) from different regions.

Element	Jinggu	Bangdong	Ning'er
Mg (µg/kg) *	4973.044 ± 1006.566 [a]	2381.777 ± 168.522 [b]	1535.505 ± 76.886 [b]
K (mg/kg) *	27.28 ± 2.41 [a]	10.85 ± 0.08	11.55 ± 0.27 [b]
Ca (µg/kg) *	66.26 ± 22.42 [a]	51.38 ± 5.59 [ab]	37.26 ± 1.24 [b]
Mn (µg/kg) **	1264 ± 46 [b]	1470 ± 40 [a]	341 ± 26 [c]
Fe (mg/kg) *	38 ± 5 [a]	32 ± 1 [a]	17 ± 1 [b]
Cu (µg/kg) *	57.2 ± 7.8 [a]	49.3 ± 1.6 [a]	18.4 ± 0.3 [b]
Zn (µg/kg) **	156.1 ± 14.7 [a]	96.9 ± 3.1 [b]	42.9 ± 2.1 [c]
Rb (µg/kg) **	134 ± 13 [a]	49 ± 4 [c]	82.36 ± 2.04 [b]
Sr (µg/kg) **	28 ± 4 [b]	36 ± 0 [a]	20 ± 1 [c]
Y (µg/kg) *	18.18 ± 1.35 [a]	11.66 ± 0.85 [b]	9.68 ± 1.80 [b]
La (µg/kg) *	40.03 ± 2.05 [a]	27.05 ± 1.64 [b]	31.82 ± 7.64 [ab]
Pr (µg/kg) *	9 ± 0 [a]	5 ± 0 [b]	6 ± 2 [b]
Nd (µg/kg) *	34.81 ± 1.35 [a]	18.09 ± 1.27 [b]	20.85 ± 7.20 [b]
Sm (µg/kg) *	7 ± 0 [a]	3 ± 0 [b]	4 ± 2 [b]
Eu (µg/kg) **	0.8 ± 0.1 [a]	0.5 ± 0.0 [b]	0.3 ± 0.0 [c]
Gd (µg/kg) *	6 ± 0 [a]	2 ± 0 [b]	3 ± 1 [b]
Tb (µg/kg) *	0.7 ± 0.1 [a]	0.3 ± 0.0 [b]	0.4 ± 0.1 [b]
Dy (µg/kg) *	4 ± 0 [a]	2 ± 0 [b]	2 ± 1 [b]
Ho (µg/kg) *	0.7 ± 0.1 [a]	0.4 ± 0.0 [b]	0.3 ± 0.1 [b]
Er (µg/kg) *	2 ± 0 [a]	1 ± 0 [b]	1 ± 0 [b]
Tm (µg/kg) **	0.2 ± 0.0 [a]	0.2 ± 0.0 [b]	0.1 ± 0.0 [c]
Yb (µg/kg) **	2 ± 0 [a]	1 ± 0 [b]	1 ± 0 [c]
Lu (µg/kg) **	0.2 ± 0.0 [a]	0.1 ± 0.0 [b]	0.1 ± 0.0 [c]

Data are shown as the mean ± standard deviation. [a–c] in the same row indicated that there are significant differences among regions at $p < 0.05$ level. * means significant difference ($p < 0.05$), ** means highly significant difference ($p < 0.01$).

As can be seen from Table 4, the canonical correlation analysis (CCA) extracted a total of 9 groups of typical variables, of which 7 groups of typical variables had a correlation coefficient of 0.317, and 8 groups of typical variables had a correlation coefficient of 0.111. As can be seen in Figure 2, when CCA1 was taken as a benchmark, the contents of Nd, La, Pr, Sm, Gd, Mn, Yb, Dy, Fe, Tm, and Ce were positively correlated with soil elemental content, and Eu, Cu, Rb, K, Se, Ca, Tb, and Y were negatively correlated with soil elemental content, of which the content of Ho in tea was weakly correlated with soil elemental content; when CCA2 was taken as a benchmark, the content of Zn, and Sr in tea was positively correlated with soil elemental content, Eu, Cu, Rb, K, Se, Ca, Tb, and Y were positively correlated with soil elemental content, and Eu, Cu, Rb, K, Se, Ca, Tb, and Y were positively correlated with soil elemental content. The contents of Eu, Cu, Rb, K, Se, Ca, Tb, and Y were negatively correlated with the soil element contents, and the content of Mg in tea was weakly negatively correlated with the soil element contents. At the same time, the soil characteristics of the different regions (pH, EC, etc.) are shown in Table 5. Among them, the highest pH value was found in Bangdong, which was significantly different from the other two regions ($p < 0.01$). The lowest EC value was found in Ning'er, which was highly significantly different from the other two regions ($p < 0.01$).

Table 4. The canonical correlation coefficients.

Canonical Variable	Correlation Coefficient
1	−0.077
2	−0.150
3	−0.069
4	−0.255
5	−0.246
6	−0.215
7	0.317
8	0.111
9	0.371

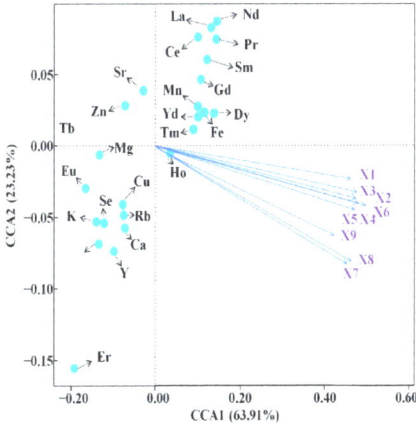

Figure 2. Canonical correlation analysis plot.

Table 5. The soil characteristics of the different regions (pH, EC, etc.).

Region	Bangdong	Jinggu	Ning'er
pH	5.48 ± 0.15 [a]	5.07 ± 0.17 [b]	5.03 ± 0.06 [b]
EC (μs/cm)	46.98 ± 0.93 [a]	34.99 ± 5.97 [b]	24.21 ± 5.64 [c]

[a–c] in the same row indicated that there are significant differences among regions at $p < 0.05$ level.

3.2. Comparison of Isotopic Ratios and Mineral Contents from Different Tree Ages

The mean values and standard deviations of mineral element contents in Pu-erh tea samples of different ages are shown in Table 6. In addition to Zn, other mineral elements (Mg, K, Ca, Mn, Fe, Cu, Rb, Sr, Y, La, Pr, Nd, Sm, Eu, Gd, Tb, Dy, Ho, Er, Tm, Yb, and Lu) and isotopes ($\delta^{13}C$ and $\delta^{15}N$) did not show any significant differences ($p > 0.05$) among tree ages. Among them, the elemental content of Zn was higher in Pu-erh tea samples aged 100~200 than in other ages. Specifically, the elemental differences among tree ages for each region are shown in Table 7. In the region of Bangdong, significant differences ($p < 0.05$) were found for $\delta^{13}C$ and the contents of Ca, Zn, Ho, and Yb in tea leaves among different tree ages. However, the contents of Ca, Pr, Nd, Sm, Eu and Gd in tea leaves had significant differences in the region of Ning'er ($p < 0.05$).

Table 6. Stable isotopes and mineral contents in Pu-erh tea from different tree ages.

Element	20~100	100~200	>200
$\delta^{13}C$ (‰)	−25.19 ± 1.27 [a]	−25.56 ± 1.07 [a]	−25.86 ± 1.37 [a]
$\delta^{15}N$ (‰)	1.82 ± 2.30 [a]	2.43 ± 2.93 [a]	2.36 ± 2.43 [a]
Mg (mg/kg)	1758.798 ± 257.603 [a]	1799.159 ± 335.310 [a]	1808.026 ± 233.497 [a]
K (mg/kg)	20,348.89 ± 1777.85 [a]	19,778.20 ± 1233.41 [a]	19,528.80 ± 1504.73 [a]
Ca (mg/kg)	4109.37 ± 567.86 [a]	3826.25 ± 757.32 [a]	4137.37 ± 431.45 [a]
Mn (μg/kg)	821 ± 481 [a]	889 ± 363 [a]	855 ± 400 [a]
Fe (mg/kg)	1171 ± 124 [a]	86 ± 50 [a]	80 ± 20 [a]
Cu (mg/kg)	13.9 ± 2.5 [a]	15.2 ± 2.5 [a]	13.4 ± 1.7 [a]
Zn (mg/kg) *	34.4 ± 4.7 [ab]	37.1 ± 5.9 [a]	32.4 ± 4.0 [b]
Rb (mg/kg)	62 ± 25 [a]	51 ± 23 [a]	55 ± 25 [a]
Sr (mg/kg)	10 ± 4 [a]	112 ± 6 [a]	12 ± 5 [a]
Y (μg/kg)	935.15 ± 137.55 [a]	942.68 ± 126.28 [a]	916.89 ± 159.38 [a]
La (μg/kg)	109.72 ± 68.93 [a]	68.80 ± 46.51 [a]	94.24 ± 74.79 [a]
Pr (μg/kg)	25 ± 16 [a]	16 ± 9 [a]	20 ± 14 [a]
Nd (μg/kg)	95.70 ± 61.48 [a]	61.80 ± 35.75 [a]	79.98 ± 55.41 [a]
Sm (μg/kg)	21 ± 13 [a]	13 ± 7 [a]	17 ± 11 [a]
Eu (μg/kg)	5.4 ± 2.6 [a]	4.3 ± 1.8 [a]	5.1 ± 2.3 [a]
Gd (μg/kg)	20 ± 13 [a]	14 ± 7 [a]	18 ± 11 [a]
Tb (μg/kg)	638.3 ± 478.3 [a]	520.7 ± 306.6 [a]	560.2 ± 351.2 [a]
Dy (μg/kg)	16 ± 10 [a]	12 ± 6 [a]	146 ± 9 [a]
Ho (μg/kg)	3.3 ± 2.0 [a]	2.5 ± 1.2 [a]	3.0 ± 1.8 [a]
Er (μg/kg)	10 ± 6 [a]	8 ± 4 [a]	9 ± 5 [a]
Tm (μg/kg)	1.4 ± 1.0 [a]	1.1 ± 0.7 [a]	1.3 ± 0.9 [a]
Yb (μg/kg)	9 ± 6 [a]	7 ± 4 [a]	9 ± 5 [a]
Lu (μg/kg)	9.9 ± 5.4 [a]	7.9 ± 3.3 [b]	9.2 ± 4.0 [c]

Data are shown as the mean ± standard deviation. [a-c] in the same row indicated that there are significant differences among tree ages at $p < 0.05$ level. * means significant difference ($p < 0.05$).

Table 7. Stable isotopes and mineral content of Pu-erh tea of different tree ages in each origin.

Element	Jinggu			Bangdong			Ning'er		
	20–100	100–200	>200	20–100	100–200	>200	20–100	100–200	>200
δ¹³C (‰) *	−24.99 ± 0.90 a	−25.46 ± 0.33 a	−25.33 ± 1.11 a	−26.97 ± 0.34 b	−26.19 ± 0.53 a	−27.15 ± 0.50 b	−24.58 ± 1.04 a	−25.09 ± 1.43 a	−25.04 ± 1.22 a
δ¹⁵N (‰)	2.53 ± 3.20 a	6.82 ± 3.29 a	5.37 ± 1.67 a	−0.53 ± 0.50 a	0.21 ± 0.88 a	−0.01 ± 0.38 a	2.33 ± 1.33 a	2.08 ± 0.88 a	2.83 ± 1.65 a
Mg (mg/kg)	1801.02 ± 210.65 a	1731.73 ± 184.49 a	1754.36 ± 161.95 a	2022.54 ± 196.35 a	2146.70 ± 150.99 a	2062.52 ± 98.59 a	1620.76 ± 220.96 a	1543.25 ± 241.60 a	1622.79 ± 125.77 a
K (mg/kg)	19,745.13 ± 1778.10 a	19,765.25 ± 1961.40 a	19,130.87 ± 1048.56 a	19,640.30 ± 794.35 a	20,228.30 ± 1420.24 a	19,235.15 ± 694.88 a	21,046.64 ± 1905.34 a	19,409.59 ± 661.17 a	19,972.49 ± 2154.85 a
Ca (mg/kg) *	4573.75 ± 567.83 a	3250.35 ± 1008.22 b	4123.57 ± 558.13 a	3886.28 ± 424.46 b	4532.52 ± 350.73 a	4133.20 ± 509.79 ab	3892.74 ± 449.67 ab	3525.65 ± 424.20 b	4147.75 ± 388.87 a
Mn (mg/kg)	345 ± 147.577 a	390 ± 162,990 a	443 ± 106,601 a	2 ± 196 a	2 ± 151 a	2 ± 99 a	1207 ± 362 a	1130 ± 299 a	1093 ± 451 a
Fe (mg/kg)	182 ± 210 a	138 ± 103 a	100 ± 32 a	76 ± 39 a	66 ± 7 a	68 ± 4 a	90 ± 25 a	76 ± 10 a	80 ± 15 a
Cu (mg/kg)	12.1 ± 2.6 a	14.5 ± 3.1 a	12.5 ± 0.9 a	15.6 ± 1.1 a	15.6 ± 0.8 a	14.4 ± 0.9 a	14.5 ± 2.3 a	15.1 ± 3.3 a	13.1 ± 2.1 a
Zn (mg/kg) *	35.5 ± 4.8 a	34.9 ± 11.0 a	32.4 ± 3.7 a	37.1 ± 3.6 ab	41.7 ± 2.2 a	33.0 ± 4.1 b	32.6 ± 4.7 a	34.5 ± 2.5 a	31.9 ± 4.6 a
Rb (mg/kg)	77 ± 21 a	62 ± 24 a	82 ± 18 a	26 ± 5 a	27 ± 8 a	32 ± 5 a	67 ± 17 a	65.477 ± 15 a	60 ± 21 a
Sr (mg/kg)	12 ± 3 a	20 ± 3 a	15 ± 2 a	7 ± 2 a	6 ± 2 a	8 ± 2 a	11 ± 4 a	10 ± 3 a	13 ± 6 a
Y (μg/kg)	882.84 ± 89.57 a	871.83 ± 76.97 a	866.40 ± 83.77 a	820.49 ± 126.44 a	891.47 ± 98.12 a	817.53 ± 144.60 a	1017.80 ± 122.24 a	1020.78 ± 135.79 a	1024.94 ± 145.27 a
La (μg/kg)	104.81 ± 28.51 a	118.79 ± 36.43 a	161.04 ± 46.52 a	22.65 ± 3.31 a	26.91 ± 6.35 a	25.70 ± 2.23 a	149.27 ± 68.38 a	78.72 ± 41.09 a	117.96 ± 75.00 a
Pr (μg/kg) *	21 ± 7 a	27 ± 7 a	29 ± 8 a	6 ± 2 a	7 ± 1 a	6 ± 1 a	36 ± 14 a	18 ± 7 b	28 ± 14 ab
Nd (μg/kg) *	77.34 ± 30.11 a	99.98 ± 26.08 a	106.19 ± 31.11 a	20.61 ± 4.17 a	26.65 ± 7.40 a	26.33 ± 5.63 a	139.23 ± 52.80 a	71.99 ± 27.79 b	111.59 ± 55.50 ab
Sm (μg/kg) *	16 ± 6 a	20 ± 6 a	21 ± 4 a	5 ± 1 a	7 ± 2 a	7 ± 2 a	30 ± 11 a	16 ± 6 b	24 ± 12 ab
Eu (μg/kg) *	4.5 ± 0.8 a	5.7 ± 2.0 a	5.6 ± 0.8 a	2.1 ± 0.4 a	2.9 ± 0.6 a	2.9 ± 1.0 a	7.4 ± 2.2 a	4.6 ± 1.7 b	6.6 ± 2.3 ab
Gd (μg/kg) *	14 ± 4 a	8 ± 6 a	17 ± 6 a	5 ± 1 a	8 ± 3 a	8 ± 4 a	31 ± 10 a	18 ± 7 b	26 ± 12 ab
Tb (μg/kg) *	1252.0 ± 207.2 a	864.3 ± 64.2 b	1036.8 ± 192.7 a	654.1 ± 115.1 a	652.9 ± 127.3 a	584.9 ± 145.2 a	222.6 ± 66.5 a	182.2 ± 100.2 a	249.6 ± 196.4 a
Dy (μg/kg)	12 ± 3 a	14 ± 5 a	14 ± 3 a	4 ± 1 a	6 ± 1 a	7 ± 3 a	24 ± 9 a	15 ± 5 a	21 ± 10 a
Ho (μg/kg) *	2.5 ± 0.6 a	3.1 ± 0.7 a	3.1 ± 0.8 a	0.9 ± 0.2 b	1.2 ± 0.2 ab	1.5 ± 0.7 a	4.8 ± 1.6 a	3.2 ± 1.1 a	4.3 ± 1.9 a
Er (μg/kg)	8 ± 2 a	1 ± 4 a	9 ± 3 a	3 ± 1 a	4 ± 2 a	4 ± 2 a	14 ± 5 a	10 ± 3 a	13 ± 5 a
Tm (μg/kg) *	1.0 ± 0.4 a	1.7 ± 0.7 a	1.3 ± 0.5 a	0.3 ± 0.1 a	0.4 ± 0.1 a	0.5 ± 0.3 a	2.2 ± 0.9 a	1.4 ± 0.5 a	2.0 ± 0.8 a
Yb (μg/kg) *	7 ± 3 a	10 ± 4 a	10 ± 3 a	2 ± 1 b	3 ± 1 ab	4 ± 2 a	14 ± 4 a	9 ± 3 a	12 ± 5 ab
Lu (μg/kg)	3.7 ± 2.7 a	3.5 ± 1.1 a	3.6 ± 1.7 a	7.6 ± 2.2 a	8.2 ± 3.4 a	9.6 ± 3.1 a	12.9 ± 4.8 a	9.8 ± 1.7 a	11.8 ± 2.6 a

Data are shown as the mean ± standard deviation. a,b in the same row indicated that there are significant differences among regions at $p < 0.05$ level. * means significant difference ($p < 0.05$).

3.3. Multi-Way Analysis of Variance for Stable Isotopic Ratios and Elements

A combined analysis of variance across three regions and three tree ages was performed using the general linear model (GLM) procedure of SPSS (Table 8). Regions and tree age were considered as fixed factors, and the effects were portioned into different sources, such as region (R), age (A), and region × age (R × A). In total, the stable isotope values (δ^{15}N and δ^{13}C) and the mineral contents (Mg, Mn, Rb, Sr, Y La, Pr, Nd, Sm, Eu, Gd, Tb, Dy, Ho, Er, Tm, Yb, and Lu) in Pu-erh tea were highly significantly influenced by region ($p < 0.01$), the contents of Fe and Zn in Pu-erh tea were significantly influenced by region ($p < 0.05$), whereas R × A had significant effects on Mn content ($p < 0.01$).

Table 8. Mean square of each stable isotope and element by analysis of variance.

Source of Variation	Region (R)	Age (A)	R × A	Error
DF	2	2	4	44
cc (‰)	16.162 **	0.453	0.783	0.918
δ^{15}N (‰)	89.32 **	4.98	3.31	3.24
Mg (mg/kg)	940,372.990 **	214.532	16,805.581	35,097.374
K (mg/kg)	320,175.52	4,407,718.36	1,902,670.37	2,576,350.83
Ca (mg/kg)	343,041.76	441,090.52	973,706.97	223,680.31
Mn (mg/kg)	212,6241 **	45,782	38,559,311 **	88,978,814
Fe (mg/kg)	28,113 *	12,679	7124	8161
Cu (mg/kg)	12,380.3	9732.2	1244.7	5492.3
Zn (mg/kg)	77,533.4 *	48,583.2	22,130.5	21,778.1
Rb (mg/kg)	7,570,777 **	208,510	230,305	211,491
Sr (mg/kg)	231,854 **	32,516	34,624	13,801
Y (mg/kg)	178.84 **	4.56	2.25	15.11
La (mg/kg)	51.79 **	2.90	2.40	2.32
Pr (µg/kg)	2357 **	82	152	95
Nd (mg/kg)	35.45 **	1.23	2.20	1.38
Sm (µg/kg)	1466 **	56	95	61
Eu (µg/kg)	60.9 **	1.3	4.9	2.7
Gd (µg/kg)	1439 **	28	97	57
Tb (mg/kg)	2068.2 **	0.0	0.0	0.0
Dy (µg/kg)	954 **	11	48	39
Ho (µg/kg)	39.5 **	0.7	1.6	1.4
Er (µg/kg)	363 **	2	18	13
Tm (µg/kg)	9.5 **	0.0	0.5	0.4
Yb (µg/kg)	364 **	5	22	13
Lu (µg/kg)	215.4 **	3.8	5.5	11.3

* means significant effect ($p < 0.05$), ** means highly significant effect ($p < 0.01$).

3.4. Principal Component Analysis of Isotope Ratios and Mineral Content of Pu-erh Tea from Different Regions

Through the above effects of region, tree age and their interaction on the isotope ratios and mineral contents of Pu-erh tea, 22 characteristic mineral elements related to the regions, including Mg, Mn, Fe, Zn, Rb, Sr, Y, La, Pr, Nd, Sm, Eu, Gd, Tb, Dy, Ho, Er, Tm, Yb, Lu, δ^{13}C and δ^{15}N were screened. The screened 22 characteristic mineral elements were subjected to principal component analysis of different regions, and the results are shown in Table S2. Four principal components were obtained with a cumulative contribution of 82.54%. Principal component 1 mainly contains δ^{13}C, δ^{15}N, Fe, Cu, Sr, Y, La, Pr, Nd, Sm, Eu, Gd, Tb, Ho, Er, Tm, Yb and Lu, and the contribution rate is 57.76%, principal component 2 mainly contains δ^{15}N, Cu, Sr, Y, Pr, Nd, Sm and Dy element information, and the contribution rate is 13.43%, principal component 3 mainly contains the information of δ^{15}N and Mg, Cu, Rb, Pr, Nd, Sm, Eu, Tb and Dy elements, and the contribution rate is 6.76%, principal component 4 mainly contains δ^{13}C, Fe, Cu, Rb, Sr and La information with a contribution rate of 4.60%. The four most important variables were Nd, Sm, Eu, Gd, Tb, Ho, Er, Tm, Yb and Lu in PC1, and δ^{15}N, Sr, Y and Dy in PC2, and Mg in PC3, respectively (Figure 3a). Meanwhile, three origin samples (Ning'er, Jinggu, Bangdong) were correctly distinguished. And they are distributed in different spatial regions. It shows that the selected mineral elements and stable isotope origin traceability fingerprint can be used to distinguish Pu-erh tea from different origins (Figure 3b). The Pu-erh tea samples from three geographical origins were distributed in different spatial distributions. The results indicated that these elements could be used for the identification of the geographical origin of Pu-erh tea.

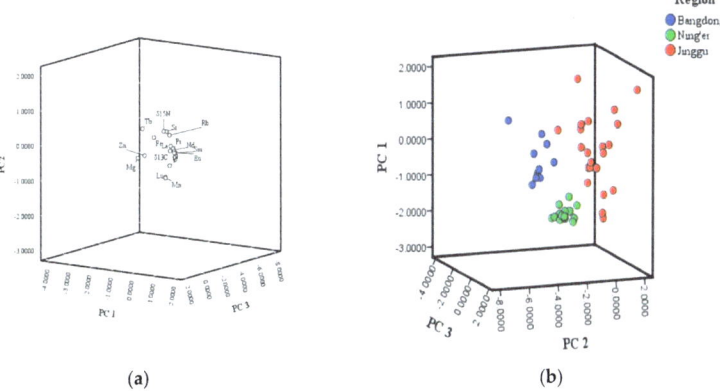

Figure 3. Discriminant function scores of Pu-erh tea of different regions. (**a**) The Pu-erh tea samples from different origin sources were plotted using principal component scores; (**b**) The scores of Pu-erh tea from different origin sources were plotted using the scores of PC1, PC2, and PC3.

3.5. Discriminant Analysis of Isotope Ratio and Mineral Element Content of Pu-erh Tea from Different Regions

Stepwise discriminant analysis was conducted on Mg, Mn, Fe, Zn, Rb, Sr, Y, La, Pr, Nd, Sm, Eu, Gd, Tb, Dy, Ho, Er, Tm, Yb, Lu, δ^{13}C and δ^{15}N, and seven indicators were selected to establish the discriminant model. The cross-validation model was also used to obtain the classification results of Pu-erh tea samples from three regions, as shown in Table S3. Based on the discriminant model using the screened elements, the classification results showed that both original and cross-validation of correct discriminant rates could reach 100%. The result indicated that a discriminative model consisting of these elements was fully capable of correctly discriminating samples.

The discrimination model formula is as follows:

$$Y_{Bangdong} = -44.943\ \delta^{13}C + 0.081\ \delta^{15}N + 0.42\ Mg + 2.863 \times 10^{-5}\ Mn + 8.186 \times 10^{-6}\ Rb + 0.175\ La + 0.101\ Tb - 675.771$$

$$Y_{Ning'er} = -48.217\ \delta^{13}C - 3.003\ \delta^{15}N + 0.054\ Mg + 4.555 \times 10^{-5}\ Mn - 3.021 \times 10^{-4}\ Rb + 0.129\ La + 0.068\ Tb - 739.961$$

$$Y_{Jinggu} = -45.218\ \delta^{13}C - 3.404\ \delta^{15}N + 0.031\ Mg + 4.504 \times 10^{-5}\ Mn - 1.039 \times 10^{-4}\ Rb + 0.220\ La + 0.034\ Tb - 621.148$$

As shown in Figure 4, the distribution of Pu-erh tea from different regions was obtained. As was seen from the figure, the Pu-erh tea samples from the three regions were completely distinguished and located in different spaces, and there was a certain spatial range between the regions, indicating that the selected indicators related to the region were accurate and effective.

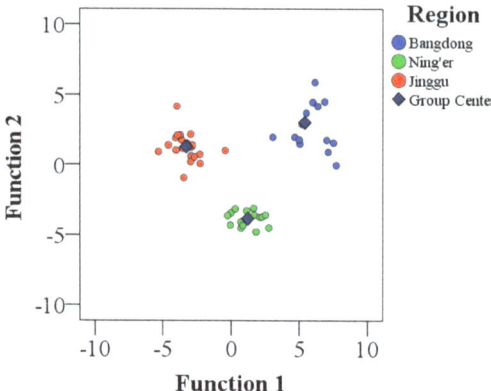

Figure 4. Discriminant function score map of Pu-erh tea from different regions.

As can be seen from Table 9, the model was validated by determining the indicators (δ^{13}C, δ^{15}N, Mg, Mn, Rb, La, and Tb) of nine Pu-erh tea samples from Bangdong. All the samples were correctly discriminated, and a correct discrimination rate of 100.00% was obtained.

Table 9. The external validation based on the indicator of new Pu-erh tea samples.

Region	δ^{13}C	δ^{15}N	Mg	Mn	Rb	La	Tb
	−26.01	1.40	2,724,050.97	1,235,282.25	90,404.89	523.63	8.20
	−25.98	2.74	2,772,521.47	1,066,798.51	86,209.27	289.25	6.09
	−27.43	3.19	2,632,641.73	1,043,034.78	96,223.16	214.16	4.73
	−27.91	2.75	2,686,877.79	916,569.28	102,914.99	367.90	6.83
Bangdong	−26.16	2.57	3,067,714.29	969,110.57	133,737.01	375.74	5.66
	−25.36	2.50	2,658,854.62	737,281.79	108,884.34	242.07	5.16
	−25.68	2.31	2,482,755.05	1,006,464.11	102,004.56	391.33	7.49
	−25.32	1.93	2,760,370.63	1,260,159.98	120,953.10	295.24	7.58
	−26.30	2.57	2,543,127.79	947,274.99	95,336.29	369.31	6.56

4. Discussion

In our study, there were significant differences in stable isotopes among the three regions. The lowest δ^{13}C value was found in Pu-erh tea leaves from the Bangdong region, while no significant difference was found between the other two regions. The δ^{13}C value in tea leaves was shown as follows: Ning'er > Jinggu > Bangdong, while the tendency of latitude for the three regions was the same, which indicated that the δ^{13}C values in tea leaves increased with the higher latitude, which is consistent with the previous results [33]. Generally, tea areas at low latitudes have high average annual temperatures and receive more light radiation on the surface of the ground. Pu-erh tea, as a C_3 plant, utilizes the Calvin photosynthetic pathway for CO_2 assimilation. The δ^{13}C values in plants have been found to correlate with the ratio of intercellular CO_2 and CO_2 from the surrounding environment (P_i/P_a) [34]. This correlation reflects the variability in CO_2 sources (both concentrations and δ^{13}C values) across different regions. Specifically, higher latitude is often associated with higher atmospheric CO_2 concentrations, which in turn results in variations in physiological processes and δ^{13}C values within Pu-erh tea. In addition, the δ^{13}C values of Pu-erh tea samples with different geographical origins ranged from −24.58‰ to −27.15‰, falling in the range of C_3 plants (−34‰ to −24‰) [35], and the result was agreed with a previous report in which δ^{13}C values for Chinese green tea varied between −28.5‰ and −24.5‰ [36]. The observed variation in δ^{15}N value was found in Pu-erh tea from the Bangdong region, while there was no significant difference in values. Numerous investigations have showcased the correlation between fertilizer application in agricultural techniques and the $\delta^{15}N$ levels in plants. Traditionally, synthetic nitrogen-based fertilizers exhibit nitrogen isotope values ranging from −4‰ to 4‰, while organic fertilizers generally manifest higher $\delta^{15}N$ values and exhibit a considerably broader spectrum (2–30‰) than their synthetic counterparts [37]. It is worth mentioning that distinct synthetic nitrogen fertilizers may also display varying $\delta^{15}N$ values.

In addition, the contents of mineral elements such as Rb, La, Pr, and Nd were lower in Pu-erh tea leaves from the Bangdong region, while no significant difference was found between the other two regions. There were significant differences in the contents of mineral elements (Fe) in Pu-erh tea leaves in the Jinggu region compared with other regions. This might be because the mineral elements in plants were closely related to the mineral contents in the regional soil [38]. The mineral contents in soils were mainly influenced by conditions such as soil-forming parent material, soil pH, climate, and precipitation, which formed the specific elemental fingerprints among different regions. The characteristics of the "soil-plant" system led to variations in the composition of trace elements in plant tissues. At the same time, compared with the previous mineral elements of Pu-erh tea, especially the Mg values of Pu-erh tea samples with different geographical origins ranged from 1797.00 to 2273.50 mg/kg, agreeing with a previous report in which Mn values for Pu-erh tea varied between 381.65 to 878.15 mg/kg [39]. For Pu-erh tea from Yunnan Province, the total amount of Eu (0.010 ± 0.002 µg/g) was close to a previous report in which the content of Eu was 6.49 ± 2.30 µg/kg, and the Yb content (0.019 ± 0.006 µg/g) was also similar with the previous report, with the Yb content was 12.25 ± 4.66 µg/kg [40]. Furthermore, the mineral element content (e.g., Zn) in Pu-erh tea is also influenced by the age of the tea trees. Differences in Zn content can arise as a result of variations in the growing environment of tea trees of different ages, given that Zn constitutes one of the vital trace elements needed for plant growth and development. However, additional comprehensive investigations are required to establish the pattern of change in the content of other mineral elements across different ages of Pu-erh tea trees.

Although previous studies have obtained good discrimination for the geographical origins of tea by using the stable isotope techniques or mineral element techniques [41,42], the combination of two techniques was used for the first time to effectively identify the origin of fresh Pu-erh tea, obtaining a high overall correct classification rate (100.0%) and cross-validation rate (100.0%).

5. Conclusions

In this study, $\delta^{13}C$ and $\delta^{15}N$ values and 24 elemental contents of Pu-erh tea samples from different regions and tree ages were comprehensively analyzed. Based on the multi-way analysis of variance, only those significantly influenced by region were screened to better distinguish between samples of different geographical origins. Using the screened elements, step-wised discriminant analysis with 100.0% correct discrimination and 100.0% cross-validation was obtained, and a discriminant model was established with only six parameters ($\delta^{13}C$, $\delta^{15}N$, Mn, Mg, La, and Tb), indicating that the elements screened in relation to origin were accurate and effective. Therefore, it is technically feasible to screen the effective stable isotope and mineral elements to discriminate the origin of Pu-erh tea. In addition, the study could also provide a reference for the establishment of a database for the traceability of Pu-erh tea's geographical origin. Because the tree age of 100 years is a variable, the data should be available for identification in the second year. However, it requires resampling for validation. Two tea plantations were chosen from each region, which were representative to a certain extent but still this is not many. Therefore, further expansion of the production areas under study is needed.

Supplementary Materials: The following supporting information can be downloaded at: https://www.mdpi.com/article/10.3390/foods13030473/s1, Table S1: Stable isotopes and mineral contents in Pu-erh tea from different tree ages; Table S2: Principal component analysis table of characteristic mineral elements; Table S3: Classification results of Pu-erh tea from different regions; Table S4:

Stable isotope and mineral element content in Pu-erh tea samples from different regions (Tree age, variety, etc.).

Author Contributions: H.-Y.L. and L.-L.Q. conceived the idea and designed the experiments. M.-M.C. and Q.-H.L. analyzed the data and wrote the manuscript draft. H.-D.Z., Y.-L.L. and Y.S. performed the experiments. Q.-H.L., Y.X., Y.L. and H.-Y.L. edited and revised the manuscript, H.-Y.L. and Z.-L.L. provided the funding. The final version of the manuscript was approved by all authors. All authors have read and agreed to the published version of the manuscript.

Funding: The National Natural Science Foundation of China (No. 32202169), the Local Financial Funds of National Agricultural Science and Technology Center, Chengdu (No. NASC2022KR06), the Agricultural Science and Technology Innovation Program (No. ASTIP-IUA-2023003), and the Open Project of China Food Flavor and Nutrition Health Innovation Center (No. CFC2023B-027).

Institutional Review Board Statement: Not Applicable.

Informed Consent Statement: Not Applicable.

Data Availability Statement: Data is contained within the article or supplementary material.

Conflicts of Interest: The authors declare no conflict of interest.

References

1. Liu, Z.; Yuan, Y.W.; Zhang, Y.Z.; Shi, Y.Z.; Hu, G.Z.; Zhu, J.H.; Rogers, K.M. Geographical traceability of Chinese green tea using stable isotope and multi-element chemometrics. *Rapid Commun. Mass Spectrom.* **2019**, *33*, 778–788. [CrossRef]
2. Chen, W.; Keita, Y.; Osamu, S.K.; Akiko, M.; Alexis, G.; Naohiro, Y. Development of a methodology using gas chromatography-combustion-isotope ratio mass spectrometry for the determination of the carbon isotope ratio of caffeine extracted from tea leaves (*Camellia sinensis*). *Rapid Commun. Mass Spectrom.* **2012**, *26*, 978–982. [CrossRef]
3. Lin, F.J.; Wei, X.L.; Liu, H.Y.; Li, H.; Xia, Y.; Wu, D.T.; Zhang, P.Z.; Gandhi, G.R.; Li, H.B.; Gan, R.Y. State-of-the-art review of dark tea: From chemistry to health benefits. *Trends Food Sci. Technol.* **2021**, *109*, 126–138. [CrossRef]
4. Huyen, T.V.; Fu, V.S.; Kun, V.T.; Haibin, S.; Gregory, A.C. Systematic characterization of the structure and radical scavenging potency of Pu-erh tea polyphenol theaflavin. *Org. Biomol. Chem.* **2019**, *17*, 9942–9950. [CrossRef]
5. Su, J.J.; Wang, X.Q.; Song, W.J.; Bai, X.L.; Li, C.W. Reducing oxidative stress and hepatoprotective effect of the water extracts from Pu-erh tea on rats fed with high-fat diet. *Food Sci. Hum. Wellness* **2016**, *5*, 199–206. [CrossRef]
6. Lv, H.P.; Zhu, Y.; Tan, J.F.; Guo, L.; Dai, W.D.; Lin, Z. Bioactive compounds from Pu-erh tea with therapy for hyperlipidaemia. *J. Funct. Foods* **2016**, *19*, 194–203. [CrossRef]
7. Huang, F.J.; Wang, S.L.; Zhao, A.H.; Zheng, X.J.; Zhang, Y.J.; Lei, S.; Ge, K.; Qu, C.; Zhao, Q.; Yan, C.; et al. Pu-erh tea regulates fatty acid metabolism in mice under high-fat diet. *Front. Pharmacol.* **2019**, *10*, 63. [CrossRef]
8. Luo, D.; Chen, X.J.; Zhu, X.; Liu, S.; Li, J.; Xu, J.P.; Zhao, J.H.; Ji, X. Pu-erh tea relaxes the thoracic aorta of rats by reducing intracellular calcium. *Front. Pharmacol.* **2019**, *10*, 1430. [CrossRef]
9. Gabriella, R.; Cristina, M.; Anita, G.; Claudia, P.; Giancarlo, A.; Marina, C.; Luca, R. Ripe and raw Pu-erh tea: LCMS profiling, antioxidant capacity and enzyme inhibition activities of aqueous and Hydro-alcoholic extracts. *Molecules* **2004**, *24*, 473–475. [CrossRef]
10. Navratilova, K.; Hrbek, V.; Kratky, F. Green tea: Authentication of geographic origin based on UHPLC-HRMS fingerprints. *J. Food Compos. Anal.* **2019**, *78*, 121–128. [CrossRef]
11. Lin, J.; Zhang, P.; Pan, Z.Q. Discrimination of oolong tea (*Camellia sinensis*) varieties based on feature extraction and selection from aromatic profiles analysed by HS-SPME/GC-MS. *Food Chem.* **2013**, *141*, 259–265. [CrossRef]
12. Kumar, V.; Roy, B.K. Population authentication of the traditional medicinal plant Cassia tora L. based on ISSR markers and FTIR analysis. *Sci. Rep.* **2018**, *8*, 10714. [CrossRef] [PubMed]
13. Kovcs, Z.; Dalmadi, I.; Lukcs, L. Geographical origin identification of pure Sri Lanka tea infusions with electronic nose, electronic tongue and sensory profile analysis. *J. Chemom.* **2009**, *24*, 121–130. [CrossRef]
14. Zhang, Y.H.; Jiang, L.; Feng, N.C.; Gao, Y.Y.; Zhu, M.L. Content Comparison of Seven Harmful Elements in Lycium barbarum Berry from the Geographical Origin Fields and Supermarkets. *Int. J. Agric. Biol.* **2020**, *6*, 1565–1572. [CrossRef]
15. Pilgrim, T.S.; Watling, R.J.; Grice, K. Application of trace element and stable isotope signatures to determine the provenance of tea (*Camellia sinensis*) samples. *Food Chem.* **2010**, *118*, 921–926. [CrossRef]
16. Fern, N.C.; Mart, N.M.J.; Pablos, F. Differentiation of tea (*Camellia sinensis*) varieties and their geographical origin according to their metal content. *J. Agric. Food Chem.* **2001**, *49*, 4775–4779. [CrossRef]
17. Budnov, G.; Vláčil, D.; Mestek, O.; Volka, K. Application of infrared spectroscopy to the assessment of authenticity of tea. *Talanta* **1998**, *47*, 255–260. [CrossRef] [PubMed]
18. Zhang, M.L.; Huang, C.W.; Zhang, J.Y. Accurate discrimination of tea from multiple geographical regions by combining multi-elements with multivariate statistical analysis. *J. Food Meas. Charact.* **2020**, *14*, 3361–3370. [CrossRef]

19. Liu, W.W.; Chen, Y.; Liao, R.X.; Zhao, J.; Yang, H.; Wang, F.H. Authentication of the geographical origin of Guizhou green tea using stable isotope and mineral element signatures combined with chemometric analysis. *Food Control* **2021**, *125*, 3–8. [CrossRef]
20. Ni, K.; Wang, J.; Zhang, Q.F.; Yi, X.Y.; Ma, L.F.; Shi, Y.Z.; Ruan, J.Y. Multi-element composition and isotopic signatures for the geographical origin discrimination of green tea in China: A case study of Xihu Longjing. *J. Food Compos. Anal.* **2018**, *67*, 104–109. [CrossRef]
21. Rashid, M.H.; Fardous, Z.; Chowdhury, M.A.Z.; Alam, M.K.; Bari, M.L.; Moniruzzaman, M.L.; Gan, S.H. Determination of heavy metals in the soils of tea plantations and in fresh and processed tea leaves: An evaluation of six digestion methods. *Chem. Cent. J.* **2016**, *10*, 7. [CrossRef]
22. Han, W.; Shi, Y.; Ma, L.; Ruan, J.; Zhao, F. Effect of liming and seasonal variation on lead concentration of tea plant (*Camellia sinensis* (L.) O. Kuntze). *Chemosphere* **2007**, *66*, 84–90. [CrossRef]
23. Du, Y.; Shin, S.; Wang, K.; Lu, J.; Liang, Y. Effect of temperature on the expression of genes related to the accumulation of chlorophylls and carotenoids in albino tea. *J. Hortic. Sci. Biotechnol.* **2015**, *84*, 365–369. [CrossRef]
24. Jayasekera, S.; Kaur, L.; Molan, A.; Garg, M.L.; Moughan, P. Effects of season and plantation on phenolic content of unfermented and fermented Sri Lankan tea. *Food Chem.* **2014**, *152*, 546–551. [CrossRef] [PubMed]
25. Zhang, J.Y.; Ma, G.C.; Chen, L.Y.; Liu, T.; Liu, X.; Lu, C.Y. Profiling elements in Pu-erh tea from Yunnan province, China. *Food Addit. Contam. Part B* **2017**, *10*, 155–164. [CrossRef]
26. Li, F.; Lu, Q.H.; Li, M.; Yang, X.M.; Xiong, C.Y.; Yang, B. Comparison and risk assessment for trace heavy metals in raw Pu-erh tea with different storage years. *Biol. Trace Elem. Res.* **2020**, *195*, 696–706. [CrossRef]
27. Zhao, H.Y.; Yang, Q.L. The suitability of rare earth elements for geographical traceability of tea leaves. *J. Sci. Food Agric.* **2019**, *99*, 6509–6514. [CrossRef]
28. Zhao, H.Y.; Yu, C.D.; Li, M. Effects of geographical origin, variety, season and their interactions on minerals in tea for traceability. *J. Food Compos. Anal.* **2017**, *63*, 15–20. [CrossRef]
29. Ding, B.; Zeng, G.F.; Wang, Z.Y.; Xie, J.J.; Wang, L.; Chen, W.R. Authenticity determination of tea drinks in the Chinese market by liquid chromatography coupled to isotope ratio mass spectrometry. *Microchem. J.* **2019**, *144*, 139–143. [CrossRef]
30. Liu, H.Y.; Wei, Y.M.; Zhang, Y.Q.; Wei, S.; Zhang, S.S.; Guo, B.L. The effectiveness of multi-element fingerprints for identifying the geographical origin of wheat. *Int. J. Food Sci. Technol.* **2017**, *52*, 1018–1025. [CrossRef]
31. GB/T 22111-2008; Geographical Indication Products Pu-erh Tea. Available online: https://www.chinesestandard.net/PDF/English.aspx/GBT22111-2008 (accessed on 8 August 2023).
32. Wold, S.; Esbensen, K.; Geladi, P. Principal component analysis. *Chemom. Intell. Lab. Syst.* **1987**, *2*, 37–52. [CrossRef]
33. Wang, J.; Li, X.; Wu, Y.; Qu, F.; Liu, L.; Wang, B.; Wang, P.; Zhang, X. HS−SPME/GC−MS Reveals the Season Effects on Volatile Compounds of Green Tea in High−Latitude Region. *Foods* **2022**, *11*, 3016. [CrossRef] [PubMed]
34. Farquhar, G.D.; O'Leary, M.H.; Berry, J.A. On the Relationship Between Carbon Isotope Discrimination and the intercellular carbon dioxide concentration in leaves. *Aust. J. Plant Physiol.* **1982**, *9*, 121–137. [CrossRef]
35. Vogel, J.C. *Fractionation of the Carbon Isotopes during Photosynthesis*; Springer: Berlin/Heidelberg, Germany, 1980; pp. 111–135. [CrossRef]
36. Deng, X.F.; Liu, Z.; Zhan, Y.; Ni, K.; Zhang, Y.Z.; Ma, W.Z.; Shao, S.Z.; Lv, X.N.; Yuan, Y.W.; Rogers, K.M. Predictive geographical authentication of green tea with protected designation of origin using a random forest model. *Food Control* **2020**, *107*, 106807. [CrossRef]
37. Kendall, C. Tracing nitrogen sources and cycling in catchments. In *Isotope Tracers in Catchment Hydrology*; Kendall, C., McDonnell, J.J., Eds.; Elsevier: Amsterdam, The Netherlands, 1998; pp. 519–576. [CrossRef]
38. Zhang, J.Y.; Nie, J.Y.; Zhang, L.B.; Xu, G.F.; Zheng, H.D.; Shen, Y.M.; Kuang, L.X.; Gao, X.Q.; Zhang, H. Multielement authentication of apples from the cold highlands in southwest China. *J. Sci. Food Agric.* **2022**, *102*, 241–249. [CrossRef]
39. Lv, H.P.; Lin, Z.; Zhang, Y.; Liang, Y.R. Study on the content of the major mineral elements in Pu-erh tea. *J. Tea Sci.* **2013**, *33*, 411–419. [CrossRef]
40. Zhu, J.Y.; Chen, L.; Chen, Y.; Rong, Y.T.; Jiang, Y.W.; Liu, F.Q.; Zhou, Q.H.; Wei, X.H.; Yuan, H.B.; Zhang, J.J.; et al. Effect of geographical origins and pile-fermentation on the multi-element profiles of ripen Pu-erh tea revealed by comprehensive elemental fingerprinting. *Food Control* **2013**, *105*, 109978. [CrossRef]
41. Lagad, R.A.; Alamelu, D.; Laskar, A.H.; Rai, V.K.; Singh, S.K.; Aggarwal, S.K. Isotope signature study of the tea samples produced at four different regions in India. *Anal. Methods* **2013**, *5*, 1604. [CrossRef]
42. Lou, Y.X.; Fu, X.S.; Yu, X.P.; Ye, Z.H.; Cui, H.F.; Zhang, Y.F. Stable isotope ratio and elemental profile combined with support vector machine for provenance discrimination of Oolong tea (Wuyi-Rock Tea). *J. Anal. Methods Chem.* **2017**, *2017*, 5454231. [CrossRef]

Disclaimer/Publisher's Note: The statements, opinions and data contained in all publications are solely those of the individual author(s) and contributor(s) and not of MDPI and/or the editor(s). MDPI and/or the editor(s) disclaim responsibility for any injury to people or property resulting from any ideas, methods, instructions or products referred to in the content.

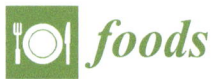

Communication

Traceability Research on *Dendrobium devonianum* Based on SWATHtoMRM

Tao Lin [1], Xinglian Chen [1], Lijuan Du [1], Jing Wang [2], Zhengxu Hu [2], Long Cheng [3], Zhenhuan Liu [1] and Hongcheng Liu [1,*]

[1] Quality Standards and Testing Technology Research Institute, Yunnan Academy of Agricultural Sciences, Kunming 650205, China; lintaonj@126.com (T.L.); chen544141152@163.com (X.C.); 15825298061@163.com (L.D.); lzh@yaas.org.cn (Z.L.)

[2] Longling Agricultural Environmental Protection Monitoring Station, Baoshan 678300, China; jingjingmichuer@163.com (J.W.); 18708755021@139.com (Z.H.)

[3] SCIEX Analytical Instrument Trading Co., Ltd., Shanghai 200335, China; long.cheng@sciex.com

* Correspondence: lhc@yaas.org.cn; Tel./Fax: +86-871-6514-9900

Abstract: SWATHtoMRM technology was used in this experiment to further identify and trace the sources of *Dendrobium devonianum* and *Dendrobium officinale* produced in the same area using TOF and MS-MRM. After the conversion of the R package of SWATHtoMRM, 191 MRM pairs of positive ions and 96 pairs of negative ions were obtained. *Dendrobium devonianum* and *Dendrobium officinale* can be separated very well using the PCA and PLS-DA analysis of MRM ion pairs; this shows that there are obvious differences in chemical composition between *Dendrobium devonianum* and *Dendrobium officinale*, which clearly proves that the pseudotargeted metabolomics method based on SWATHtoMRM can be used for traceability identification research. A total of 146 characteristic compounds were obtained, with 20 characteristic compounds in *Dendrobium devonianum*. The enrichment pathways of the characteristic compounds were mainly concentrated in lipids and atherosclerosis, chagas disease, fluid shear stress and atherosclerosis, proteoglycans in cancer, the IL-17 signaling pathway, the sphingolipid signaling pathway, diabetic cardiomyopathy, arginine and proline metabolism, etc., among which the lipid and atherosclerosis pathways were more enriched, and 11 characteristic compounds affected the expression levels of IL-1, TNFα, CD36, IL-1β, etc. These can be used as a reference for research on variety improvement and active substance accumulation in *Dendrobium devonianum* and *Dendrobium officinale*.

Keywords: time-of-flight mass spectrometry; identification; *Dendrobium devonianum*; Longling area

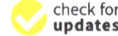

Citation: Lin, T.; Chen, X.; Du, L.; Wang, J.; Hu, Z.; Cheng, L.; Liu, Z.; Liu, H. Traceability Research on *Dendrobium devonianum* Based on SWATHtoMRM. *Foods* **2023**, *12*, 3608. https://doi.org/10.3390/foods12193608

Academic Editor: Emilio Alvarez-Parrilla

Received: 30 August 2023
Revised: 25 September 2023
Accepted: 27 September 2023
Published: 28 September 2023

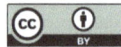

Copyright: © 2023 by the authors. Licensee MDPI, Basel, Switzerland. This article is an open access article distributed under the terms and conditions of the Creative Commons Attribution (CC BY) license (https:// creativecommons.org/licenses/by/ 4.0/).

1. Introduction

Dendrobium devonianum is a characteristic Chinese herbal medicine produced in the Longling area of Yunnan, China, and it is also a Chinese plant that can be eaten as food [1–3]. *Dendrobium devonianum* has good biological health effects [4,5], and the geographical location where it grows has a large impact on it. Among them, the Longling area produces nationally important products, but the *Dendrobium devonianum* that grows in other parts of Yunnan is not a notable product [6]. In order to counterfeit *Dendrobium devonianum* produced in the Longling area of Yunnan, *Dendrobium officinale* is often planted in the Longling area and sold as *Dendrobium devonianum*. Although the appearance and shape of *Dendrobium devonianum* and *Dendrobium officinale* produced in the Longling area are different, it is difficult to identify when it is dried or crushed into a powder, which seriously affects the quality evaluation and origin traceability of *Dendrobium devonianum* [7]. Therefore, it is essential to establish an effective *Dendrobium devonianum* traceability technology.

High-resolution mass spectrometry is one of the commonly used and effective traceability technologies [8–11]. In our laboratory, TOF and UPLC-PDA have also been used to trace the origins of *Dendrobium devonianum* and *Dendrobium officinale* produced in the same area; *Dendrobium devonianum* and *Dendrobium officinale* can be better distinguished through relevant PCA and VIP analyses, etc., but the number of confirmed differential markers obtained was small, and the amount of characteristic information about the differential markers was low [7,12]. This also shows that, although they have a wide coverage, TOF or UPLC-PDA have a dynamic range, quantitative accuracy, and significantly reduced sensitivity, and the final characteristic information total obtained is less [13–15].

With the emergence of sequential windowed acquisition of all theoretical fragment ions to multiple reaction monitoring (SWATHtoMRM) technology, the problems of the low sensitivity of mass spectrometry in full scan mode and accuracy and reliability in the process of structure identification have been effectively solved. Through a non-targeted analysis of SWATH data, the generation of MRM ion pair information, and the targeted analysis of each correlated MRM ion pair, SWATHtoMRM technology combines the powerful qualitative ability of SWATH technology with the precise quantitative ability of MRM technology to achieve high coverage and accurate quantification of known and unknown metabolites detected in a non-targeted analysis [16]. At present, this has been widely used in metabolomics, foodomics, etc. [17–19].

In order to obtain as much information as possible about the characteristic compounds in *Dendrobium devonianum* produced in the Longling area of Yunnan, SWATHtoMRM technology was used in this experiment to further identify and trace the sources of *Dendrobium devonianum* and *Dendrobium officinale* produced in the same area using TOF and MS-MRM to analyze the known and unknown metabolites in *Dendrobium devonianum* and *Dendrobium officinale* to obtain more information on the characteristic metabolites in *Dendrobium devonianum*.

2. Materials and Methods

2.1. Sample Collection and Preparation

Twenty-six samples of *Dendrobium devonianum* and *Dendrobium officinale*, thirteen each, were collected from the Longling area of Yunnan, China, in 2020. Each collected sample was composed of 10 fresh branches, kept under the same growth condition. The branches were cut into lengths of about 5 cm, dried at 60 °C, crushed at a high speed, passed through a 0.28 μm sample sieve, and stored in the laboratory at 4 °C in the dark.

2.2. Chemicals and Reagents

HPLC-grade acetonitrile, isopropanol, and methanol were purchased from Merck (Darmstadt, Germany). HPLC-grade ammonium acetate and formic acid were purchased from DiKMA Technologies (Beijing, China). Ultrapure water was prepared using Elga's water system (Wycombe, UK).

2.3. Sample Preparation and Analysis

2.3.1. Sample Preparation and Instrumental Method

First, 2 g of sample was placed into a 50 mL centrifuge tube, 20 mL of methanol–water solution (V:V = 90:10) was added and vortexed for 1 min, then ultrasonic was extracted for 30 min and centrifuged at 5000 r/min for 5 min, and the supernatant was filtered through a 0.22 μm filter membrane.

The SCIEX X500R QTOF system (Framingham, MS, USA) used was equipped with an ExionLC AD ultra-high-performance liquid chromatography (Framingham, MS, USA) and Waters ACQUITY UPLC BEH C18 column (2.1 × 100 mm, 1.7 μm, Waters, Milford, MA, USA). Referring to the relevant parameters in reference [7]: solvent A was 2 mM ammonium acetate in ultrapure water with 0.01% formic acid, and B was the mixed solution of acetonitrile, isopropanol, and water (V:V:V = 47.5:47.5:5) containing 2 mM formic acid and 0.01% formic acid. The flow rate for UPLC was 0.4 mL/min with the following gradients: 10% B (0~5.0 min), 10% B~50% B (5.0~6.0 min), 50% B~95% B (6.0~15.0 min), 95% B~100% B (15.0~20.0 min), 100% B (20.0~35.0 min), 100% B~5% B (35.0~35.1 min), and 5% B (35.1~40.0 min). The injection volume was 5 μL. Data were collected using primary and secondary mass spectrometry, among which the MS scan range was 100~1500 m/z, and the MS IDA scan range was 50~1500 m/z, CE = ± 30 V.

2.3.2. MRM Data Collection

The wiff format of the sample data collected via TOF was converted to the mzXML format using MSConvert software (3.0.4140), and the R package (4.3.1) of SWATHtoMRM was used for the conversion of MRM transitions. Twenty-six samples were analyzed using the AB SCIEX 4500 system (Framingham, MS, USA). The same chromatographic column and gradient elution conditions as in QTOF-MS data collection were used, along with the converted MRM transition and schedule mode (MRM detection window: 50 s), where the DP was uniformly ± 50 V and the collision energy was uniformly ± 40 V. At the same time, the same volume of the extraction solution of each sample in this experiment was drawn and mixed to make a quality control sample (QC). During the sample analysis process, the analysis of QC samples was performed after every 5 samples to monitor the sensitivity and stability of the instrument and to perform a subsequent data analysis and correction.

2.3.3. Data Processing and Statistical Analysis

The ions whose response peak area was lower than 10^2 were deleted, and the ion pairs with a high response intensity were retained, which were analyzed using the peak area response of each ion pair of the QC sample. Lists of peak areas corresponding to MRM were imported into MetaboAnalyst (https://www.metaboanalyst.ca/ (accessed on 7 July 2023)) for a principal component analysis (PCA), ANOVA, false discovery rate (FDR), and VIP analysis to find differential MRM ion pairs. Differential MRM ion pairs were compared to TOF data using ion pair information and the peak time to obtain primary and secondary mass spectrum information of differential compounds, and the chemical structure was identified using the Natural Product s-TCM Library_1.0 established by SCIEX and the online ChemSpider database (HMDB, Massbank, Pubmed, etc.). In order to further analyze the possible signaling pathways affecting differential metabolites, the differential metabolites were imported into the MetaboAnalyst5.0 (https://www.metaboanalyst.ca/ (accessed on 7 July 2023)) online website to analyze the main enriched KEGG biosynthetic pathways.

3. Results

3.1. Analytical Characteristics of SWATHtoMRM Method

After the conversion of the R package of SWATHtoMRM, the ion pairs were obtained, in which the positive ions totaled 2439 pairs of MRMs and the negative ions totaled 601 pairs of MRMs (Supplementary File S1). From the m/z distribution of the parent ions in Figure 1, it can be seen that the MRM of the positive ions was mainly concentrated in the range of 300–600. After screening the ion pairs with the low-level response QC samples, 191 MRM pairs of positive ions and 96 pairs of negative ions were obtained (Supplementary File S2).

3.2. MRM Data Analysis

As can be seen from Figure 2, the MRM ion pairs obtained after screening were analyzed using a PCA, and the degree of polymerization of the QC was high, indicating that the data were stable and the quality was guaranteed. It can be seen that *Dendrobium devonianum* and *Dendrobium officinale* can be separated very well using a PCA analysis; this shows that there are obvious differences in the chemical composition between *Dendrobium devonianum* and *Dendrobium officinale*.

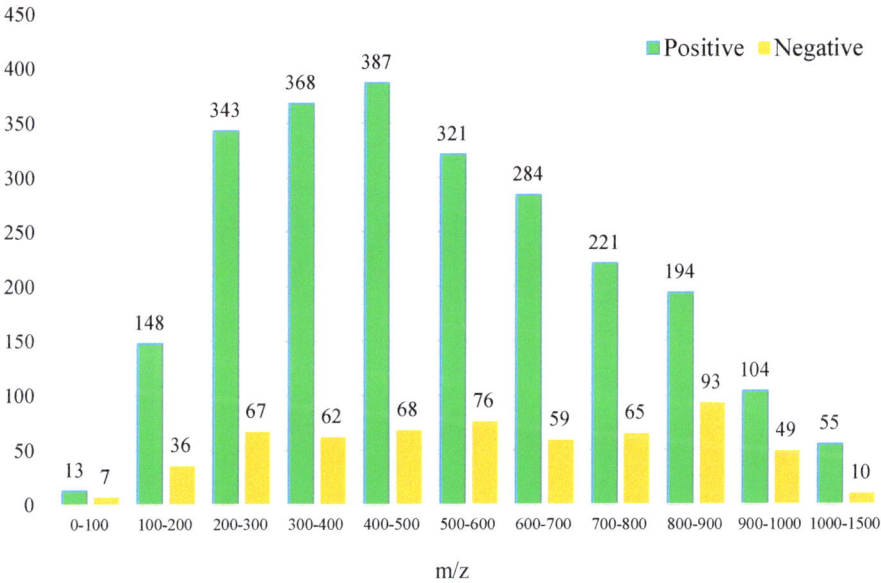

Figure 1. Molecular weight distribution of compounds converted using SWATHtoMRM.

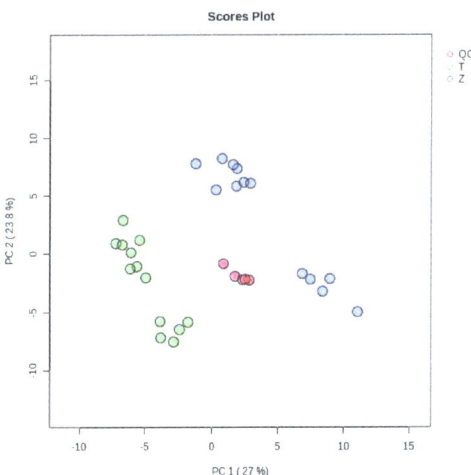

Figure 2. Loading plots of PCA of *Dendrobium devonianum* and *Dendrobium officinale* (T: *Dendrobium officinale*, Z: *Dendrobium devonianum*, QC: QC samples).

The difference in the comparisons in this experiment is mainly reflected in the difference in the peak areas of the common components contained in *Dendrobium devonianum* and *Dendrobium officinale*. The two principal components, PC1 and PC2, accounted for 27.0% and 23.8% of the total difference, respectively, indicating that by comparing the difference in the peak area of the common components in *Dendrobium devonianum* and *Dendrobium officinale*, it is possible to effectively distinguish *Dendrobium devonianum* and *Dendrobium officinale*. It also shows that the ion pairs converted using SWATHtoMRM were analyzed via PCA, and the two *Dendrobium* samples were densely gathered together, which clearly proves that the pseudotargeted metabolomics method based on SWATHtoMRM can be used for traceability identification research.

On the other hand, PLS-DA was also used for the analysis, and the analysis results were consistent with the PCA, and *Dendrobium devonianum* and *Dendrobium officinale* can be separated well (Figure 3), as can be seen in the PLS-DA cross-validation data (Figure 4). R2 is the correlation coefficient of cross validation, and the values of components of 1–5 were 0.96224, 0.98362, 0.99473, 0.99767, and 0.99929, respectively, which were close to 1, indicating that their fitting degree was good. Q2 represents the predictive performance of the PLS-DA model, and Q2 was higher than 0.9, so it can be considered a very good model in this experiment.

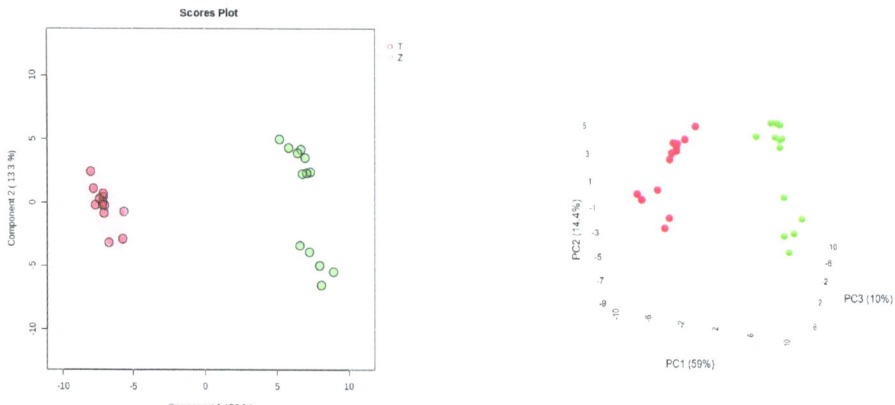

Figure 3. PLS-DA score chart and model diagram of *Dendrobium devonianum* and *Dendrobium officinale* (T: *Dendrobium officinale*, red range; Z: *Dendrobium devonianum*, green range).

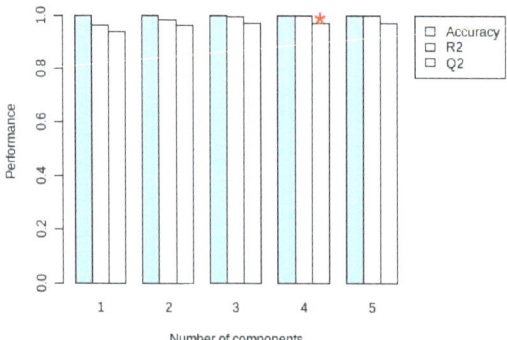

Figure 4. PLS-DA cross validation details of *Dendrobium devonianum* and *Dendrobium officinale*. (* The Q2 value was 0.96961, which was also the largest).

3.3. ANOVA, FDR, and VIP Analysis

ANOVA, FDR, and VIP analyses were performed on the obtained MRM ion pairs, and the MRM ion pairs with a p-value < 0.01, FDR < 0.05, and VIP > 1 were selected as the ion pairs with large differences. A total of 146 characteristic compounds were obtained (Supplementary File S3).

As shown in Figures 5 and 6, the retention time of the 146 characteristic compounds was mainly the range of 6–20 min, and the molecular weight was mainly concentrated between 200 and 300 and 500 and 700. According to the chromatographic conditions in

Section 2.3.1, during a time period of 6–15 min, the organic phase was from 50 to 95%, and at 15–20 min, the organic phase was from 95 to 100%. The main elution components were medium and medium-to-small polar compounds, which were the same as the main components in *Dendrobium*, which were consistent with alkaloids, flavonoids, phenanthrenes, and bibenzyls [20].

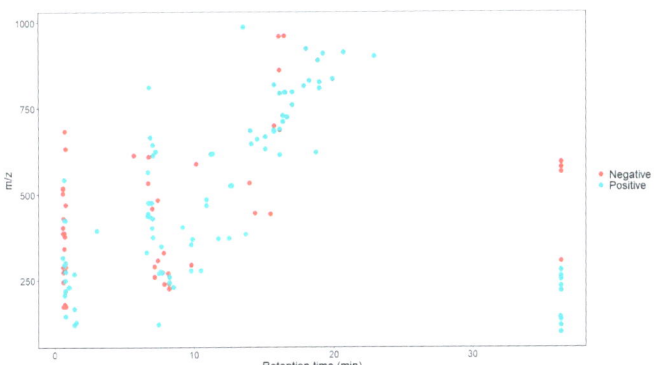

Figure 5. Scatter plot of 146 characteristic compounds.

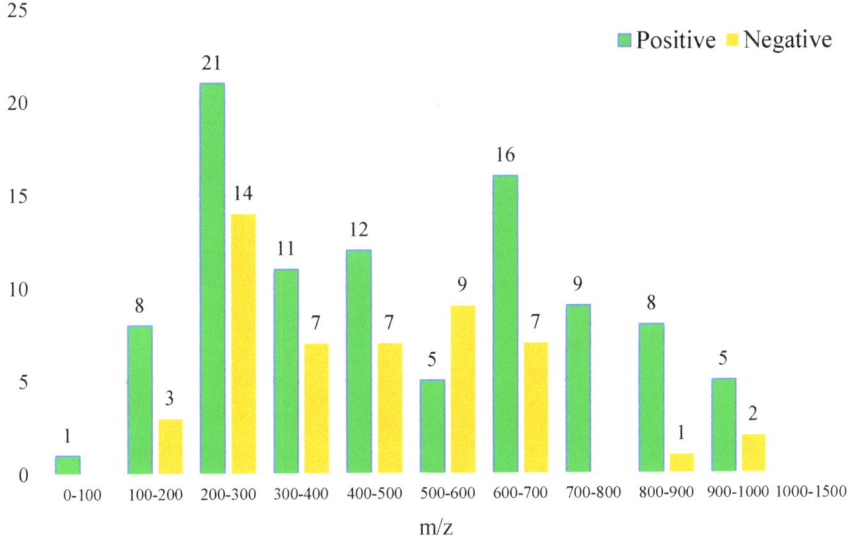

Figure 6. Molecular weight distribution of 146 characteristic compounds (the numbers on the bar graph represent the number of characteristic compounds in that molecular weight range).

It can be seen from the analysis of the VIP scores (Figure 7), volcano map (Figure 8), and heat map (Figure 9) of the 50 compounds with large differences that, as shown in Table 1, there were 20 characteristic compounds in *Dendrobium devonianum*, the content of *Dendrobium devonianum* was larger than that of *Dendrobium officinale*, and the content of 30 characteristic compounds was smaller than that of *Dendrobium officinale*. The difference in the contents of the common compounds was the largest ($p = 6.32 \times 10^{-17}$), which may be the characteristic component of *Dendrobium devonianum*; the three differential compounds with a reduced content may be the characteristic components of *Dendrobium officinale*.

As shown in Figure 10, the contents of the five characteristic compounds of *Dendrobium devonianum* and *Dendrobium officinale* were very different. The normalized concentrations of the five characteristic compounds were close to +1 and −1, respectively, and the difference can be clearly seen after normalization.

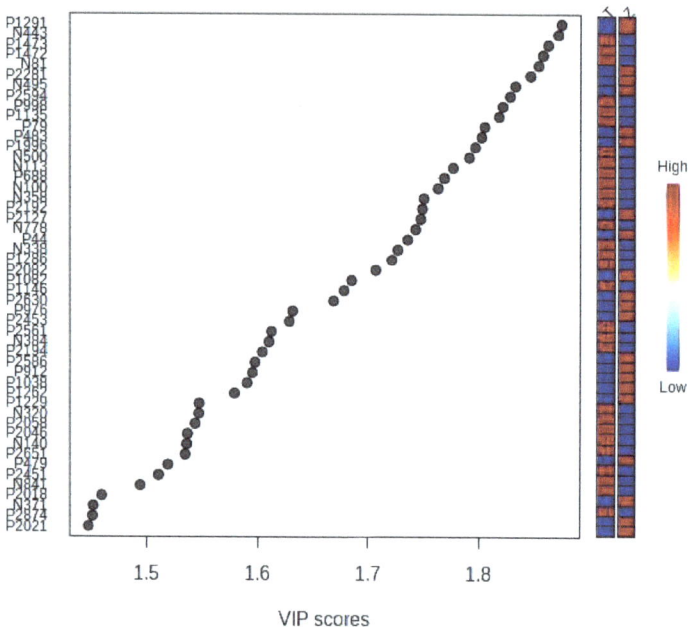

Figure 7. The VIP scores of *Dendrobium devonianum* and *Dendrobium officinale* (T: *Dendrobium officinale*, Z: *Dendrobium devonianum*).

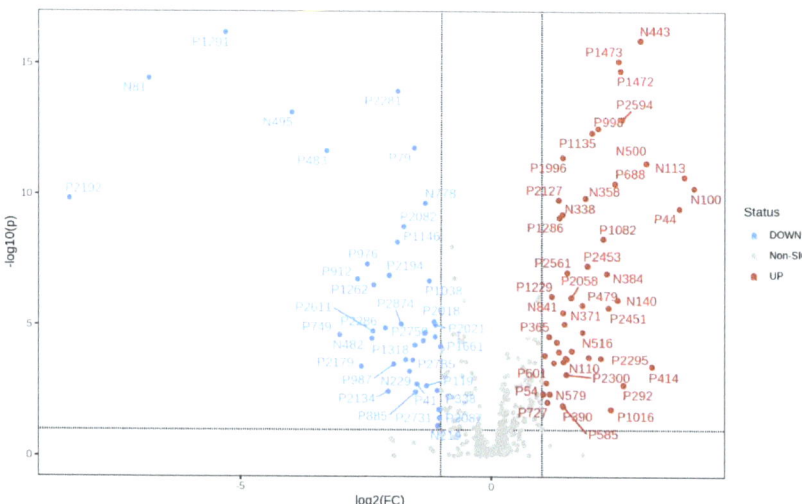

Figure 8. A volcano plot of *Dendrobium devonianum* and *Dendrobium officinale*.

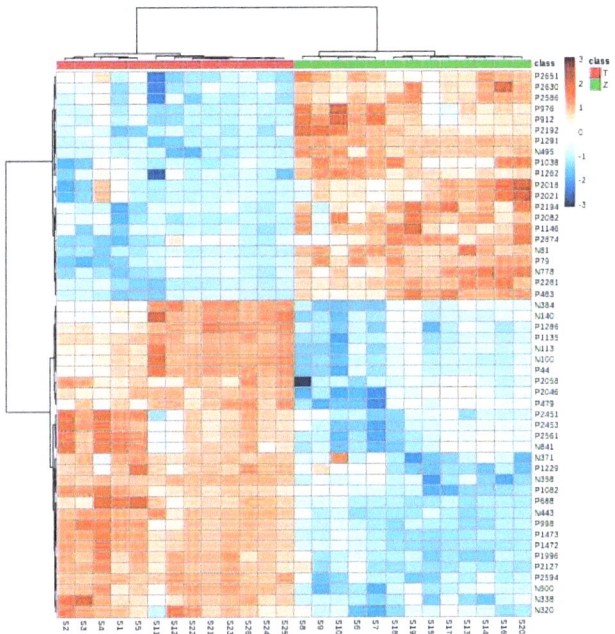

Figure 9. A heatmap of *Dendrobium devonianum* (Z) and *Dendrobium officinale* (T).

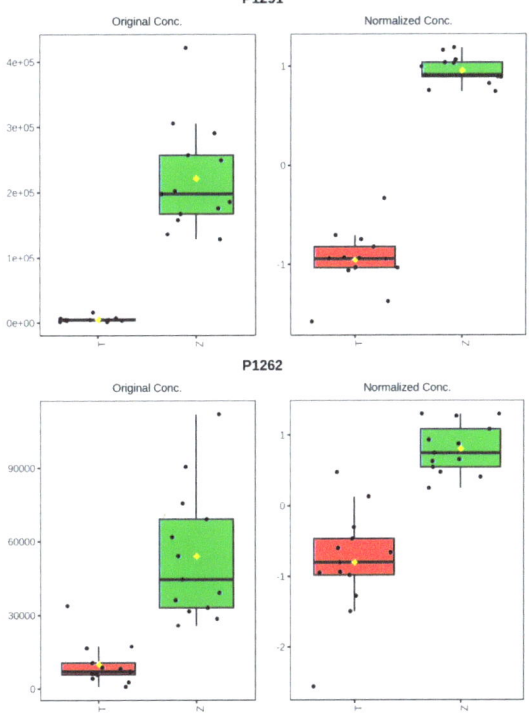

Figure 10. *Cont.*

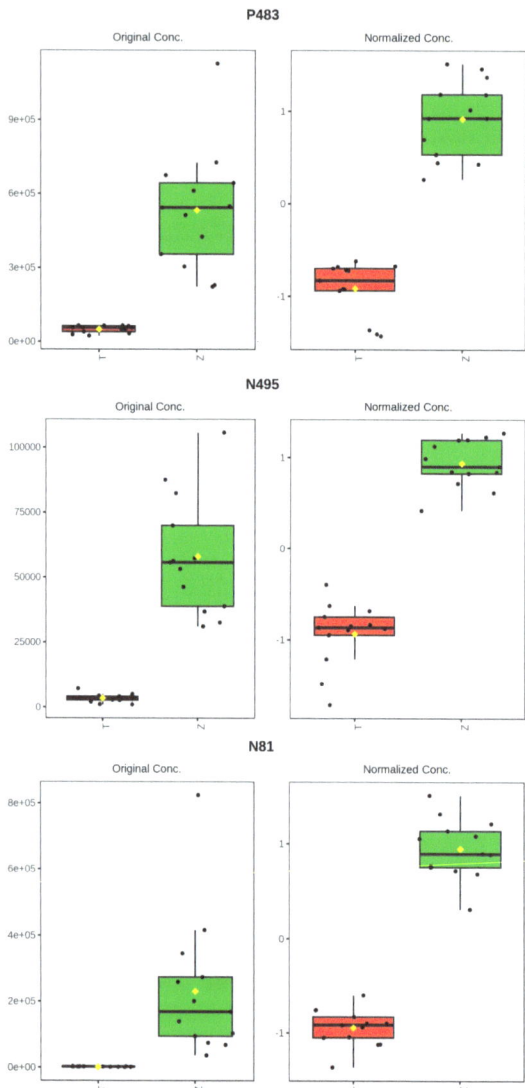

Figure 10. Box plot of the five characteristic compounds (T: *Dendrobium officinale*, red range; Z: *Dendrobium devonianum*, green range).

Table 1. Information on characteristic compounds.

Compound Code	Precursor Ion (m/z)	Product Ion (m/z)	Retention Time (min)	p Value	FDR	VIP	Changes in Content	
							Dendrobium devonianum	*Dendrobium officinale*
P1291	438.2390	70.0651	6.60	6.32×10^{-17}	2.20×10^{-14}	1.8749	↑	↓
N443	533.1296	124.9909	6.64	1.24×10^{-16}	2.20×10^{-14}	1.8719	↓	↑
P1473	476.2134	137.0597	6.90	7.73×10^{-16}	9.17×10^{-14}	1.8630	↓	↑
P1472	476.1928	137.0236	6.67	1.81×10^{-15}	1.61×10^{-13}	1.8583	↓	↑
N81	239.0707	196.0524	7.79	3.52×10^{-15}	2.50×10^{-13}	1.8544	↓	↑
P2281	682.5257	248.2375	15.73	1.11×10^{-14}	6.57×10^{-13}	1.8472	↑	↓

Table 1. Cont.

Compound Code	Precursor Ion (m/z)	Product Ion (m/z)	Retention Time (min)	p Value	FDR	VIP	Changes in Content Dendrobium devonianum	Changes in Content Dendrobium officinale
N495	609.1449	311.0557	6.66	7.31×10^{-14}	3.72×10^{-12}	1.8335	↑	↓
P2594	811.6109	235.0970	6.69	1.34×10^{-13}	5.97×10^{-12}	1.8287	↓	↑
P998	374.1813	154.0624	7.00	2.92×10^{-13}	1.16×10^{-11}	1.8220	↓	↑
P1135	401.1601	167.0706	6.93	4.30×10^{-13}	1.53×10^{-11}	1.8185	↓	↑
P79	144.1019	70.0650	0.73	1.68×10^{-12}	5.43×10^{-11}	1.8053	↑	↓
P483	272.2222	105.0698	7.66	2.19×10^{-12}	6.49×10^{-11}	1.8026	↑	↓
P1996	613.2288	167.0703	6.99	3.79×10^{-12}	1.04×10^{-10}	1.7966	↓	↑
N500	614.2169	61.9883	5.61	6.18×10^{-12}	1.57×10^{-10}	1.7911	↓	↑
N113	273.1128	137.0238	7.68	2.06×10^{-11}	4.89×10^{-10}	1.7764	↓	↑
P688	315.9915	119.0186	0.56	3.73×10^{-11}	8.29×10^{-10}	1.7686	↓	↑
N100	271.0969	213.0553	8.07	5.57×10^{-11}	1.17×10^{-9}	1.7630	↓	↑
N358	459.1506	149.0598	6.94	1.32×10^{-10}	2.61×10^{-9}	1.7504	↓	↑
P2192	665.1730	271.0600	6.80	1.44×10^{-10}	2.71×10^{-9}	1.7490	↑	↓
P2127	643.2394	167.0702	6.97	1.58×10^{-10}	2.82×10^{-9}	1.7476	↓	↑
N778	861.5465	279.2321	16.08	2.15×10^{-10}	3.64×10^{-9}	1.7429	↓	↑
P44	121.0647	78.0463	7.39	3.33×10^{-10}	5.39×10^{-9}	1.7357	↓	↑
N338	443.3365	309.3152	15.45	5.58×10^{-10}	8.63×10^{-9}	1.7270	↓	↑
P1286	436.2185	219.0805	6.72	7.55×10^{-10}	1.12×10^{-8}	1.7217	↓	↑
P2082	631.4929	81.0186	15.11	1.66×10^{-9}	2.36×10^{-8}	1.7072	↑	↓
P1082	393.2233	107.0491	3.00	4.90×10^{-9}	6.71×10^{-8}	1.6853	↓	↑
P1146	404.1015	93.0698	9.13	6.77×10^{-9}	8.93×10^{-8}	1.6783	↑	↓
P2630	826.6767	262.2528	18.95	1.03×10^{-8}	1.31×10^{-7}	1.6689	↑	↓
P976	369.2637	277.2160	9.85	4.70×10^{-8}	5.77×10^{-7}	1.6318	↓	↑
P2453	760.5814	299.0617	17.01	5.26×10^{-8}	6.24×10^{-7}	1.6289	↓	↑
P2561	798.6059	601.5166	17.00	9.51×10^{-8}	1.09×10^{-6}	1.6126	↓	↑
N384	483.1995	134.0368	7.33	1.03×10^{-7}	1.15×10^{-6}	1.6103	↓	↑
P2194	666.5303	531.4039	15.11	1.27×10^{-7}	1.37×10^{-6}	1.6043	↑	↓
P2586	808.6658	262.2528	18.95	1.60×10^{-7}	1.68×10^{-6}	1.5976	↑	↓
P912	353.2686	93.0697	9.75	1.73×10^{-7}	1.76×10^{-6}	1.5953	↑	↓
P1038	384.3474	69.0697	13.67	2.04×10^{-7}	2.01×10^{-6}	1.5904	↑	↓
P1262	430.1715	145.0284	6.97	2.95×10^{-7}	2.84×10^{-6}	1.5789	↓	↑
P1229	425.1161	245.0510	0.65	7.76×10^{-7}	7.14×10^{-6}	1.5470	↓	↑
N320	430.9467	114.9882	0.57	7.83×10^{-7}	7.14×10^{-6}	1.5467	↓	↑
P2058	625.2548	421.1464	7.20	8.59×10^{-7}	7.64×10^{-6}	1.5434	↓	↑
P2046	621.5454	147.1170	18.71	1.05×10^{-6}	9.01×10^{-6}	1.5364	↓	↑
N140	289.1076	137.0239	7.10	1.06×10^{-6}	9.01×10^{-6}	1.5359	↓	↑
P2651	836.6972	262.2531	19.89	1.11×10^{-6}	9.16×10^{-6}	1.5344	↑	↓
P479	271.0966	182.0728	7.44	1.68×10^{-6}	1.36×10^{-5}	1.5190	↓	↑
P2451	760.5056	299.0617	17.01	2.10×10^{-6}	1.66×10^{-5}	1.5106	↓	↑
N841	961.6075	112.9853	16.45	3.22×10^{-6}	2.49×10^{-5}	1.4939	↓	↑
P2018	616.3460	313.2734	11.22	7.40×10^{-6}	5.61×10^{-5}	1.4588	↑	↓
N371	470.1507	128.0353	0.75	8.85×10^{-6}	6.51×10^{-5}	1.4509	↓	↑
P2874	986.6047	611.4668	13.52	8.96×10^{-6}	6.51×10^{-5}	1.4504	↑	↓
P2021	617.3496	313.2734	11.35	9.75×10^{-6}	6.95×10^{-5}	1.4465	↑	↓

P: positive; N: negative; ↑: content went up; ↓: content went down.

3.4. Structural Identification of Characteristic Compounds

Using the Natural Products s-TCM Library_1.0 and online ChemSpider database, a total of 34 characteristic compounds were identified, including 20 in the positive ion mode and 14 in the negative ion mode, as shown in Table 2.

Table 2. Information on characteristic compounds identified.

Compound Code	Compound Name	Molecular Formula	Adduct Ion	Mass Error (ppm)	References
P44 *	4-Hydroxybenzoic acid	$C_7H_6O_3$	$[M - H_2O + H]^+$	0.8	[21]
P79 *	Stachydrine	$C_7H_{13}NO_2$	$[M + H]^+$	−0.2	[22]
P119	Phenylalanine	$C_9H_{11}NO_2$	$[M + H]^+$	0.6	[23]
P215	2-(Acetylamino)-2,6-dideoxy-α-L-galactose	$C_8H_{15}NO_5$	$[M + H]^+$	0.6	[24]

Table 2. Cont.

Compound Code	Compound Name	Molecular Formula	Adduct Ion	Mass Error (ppm)	References
P296	4-[(5-Hydroxy-3-methyl-1-oxo-2penten-1-yl)amino]-butanoic acid methyl ester	$C_{11}H_{19}NO_4$	$[M + H]^+$	−0.4	–
P338	Pinostilbene	$C_{15}H_{14}O_3$	$[M + H]^+$	−0.4	[25]
P365	Linamarin	$C_{10}H_{17}NO_6$	$[M + H]^+$	−0.2	[26]
P414	3-hydroxy-4′, 5-dimethoxybibenzyl	$C_{16}H_{18}O_3$	$[M + H]^+$	−0.4	[27]
P465	Adenosine	$C_{10}H_{13}N_5O_4$	$[M + H]^+$	0.5	[28]
P483 *	Naringenin	$C_{15}H_{12}O_5$	$[M + H]^+$	0	[29,30]
P495	Palmitic acid	$C_{16}H_{32}O_2$	$[M + NH_4]^+$	0.4	[31]
P508	Dendrobin A	$C_{16}H_{18}O_4$	$[M + H]^+$	0.5	[32]
P522	Stearidonic acid	$C_{18}H_{28}O_2$	$[M + H]^+$	−0.5	[33,34]
P688 *	Vanilloside	$C_{14}H_{18}O_8$	$[M + H]^+$	1	[35]
P987	Tetradecanoyl-L-Carnitine	$C_{21}H_{41}NO_4$	$[M + H]^+$	−0.1	[36,37]
P998 *	N-(3,4,6-Tri-O-acetyl-β-D-glucopyranosyl) piperidine	$C_{17}H_{27}NO_8$	$[M + H]^+$	0.1	–
P1291 *	2-Propen-1-yl-2-(acetylamino)-2-deoxy-3-O-β-D-galactopyranosyl-6-Omethyl-α-D-galactopyranoside	$C_{18}H_{31}NO_{11}$	$[M + H]^+$	0.5	–
P1799	Dendronobiloside A	$C_{27}H_{48}O_{12}$	$[M + H]^+$	−0.9	[38]
P2058	Heytrijumalin I	$C_{34}H_{40}O_{11}$	$[M + H]^+$	0.2	[39]
P2453	Acanthoside D	$C_{34}H_{46}O_{18}$	$[M + H]^+$	−0.5	[40,41]
N45	Shikimic acid	$C_7H_{10}O_5$	$[M − H]^−$	0.6	[42,43]
N50	D-Galactose	$C_6H_{12}O_6$	$[M − H]^−$	2.7	[44,45]
N81 *	Moscatin	$C_{15}H_{12}O_3$	$[M − H]^−$	1.4	[46,47]
N100 *	Tristin	$C_{15}H_{16}O_4$	$[M − H]^−$	0.3	[48,49]
N110	Erianthridin	$C_{16}H_{16}O_4$	$[M − H]^−$	1.7	[50,51]
N113 *	Dendrophenol	$C_{16}H_{18}O_4$	$[M − H]^−$	1.4	[52,53]
N141	Dendroxine	$C_{17}H_{25}NO_3$	$[M − H]^−$	2.1	[54,55]
N229	Pinellic acid	$C_{18}H_{34}O_5$	$[M − H]^−$	2.5	[56,57]
N241	D-(+)-Trehalose	$C_{12}H_{22}O_{11}$	$[M − H]^−$	1.7	[58]
N341	Dendroside G	$C_{21}H_{34}O_{10}$	$[M − H]^−$	0.4	[59,60]
N358 *	Dendromoniliside B	$C_{21}H_{32}O_{11}$	$[M − H]^−$	0.3	[61]
N404	Raffinose	$C_{18}H_{32}O_{16}$	$[M − H]^−$	1	[62,63]
N484	Vicenin-2	$C_{27}H_{30}O_{15}$	$[M − H]^−$	0.5	[64,65]
N495 *	Rutin	$C_{27}H_{30}O_{16}$	$[M − H]^−$	1	[66]

* The difference value was the compound before rank 50.

3.5. KEGG Pathway Analysis of Dendrobium devonianum and Dendrobium officinale

According to the 11 of the top 50 characteristic compounds with a confirmed chemical structure obtained above, a KEGG pathway analysis was performed, and the top 20 pathways with $p \leq 0.05$ were selected for visual depiction. As shown in Figure 11, the enrichment pathways of the characteristic compounds were mainly concentrated in the lipids and atherosclerosis, chagas disease, fluid shear stress and atherosclerosis, proteoglycans in cancer, IL-17 signaling pathway, sphingolipid signaling pathway, diabetic cardiomyopathy, arginine and proline metabolism, etc., among which the lipid and atherosclerosis pathways were more enriched and 11 characteristic compounds could better affect the expression levels of IL-1, TNFα, CD36, IL-1β, etc. (Figure 12). On the other hand, this also proved that the metabolic processes of lipids and atherosclerosis can be better regulated by *Dendrobium devonianum*, which is consistent with the biological health effects of *Dendrobium nobile* reported in the literature [67–69], which can be used as a reference for future research on variety improvement and active substance accumulation in *Dendrobium devonianum* and *Dendrobium officinale*.

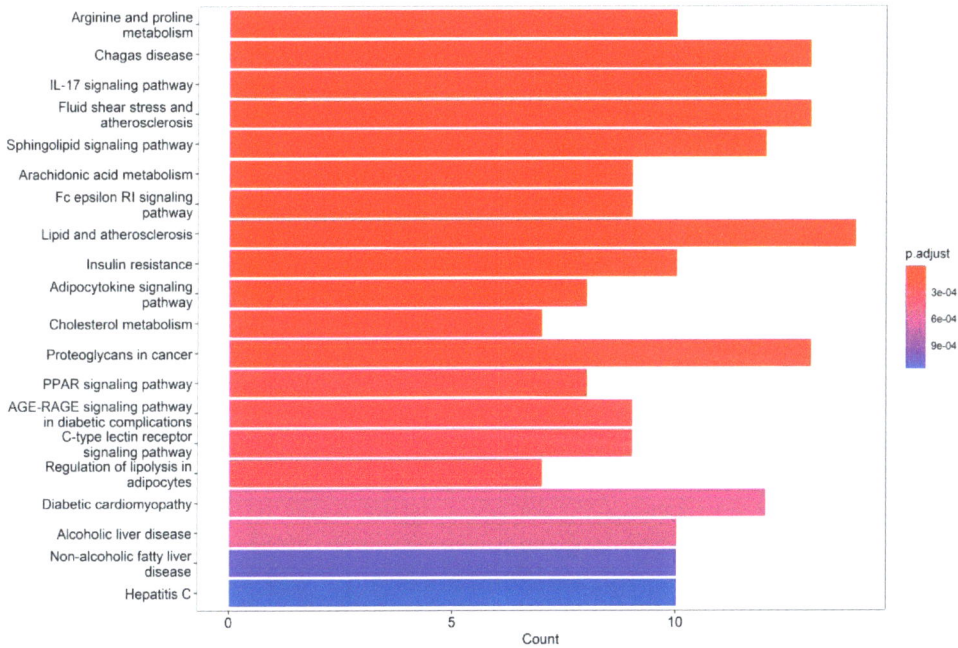

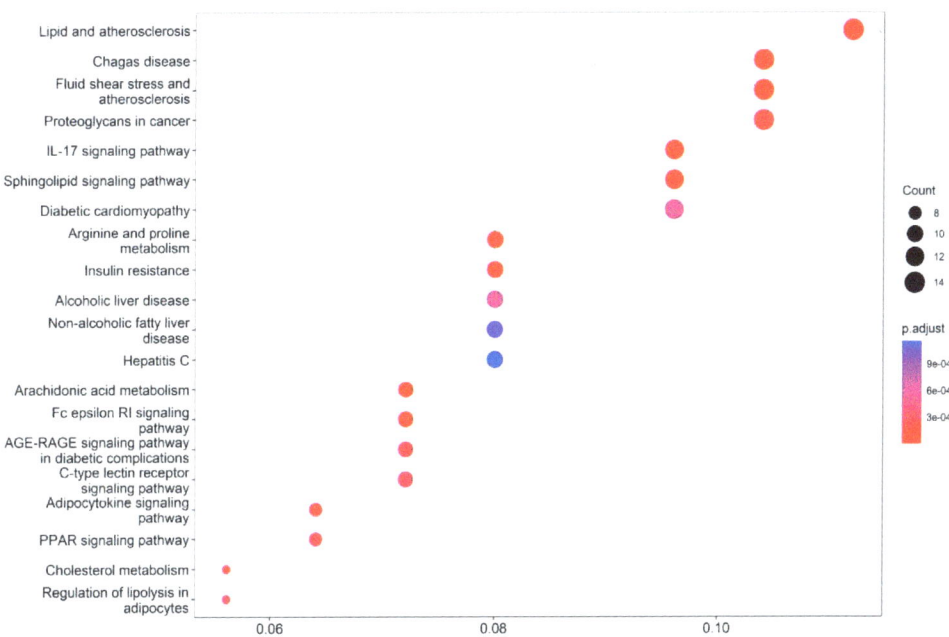

Figure 11. Barplot and dotplot of the top 20 KEGG enrichment pathways based on 11 characteristic compounds.

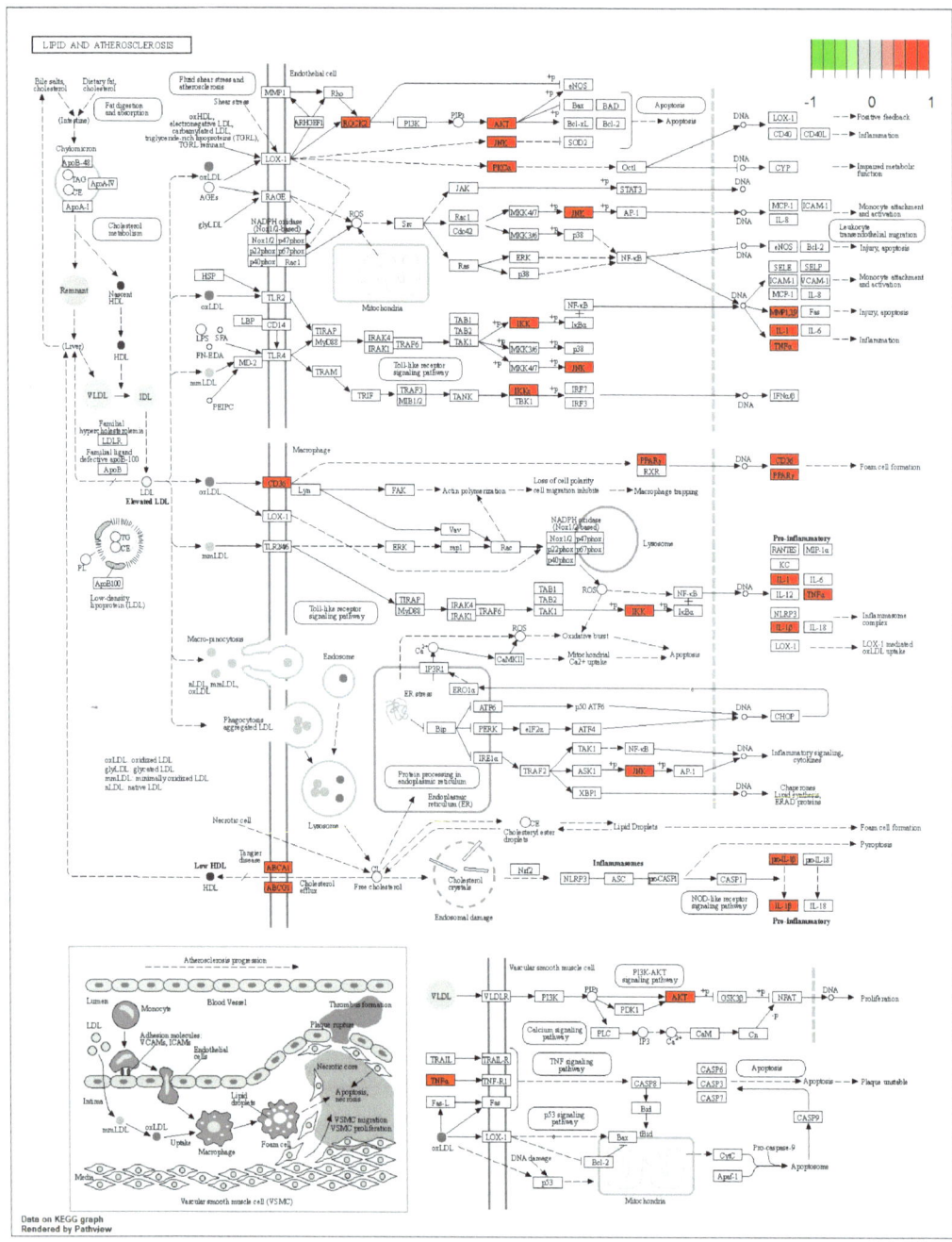

Figure 12. Lipid and atherosclerosis metabolic pathway.

4. Conclusions

In this study, SWATHtoMRM technology was used in this experiment to further identify and trace the sources of *Dendrobium devonianum* and *Dendrobium officinale* produced in the same area using TOF and MS-MRM. After the conversion of the R package of SWATHtoMRM, the ion pairs were obtained, in which the positive ions totaled 2439 pairs of MRMs, and the negative ions totaled 601 pairs of MRMs. After screening the ion pairs with low-level response QC samples, 191 MRM pairs of positive ions and 96 pairs of negative ions were obtained. *Dendrobium devonianum* and *Dendrobium officinale* can be separated very well via a PCA analysis of MRM ion pairs; this shows that there are obvious differences in chemical composition between *Dendrobium devonianum* and *Dendrobium officinale*. The difference in the comparisons in this experiment mainly reflect the differences in the peak areas of the common components contained in *Dendrobium devonianum* and *Dendrobium officinale*. This also shows that the ion pairs converted using SWATHtoMRM were analyzed via PCA, and the two *Dendrobium* samples were densely gathered together, which clearly proves that the pseudotargeted metabolomics method based on SWATHtoMRM can be used for traceability identification research. On the other hand, *Dendrobium devonianum* and *Dendrobium officinale* can be separated well via PLS-DA, as can be seen through PLS-DA cross validation. The R2 values of components 1–5 were 0.96224, 0.98362, 0.99473, 0.99767, and 0.99929, respectively, which were close to 1, indicating that their fitting degree was good, and the Q2 was above 0.9, which indicates a very good model.

The ANOVA FDR and VIP analyses were performed on the obtained MRM ion pairs. A total of 146 characteristic compounds were obtained. There were 20 characteristic compounds in *Dendrobium devonianum*; the content of *Dendrobium devonianum* was larger than that of *Dendrobium officinale*; and the content of 30 characteristic compounds was smaller than that of *Dendrobium officinale*. The difference in the contents of the most common compounds was the largest ($p = 6.32 \times 10^{-17}$), which may represent the characteristic component of *Dendrobium devonianum*; three differential compounds with reduced contents may be the characteristic components of *Dendrobium officinale*. The enrichment pathways of the characteristic compounds were mainly concentrated in the lipids and atherosclerosis, chagas disease, fluid shear stress and atherosclerosis, proteoglycans in cancer, IL-17 signaling pathway, sphingolipid signaling pathway, diabetic cardiomyopathy, arginine and proline metabolism, etc., among which the lipid and atherosclerosis pathways were more enriched and 11 characteristic compounds could better affect the expression levels of IL-1, TNFα, CD36, IL-1β, etc., which can be used as a reference for future research on variety improvement and active substance accumulation in *Dendrobium devonianum* and *Dendrobium officinale*.

Supplementary Materials: The following supporting information can be downloaded at https://www.mdpi.com/article/10.3390/foods12193608/s1: Supplementary File S1: MRMTransition; Supplementary File S2: MRMTransition peak area; Supplementary File S3: Differential MRM.

Author Contributions: Conceptualization, T.L. and H.L.; methodology, T.L. and X.C.; software, L.C. and J.W.; validation, L.D. and Z.H.; formal analysis, X.C.; investigation, Z.L.; resources, J.W. and Z.H.; data curation, L.C.; writing—original draft preparation, T.L.; writing—review and editing, H.L. and Z.L.; supervision, H.L. and Z.L.; funding acquisition. All authors have read and agreed to the published version of the manuscript.

Funding: This study was funded by General Program of Natural Science Foundation of Yunnan Province, grant number 202001AT070017, Yunnan Province Agricultural Basic Research Joint Special Project, grant number 202301BD070001-049, Yunnan Academician Expert Workstation, grant number 202305AF150015, and Yunnan Key Research and Development, grant number 202102AE090021.

Data Availability Statement: The data used to support the findings of this study can be made available by the corresponding author upon request.

Conflicts of Interest: Author Long Cheng was employed by the company SCIEX Analytical Instrument Trading Co., Ltd., which had the role of mass spectrometry detection and data analysis in this study, without any potential conflict. The remaining authors declare that the research was conducted in the absence of any commercial or financial relationship that could be construed as a potential conflict of interest.

References

1. Wu, B.-L.; Zhao, Z.-R.; Liu, H.; Jiao, D.; Wu, Y.-G. Research progress of *Dendrobium devonianum*. *Chin. Tradit. Pat. Med.* **2020**, *42*, 2990–2998.
2. Wu, L.-L.; Ding, Y.-L.; Xie, Y.-F.; Chen, D.-Q.; Xu, H. Research on bibenzyl constituents and TLC identification of the stem of *Dendrobium devoninum*. *Northwest Pharm. J.* **2020**, *35*, 791–795.
3. Available online: http://www.pbh.yn.gov.cn/wjwWebsite/web/doc/UU151669310662159294 (accessed on 7 July 2023).
4. Zhan, R.; Zhang, X.-Y.; Li, Z.-Y.; Liu, B.; Chen, Y.-G. Immunosuppressive bibenzyl-phenylpropane hybrids from *Dendrobium devonianum*. *Chem. Biodivers.* **2023**, *20*, e202201185. [CrossRef]
5. Li, J.; Zhang, X.; Li, Y.; Liu, B.; Zhan, R. Bibenzyls and lignans from *Dendrobium devonianum* and their immunosuppressive activities. *Phytochem. Lett.* **2023**, *54*, 137–140. [CrossRef]
6. *Geographical Indication Products-Dendrobium devonianum from Longling*; Yunnan Provincial Bureau of Quality and Technical Supervision: Baoshan, China, 2014.
7. Lin, T.; Chen, X.-L.; Wang, J.; Hu, Z.-X.; Wu, G.-W.; Sha, L.-J.; Cheng, L.; Liu, H.-C. Application of time of flight mass spectrometry in the identification of *Dendrobium devonianum* Paxt and *Dendrobium officinale* Kimura et Migo Grown in Longling Area of Yunnan, China. *Separations* **2022**, *9*, 108. [CrossRef]
8. Dou, X.; Zhang, L.; Yang, R.; Wang, X.; Yu, L.; Yue, X.; Ma, F.; Mao, J.; Wang, X.; Zhang, W.; et al. Mass spectrometry in food authentication and origin traceability. *Mass Spectrom. Rev.* **2022**, *42*, 1772–1807. [CrossRef]
9. Li, Q.; Yang, S.; Li, B.; Zhang, C.; Li, Y.; Li, J. Exploring critical metabolites of honey peach (*Prunus persica* (L.) Batsch) from five main cultivation regions in the north of China by UPLC-Q-TOF/MS combined with chemometrics and modeling. *Food Res. Int.* **2022**, *157*, 111213. [CrossRef]
10. Liu, X.; Zhong, C.; Xie, J.; Liu, H.; Xie, Z.; Zhang, S.; Jin, J. Geographical region traceability of *Poria cocos* and correlation between environmental factors and biomarkers based on a metabolomic approach. *Food Chem.* **2023**, *417*, 135817. [CrossRef]
11. Ye, Z.; Dai, J.-R.; Zhang, C.-G.; Lu, Y.; Wu, L.-L.; Gong, A.G.W.; Xu, H.; Tsim, K.W.K.; Wang, Z.-T. Chemical differentiation of *Dendrobium officinale* and *Dendrobium devonianum* by using HPLC fingerprints, HPLC-ESI-MS, and HPTLC analyses. *Evid.-Based Complement Alternat. Med.* **2017**, *2017*, 8647212. [CrossRef]
12. Lin, T.; Chen, X.-L.; Wu, G.-W.; Sha, L.-J.; Wang, J.; Hu, Z.-X.; Liu, H.-C. A simple method for distinguishing *Dendrobium devonianum* and *Dendrobium officinale* by ultra performance liquid chromatography-photo diode array detector. *Food Sci. Technol.* **2023**, *43*, e110122. [CrossRef]
13. Simonnet-Laprade, C.; Bayen, S.; McGoldrick, D.; McDaniel, T.; Hutinet, S.; Marchand, P.; Vénisseau, A.; Cariou, R.; Le Bizec, B.; Dervilly, G.J.C. Evidence of complementarity between targeted and non-targeted analysis based on liquid and gas-phase chromatography coupled to mass spectrometry for screening halogenated persistent organic pollutants in environmental matrices. *Chemosphere* **2022**, *293*, 133615. [CrossRef]
14. Crimmins, B.S.; Holsen, T.M. Non-targeted screening in environmental monitoring programs. In *Advancements of Mass Spectrometry in Biomedical Research*; Woods, A.G., Darie, C.C., Eds.; Springer International Publishing: Cham, Switzerland, 2019; pp. 731–741.
15. Martínez-Bueno, M.; Ramos, M.G.; Bauer, A.; Fernández-Alba, A. An overview of non-targeted screening strategies based on high resolution accurate mass spectrometry for the identification of migrants coming from plastic food packaging materials. *TrAC Trends Anal. Chem.* **2019**, *110*, 191–203. [CrossRef]
16. Zha, H.; Cai, Y.; Yin, Y.; Wang, Z.; Li, K.; Zhu, Z.-J. SWATHtoMRM: Development of high-coverage targeted metabolomics method using SWATH technology for biomarker discovery. *Anal. Chem.* **2018**, *90*, 4062–4070. [CrossRef]
17. Song, J.; Wang, X.; Guo, Y.; Yang, Y.; Xu, K.; Wang, T.; Sa, Y.; Yuan, L.; Jiang, H.; Guo, J. Novel high-coverage targeted metabolomics method (SWATHtoMRM) for exploring follicular fluid metabolome alterations in women with recurrent spontaneous abortion undergoing in vitro fertilization. *Sci. Rep.* **2019**, *9*, 10873. [CrossRef]
18. Xu, L.; Xu, Z.; Wang, X.; Wang, B.; Liao, X. The application of pseudotargeted metabolomics method for fruit juices discrimination. *Food Chem.* **2020**, *316*, 126278. [CrossRef]
19. Song, J.; Xiang, S.; Pang, C.; Guo, J.; Sun, Z. Metabolomic alternations of follicular fluid of obese women undergoing in-vitro fertilization treatment. *Sci. Rep.* **2020**, *10*, 5968. [CrossRef]
20. Tao, Z.; Lu, N.; Wu, X.; Huang, Y.; Xiao, Y.; Wang, X. Research progress on chemical constituents and pharmacological action of *Dendrobium*. *J. Pharm. Res.* **2021**, *40*, 44–51+70.
21. Rao, D.; Zhao, R.; Hu, Y.; Li, H.; Chun, Z.; Zheng, S. Revealing of intracellular antioxidants in *Dendrobium nobile* by high performance liquid chromatography-tandem mass spectrometry. *Metabolites* **2023**, *13*, 702. [CrossRef]
22. He, C.; Peng, C.; Dai, O.; Yang, L.; Liu, J.; Guo, L.; Xiong, L.; Liu, Z. Chemical constituents from *Leonurus japonicus* Injection. *Chin. Tradit. Herb. Drugs* **2014**, *45*, 3048–3052.
23. Zhang, J.; Xu, H.-X.; Zhao, Z.-L.; Xian, Y.-F.; Lin, Z.-X. *Dendrobium nobile* Lindl: A review on its chemical constituents and pharmacological effects. *Chin. Med. Cult.* **2021**, *4*, 235–242. [CrossRef]
24. Horton, D.; Rodemeyer, G.; Haskell, T.H. Analytical characterization of lipopolysaccharide antigens from seven strains of *Pseudomonas aeruginosa*. *Carbohydr. Res.* **1977**, *55*, 35–47. [CrossRef]
25. Chen, W.; Yeo, S.C.M.; Chuang, X.F.; Lin, H.-S. Determination of pinostilbene in rat plasma by LC–MS/MS: Application to a pharmacokinetic study. *J. Pharm. Biomed. Anal.* **2016**, *120*, 316–321. [CrossRef]

26. Kato, Y.; Terada, H. Determination method of linamarin in cassava products and beans by ultra high performance liquid chromatography with tandem mass spectrometry. *Shokuhin Eiseigaku Zasshi J. Food Hyg. Soc. Jpn.* **2014**, *55*, 162–166. [CrossRef]
27. Yang, X.-B.; Yan, S.; Hu, J.-M.; Zhou, J. Chemical constituents from *Dendrobium heterocarpum* Lindl. *Nat. Prod. Res. Dev.* **2019**, *31*, 1745–1752.
28. Song, C.; Zhang, Y.; Manzoor, M.A.; Li, G. Identification of alkaloids and related intermediates of *Dendrobium officinale* by solid-phase extraction coupled with high-performance liquid chromatography tandem mass spectrometry. *Front. Plant Sci.* **2022**, *13*, 952051. [CrossRef]
29. Ma, Y.; Li, P.; Chen, D.; Fang, T.; Li, H.; Su, W. LC/MS/MS quantitation assay for pharmacokinetics of naringenin and double peaks phenomenon in rats plasma. *Int. J. Pharm.* **2006**, *307*, 292–299. [CrossRef]
30. Katsumata, S.; Hamana, K.; Horie, K.; Toshima, H.; Hasegawa, M. Identification of sternbin and naringenin as detoxified metabolites from the rice flavanone phytoalexin sakuranetin by pyricularia oryzae. *Chem. Biodivers.* **2017**, *14*, e1600240. [CrossRef]
31. Bulama, J.; Dangoggo, S.; Halilu, M.; Tsafe, A.; Hassan, S. Isolation and characterization of palmitic acid from ethyl acetate extract of root bark of *Terminalia glaucescens*. *Chem. Mater. Res.* **2014**, *6*, 140–143.
32. Ye, Q.; Zhao, W. New alloaromadendrane, cadinene and cyclocopacamphane type sesquiterpene derivatives and bibenzyls from *Dendrobium nobile*. *Planta Medica* **2002**, *68*, 723–729. [CrossRef]
33. Zhu, Y.; Feng, Y.; Shen, L.; Xu, D.; Wang, B.; Ruan, K.; Cong, W. Effect of metformin on the urinary metabolites of diet-induced-obese mice studied by ultra performance liquid chromatography coupled to time-of-flight mass spectrometry (UPLC-TOF/MS). *J. Chromatogr. B* **2013**, *925*, 110–116. [CrossRef]
34. Wei, M.; Liu, Z.; Liu, Y.; Li, S.; Hu, M.; Yue, K.; Liu, T.; He, Y.; Pi, Z.; Liu, Z.; et al. Urinary and plasmatic metabolomics strategy to explore the holistic mechanism of lignans in S. chinensis in treating Alzheimer's disease using UPLC-Q-TOF-MS. *Food Funct.* **2019**, *10*, 5656–5668. [CrossRef] [PubMed]
35. Yang, J.; Han, X.; Wang, H.-Y.; Yang, J.; Kuang, Y.; Ji, K.-Y.; Yang, Y.; Pang, K.; Yang, S.-X.; Qin, J.-C.; et al. Comparison of metabolomics of Dendrobium officinale in different habitats by UPLC-Q-TOF-MS. *Biochem. Syst. Ecol.* **2020**, *89*, 104007. [CrossRef]
36. Wu, D.; Li, X.; Zhang, X.; Han, F.; Lu, X.; Liu, L.; Zhang, J.; Dong, M.; Yang, H.; Li, H. Pharmacometabolomics Identifies 3-Hydroxyadipic Acid, d-Galactose, Lysophosphatidylcholine (P-16:0), and Tetradecenoyl-l-Carnitine as Potential Predictive Indicators of Gemcitabine Efficacy in Pancreatic Cancer Patients. *Front. Oncol.* **2020**, *9*, 1524. [CrossRef]
37. Lu, X.; Zhang, X.; Zhang, Y.; Zhang, K.; Zhan, C.; Shi, X.; Li, Y.; Zhao, J.; Bai, Y.; Wang, Y.; et al. Metabolic profiling analysis upon acylcarnitines in tissues of hepatocellular carcinoma revealed the inhibited carnitine shuttle system caused by the downregulated carnitine palmitoyltransferase 2. *Mol. Carcinog.* **2019**, *58*, 749–759. [CrossRef]
38. Zhao, W.; Ye, Q.; Tan, X.; Jiang, H.; Li, X.; Chen, K.; Kinghorn, A.D. Three New Sesquiterpene Glycosides from *Dendrobium nobile* with Immunomodulatory Activity. *J. Nat. Prod.* **2001**, *64*, 1196–1200. [CrossRef]
39. Yang, W.; Kong, L.; Zhang, Y.; Tang, G.; Zhu, F.; Li, S.; Guo, L.; Cheng, Y.; Hao, X.; He, H. Phragmalin-type Limonoids from *Heynea trijuga*. *Planta Med.* **2012**, *78*, 1676–1682. [CrossRef]
40. Zhao, D.; Xie, L.; Yu, L.; An, N.; Na, W.; Chen, F.; Li, Y.; Tan, Y.; Zhang, X. New 2-Benzoxazolinone Derivatives with Cytotoxic Activities from the Roots of *Acanthus Ilicifolius* *Chem. Pharm. Bull.* **2015**, *63*, 1087–1090. [CrossRef]
41. Xiang, Y.; Li, Y.-B.; Zhang, J.; Li, P.; Yao, Y.-z. Studies on chemical constituents of *Salsola collina*. *China J. Chin. Mater. Medica* **2007**, *32*, 409–413.
42. Avula, B.; Wang, Y.-H.; Smillie, T.J.; Khan, I.A. Determination of Shikimic Acid in Fruits of *Illicium* Species and Various Other Plant Samples by LC–UV and LC–ESI–MS. *Chromatographia* **2009**, *69*, 307–314. [CrossRef]
43. Zhuang, B.; Bi, Z.-M.; Wang, Z.-Y.; Duan, L.; Lai, C.-J.-S.; Liu, E.H. Chemical profiling and quantitation of bioactive compounds in Platycladi Cacumen by UPLC-Q-TOF-MS/MS and UPLC-DAD. *J. Pharm. Biomed. Anal.* **2018**, *154*, 207–215. [CrossRef]
44. Wu, C.; Wang, J.; Zhang, C.; Wang, D.; Zhang, L.; Cao, M.; Wang, Y.; Li, Q. Determination of Four Sugars in Infant Formula Milk Powder and Dairy Products by Ion Chromatography-Mass Spectrometry. *Food Sci. Technol.* **2020**, *45*, 264–268.
45. Lan, Y.; Zhang, J.; Ll, O.; Feng, J. Determination of Three Monosaccharides in *Dendrobium denneanum* and *D.officinale* by UPLC-QQQ-MS. *Guangzhou Chem. Ind.* **2022**, *50*, 143–145.
46. Chen, Y.; Yu, H.; Lian, X. Isolation of stilbenoids and lignans from *Dendrobium hongdie*. *Trop. J. Pharm. Res.* **2015**, *14*, 2055–2059. [CrossRef]
47. Yang, L.; Wang, Y.; Zhang, G.; Zhang, F.; Zhang, Z.; Wang, Z.; Xu, L. Simultaneous quantitative and qualitative analysis of bioactive phenols in *Dendrobium aurantiacum* var. *denneanum* by high-performance liquid chromatography coupled with mass spectrometry and diode array detection. *Biomed. Chromatogr.* **2007**, *21*, 687–694. [CrossRef] [PubMed]
48. Zhu, A.-L.; Hao, J.-W.; Liu, L.; Wang, Q.; Chen, N.-D.; Wang, G.-L.; Liu, X.-Q.; Li, Q.; Xu, H.-M.; Yang, W.-H. Simultaneous Quantification of 11 Phenolic Compounds and Consistency Evaluation in Four *Dendrobium* Species Used as Ingredients of the Traditional Chinese Medicine Shihu. *Front. Nutr.* **2021**, *8*, 771078. [CrossRef] [PubMed]
49. Wang, Y.; Han, B.; Li, Z.; Nie, X.; Yang, M.; Wang, W.; Sun, Z. Determination of the Compounds of *Dendrobium pendulum* Roxb. by UPLC-Q-TOF-MS. *Chin. Pharm. J.* **2021**, *56*, 708–714.
50. Tezuka, Y.; Hirano, H.; Kikuchi, T.; Xu, G.-J. Constituents of *Ephemerantha lonchophylla*; isolation and structure elucidation of new phenolic compounds, ephemeranthol-A, ephemeranthol-B, and ephemeranthoquinone, and of a new diterpene glucoside, ephemeranthoside. *Chem. Pharm. Bull.* **1991**, *39*, 593–598. [CrossRef]

51. Yang, H.; Gong, Y.; Wang, Z.; Xu, L.; Hu, Z.; Xu, G. Studies on chemical constituents of *Dendrobium chrysotoxum*. *Chin. Tradit. Herb. Drugs* **2001**, *32*, 972–974.
52. Kaganda, N.; Adesanya, S. A new dihydrostilbene from diseased *Dioscorea mangenotiana*. *J. Nat. Prod.* **1990**, *53*, 1345–1346. [CrossRef]
53. Li, Y.; Wang, C.-L.; Guo, S.-X.; Yang, J.-S.; Xiao, P.-G. Two new compounds from *Dendrobium candidum*. *Chem. Pharm. Bull.* **2008**, *56*, 1477–1479. [CrossRef]
54. Okamoto, T.; Natsume, M.; Onaka, T.; Uchimaru, F.; Shimizu, M. The structure of dendroxine the third alkaloid from *Dendrobium nobile*. *Chem. Pharm. Bull.* **1966**, *14*, 672–675. [CrossRef] [PubMed]
55. Wang, Y.-H.; Avula, B.; Abe, N.; Wei, F.; Wang, M.; Ma, S.-C.; Ali, Z.; Elsohly, M.A.; Khan, I.A. Tandem Mass Spectrometry for Structural Identification of Sesquiterpene Alkaloids from the Stems of *Dendrobium nobile* Using LC-QToF. *Planta Medica* **2016**, *82*, 662–670. [CrossRef] [PubMed]
56. Nagai, T.; Kiyohara, H.; Munakata, K.; Shirahata, T.; Sunazuka, T.; Harigaya, Y.; Yamada, H. Pinellic acid from the tuber of *Pinellia ternata* Breitenbach as an effective oral adjuvant for nasal influenza vaccine. *Int. Immunopharmacol.* **2002**, *2*, 1183–1193. [CrossRef]
57. Cong, W.; Schwartz, E.; Peterson, D.G. Identification of inhibitors of pinellic acid generation in whole wheat bread. *Food Chem.* **2021**, *351*, 129291. [CrossRef]
58. Fujimoto, T.; Oku, K.; Tashiro, M.; Machinami, T. Crystal Structure of α,α-Trehalose–Calcium Chloride Monohydrate Complex. *J. Carbohydr. Chem.* **2006**, *25*, 521–532. [CrossRef]
59. Tan, D.; Song, Y.; Wang, J.; Gao, C.; Qin, L.; Zhao, Y.; Lu, Y.; Yang, Z.; He, Y. Identification of sesquiterpene glycosides from *Dendrobium nobile* and their α-glycosidase and α-amylase inhibitory activities. *Food Sci. Technol.* **2022**, *43*, e99782. [CrossRef]
60. Ye, Q.; Qin, G.; Zhao, W. Immunomodulatory sesquiterpene glycosides from *Dendrobium nobile*. *Phytochemistry* **2002**, *61*, 885–890. [CrossRef]
61. Zhao, C.; Liu, Q.; Halaweish, F.; Shao, B.; Ye, Y.; Zhao, W. Copacamphane, Picrotoxane, and Alloaromadendrane Sesquiterpene Glycosides and Phenolic Glycosides from *Dendrobium moniliforme*. *J. Nat. Prod.* **2003**, *66*, 1140–1143. [CrossRef]
62. Lijina, P.; Gnanesh Kumar, B.S. Discrimination of raffinose and planteose based on porous graphitic carbon chromatography in combination with mass spectrometry. *J. Chromatogr. B* **2023**, *1224*, 123758. [CrossRef]
63. Huang, Y.P.; Robinson, R.C.; Barile, D. Food glycomics: Dealing with unexpected degradation of oligosaccharides during sample preparation and analysis. *J. Food Drug Anal.* **2022**, *30*, 62–76. [CrossRef]
64. Han, J.; Ye, M.; Qiao, X.; Xu, M.; Wang, B.-R.; Guo, D.-A. Characterization of phenolic compounds in the Chinese herbal drug *Artemisia annua* by liquid chromatography coupled to electrospray ionization mass spectrometry. *J. Pharm. Biomed. Anal.* **2008**, *47*, 516–525. [CrossRef] [PubMed]
65. Silva, D.B.; Turatti, I.C.C.; Gouveia, D.R.; Ernst, M.; Teixeira, S.P.; Lopes, N.P. Mass Spectrometry of Flavonoid Vicenin-2, Based Sunlight Barriers in *Lychnophora* species. *Sci. Rep.* **2014**, *4*, 4309. [CrossRef] [PubMed]
66. Yang, J.; Qian, D.; Jiang, S.; Shang, E.-X.; Guo, J.; Duan, J.-A. Identification of rutin deglycosylated metabolites produced by human intestinal bacteria using UPLC–Q-TOF/MS. *J. Chromatogr. B* **2012**, *898*, 95–100. [CrossRef] [PubMed]
67. Oskouei, Z.; Rahbardar, M.G.; Hosseinzadeh, H. The effects of Dendrobium species on the metabolic syndrome: A review. *Iran. J. Basic Med. Sci.* **2023**, *26*, 738. [PubMed]
68. Zhou, X.; Wang, X.; Sun, Q.; Zhang, W.; Liu, C.; Ma, W.; Sun, C. Natural compounds: A new perspective on targeting polarization and infiltration of tumor-associated macrophages in lung cancer. *Biomed. Pharmacother.* **2022**, *151*, 113096. [CrossRef]
69. Inthongkaew, P.; Chatsumpun, N.; Supasuteekul, C.; Kitisripanya, T.; Putalun, W.; Likhitwitayawuid, K.; Sritularak, B. α-Glucosidase and pancreatic lipase inhibitory activities and glucose uptake stimulatory effect of phenolic compounds from *Dendrobium formosum*. *Rev. Bras. Farmacogn.* **2017**, *27*, 480–487. [CrossRef]

Disclaimer/Publisher's Note: The statements, opinions and data contained in all publications are solely those of the individual author(s) and contributor(s) and not of MDPI and/or the editor(s). MDPI and/or the editor(s) disclaim responsibility for any injury to people or property resulting from any ideas, methods, instructions or products referred to in the content.

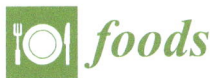

Communication

Cuttlefish Species Authentication: Advancing Label Control through Near-Infrared Spectroscopy as Rapid, Eco-Friendly, and Robust Approach

Sarah Currò, Stefania Balzan *, Enrico Novelli and Luca Fasolato

Department of Comparative Biomedicine and Food Science, University of Padova, Agripolis, Viale dell'Università 16, 35020 Legnaro, Italy; sarah.curro@unipd.it (S.C.); enrico.novelli@unipd.it (E.N.); luca.fasolato@unipd.it (L.F.)
* Correspondence: stefania.balzan@unipd.it

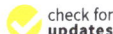

Citation: Currò, S.; Balzan, S.; Novelli, E.; Fasolato, L. Cuttlefish Species Authentication: Advancing Label Control through Near-Infrared Spectroscopy as Rapid, Eco-Friendly, and Robust Approach. *Foods* **2023**, *12*, 2973. https://doi.org/10.3390/foods12152973

Academic Editors: Hongyan Liu, Hongtao Lei, Boli Guo and Ren-You Gan

Received: 10 July 2023
Revised: 3 August 2023
Accepted: 4 August 2023
Published: 7 August 2023

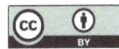

Copyright: © 2023 by the authors. Licensee MDPI, Basel, Switzerland. This article is an open access article distributed under the terms and conditions of the Creative Commons Attribution (CC BY) license (https://creativecommons.org/licenses/by/4.0/).

Abstract: Accurate species identification, especially in the fishery sector, is critical for ensuring food safety, consumer protection and to prevent economic losses. In this study, a total of 93 individual frozen–thawed cuttlefish samples from four different species (*S. officinalis*, *S. bertheloti*, *S. aculeata*, and *Sepiella inermis*) were collected from two wholesale fish plants in Chioggia, Italy. Species identification was carried out by inspection through morphological features using dichotomic keys and then through near-infrared spectroscopy (NIRS) measurements. The NIRS data were collected using a handled-portable spectrophotometer, and the spectral range scanned was from 900–1680 nm. The collected spectra were processed using principal component analysis for unsupervised analysis and a support vector machine for supervised analysis to evaluate the species identification capability. The results showed that NIRS classification had a high overall accuracy of 93% in identifying the cuttlefish species. This finding highlights the robustness and effectiveness of spectral analysis as a tool for species identification, even in complex spatial contexts. The findings emphasize the potential of NIRS as a valuable tool in the field of fishery product authentication, offering a rapid and eco-friendly approach to species identification in the post-processing stages.

Keywords: chemometrics; support vector machine; untargeted method; food inspection; seafood

1. Introduction

The genus Sepia, as classified by Linnaeus in 1758, represents a group of considerable commercial importance, encompassing approximately 100 species [1]. This genus stands as the largest among the three genera identified within the *Sepiidae* family, as established by Leach in 1817. Among the European cuttlefish species, *Sepia officinalis* holds a significant position as the prevailing genus in the Mediterranean Sea (FAO fishing area 37). Nevertheless, its presence extends further to encompass the Eastern North and Central Atlantic Oceans (FAO fishing areas 27 and 34, respectively) [2].

Accurate species identification, especially in the fishery sector, is critical for ensuring food safety by detecting harmful toxins (i.e., domoic acid) or parasites (i.e., *Dicyemid* parasite) that may be present in certain cephalopods species [3,4]. Dichotomous keys serve as valuable tools utilized by scientists and professionals in the food industry to enable rigorous classification and taxonomy, ensuring accuracy and reliability in species identification for scientific investigations and commercial applications alike. Species identification is generally conducted on unprocessed products by an official authority and food business operator through visual analysis by examining the morphological characteristics of cuttlefish, i.e., coat color, corneal membrane, horny beak, and siphon structure. The anatomical complexity of these structures necessitates highly skilled personnel and specialized techniques to ensure accurate identification [5]. However, current identification techniques have notable limitations. In particular, the taxonomic approach is not applicable when morphological characteristics have been removed (i.e., cuttlebone, statoliths, beaks, and radula [6]), and the dichotomous keys employment are difficult to consider due to inconsistent description of the catalog proposed. However, molecular analysis for identification purposes overcomes these limitations applying to whole or prepared products; indeed, despite the significant accuracy provided by molecular methods, it is crucial to acknowledge that these techniques often rely on a limited sample size. This is primarily attributed to the resource-intensive nature of molecular analyses, which require specific reagents, laboratory infrastructure, and skilled personnel, making them expensive and time-consuming processes [7]. Additionally, the primary DNA-based methods utilized, such as PCR and DNA sequencing, due to the long preparation step of the sample, are not conducive to rapid and cost-effective species identification in field settings.

A strategic, economic, non-destructive, rapid, and easy alternative approach applicable in every phase of the supply chain can be represented by the Near-InfraRed Spectroscopy (NIRS) technology for food control purposes [8–11]. Indeed, the Commission Implementing Regulation (EU) 2022/2503 has recently recognized the value of untargeted analysis (NIRS/UV-VIS) as a supporting device in assessing the physical status (fresh/frozen–thawed) of fishery products during official control [12]. The implementation of a fast and suitable technique to identify fishery species meets the need of food regulatory demand to comply with the labeling laws but also to protect the interest of the seafood business operator and consumers, guaranteeing the truthfulness of the supply chain in seafood products without the sample destruction [13]. To the best of our knowledge, studies on species identification using InfraRed Spectroscopy have primarily concentrated within the Teleost infraclass, and there is a lack of research specifically targeting cephalopod species identification using handheld-portable Near-Infrared Spectroscopy devices. In light of this, the present study aims to address this gap by focusing on four distinct cuttlefish species. Therefore, the primary aim is to assess the significant potential of Near-Infrared Spectroscopy (NIRS) in precisely identifying these prepared cuttlefish species at the initial stages of the complex supply chain.

2. Materials and Methods

2.1. Cuttlefish Sampling and Species Identification

A total of 93 individual frozen–thawed cuttlefishes of 4 species were collected in June 2022 from two wholesale fish plants in Chioggia (Venice, Italia). The species identification was performed prior to product processing as part of the company's self-monitoring process. The procedure involved evaluating the morphological features of the cuttlefish species, which were obtained prior to the sample preparation methods, adhering to the standardized protocols of the company. The species considered included *S. officinalis* (3 batches; $n = 31$ and $n = 9$ samples fished in 27.7 and in 34 FAO fishing areas, respectively), *S. bertheloti* (1 batch; $n = 9$ samples fished in 34 FAO fishing areas), *S. aculeata* (1 batch; $n = 10$ samples fished in the 51 FAO fishing area), and *Sepiella inermis* (2 batches; $n = 19$ and $n = 15$ samples fished in the 57 and 71 FAO fishing areas, respectively).

2.2. NIR Data Collection

The whole and refrigerated cuttlefish samples were subjected to NIRS measurement after the company's standard procedures, which involved removing the skin, gut, and bones and storing the samples on ice. A PoliSPEC NIR (ITPhotonics in Breganze, Italy) portable spectrophotometer was used to obtain spectral data from each sample through a round scanning window of 3.2 cm^2 placed in direct contact with the surface of the sample and scanning along the mantle. The spectral range scanned was from 900–1680 nm with a resolution of 2 nm. The individual spectrum of each cuttlefish was obtained by averaging the scans collected continuously for 5 s. The spectral data were recorded in reflectance units (R) and subsequently converted to absorbance units using the poliDATA 3.0.1 software (ITPhotonics in Breganze, Italy) by taking the logarithm of the reciprocal of R.

2.3. Identification Species Model

In the study, spectral data from cuttlefishes were analyzed in two forms: untreated and treated using different methods, namely standard normal variate (SNV), Savitzky–Golay, and derivative (none, first, and second). The investigation aimed to evaluate the best results and assess the effects of these treatments on the cuttlefish spectral data. The NIRS spectral data were processed using R software version 4.0.2 (R Core Team, 2020) for both unsupervised and supervised methods. For the unsupervised analysis, Principal Component Analysis (PCA) was employed as a descriptive tool to visualize the data distribution. On the other hand, the supervised approach involved utilizing Support Vector Machine (SVM), as reported in the works of Currò et al. [8,14]. Concisely, the SVM model was developed using the 'caret' package, employing both the svmLinear and svmRadial kernels. The training dataset underwent repeated hold-out-validation. For multi-class classification (classes > 3), the 'one-against-one' approach was utilized, entailing training k $(k - 1)/2$ binary classifiers and determining the appropriate class through a voting scheme. To improve the SVM performance, a grid search was conducted to fine-tune the C-value (Cost) in the Linear classifier and the Radial Basis Function sigma. This process involved exploring different combinations of these parameters to identify the most suitable model configuration. The SVM was employed in the development of the calibration model to assess the NIRS classification potential for species identification. Briefly, the complete dataset was divided into two sets: a training set and a testing set. The training set, which accounted for 70% of the samples ($n = 66$), was used to develop discrimination models. The testing set, representing 30% of the samples ($n = 27$), was employed to evaluate and validate the developed model. To validate the model, a hold-out validation approach was utilized. The dataset was split again, with 70% allocated to the training set for repeated cross-validation (with 10 settings and 5 repeats) and the remaining 30% forming the testing set. Table 1 provides a comprehensive breakdown of all sampled cuttlefish, along with their distribution into training and testing sets, including their respective varieties and the FAO fishing area of origin.

Table 1. Sample description according to the training and testing sets used in the hold-out validation.

	n. of Samples	n. Per Species	FAO Fishing Area
Training	66	*S. bertheloti*, n. 7 *S. officinalis*, n. 28 *S. aculeata*, n. 7 *Sepiella inermis*, n. 24	34 27.7 (*n.* 22); 34 (*n.* 6) 51 57 (*n.* 13), 71 (*n.* 11)
Testing	27	*S. bertheloti*, n. 2 *S. officinalis*, n. 12 *S. aculeata*, n. 3 *Sepiella inermis*, n. 10	34 27.7 (*n.* 9); 34 (*n.* 3) 51 57 (*n.* 6); 71 (*n.* 4)

3. Results and Discussion

Species substitution in the fish industry is a widespread issue, particularly aggravated in post-processing stages at retailers and supermarkets. The deliberate substitution of high-value species with lower-quality alternatives is the most commonly observed form of fish fraud [15]. However, accidental substitution can also occur when species closely resemble each other, leading to mistaken identities. This practice primarily affects processed products and fillets that are challenging to identify using traditional morphological analysis. The inherent complexities in species identification significantly contribute to the prevalence of this problem, especially in retail settings.

Among the results observed using untreated and treated data, the best performances were obtained for raw spectral data and were described in the following sections.

3.1. Exploratory Results

Principal Component Analysis (PCA) was employed as an unsupervised method to qualitatively visualize differences among cuttlefish samples related to the different species offering a straightforward means of identifying potential clusters of samples [16]. In particular, Figure 1 depicts the score plots of the first three PCs of the groups of cuttlefish species. Notably, PC1, PC2, and PC3 explained 68%, 28%, and 3% of the total variance.

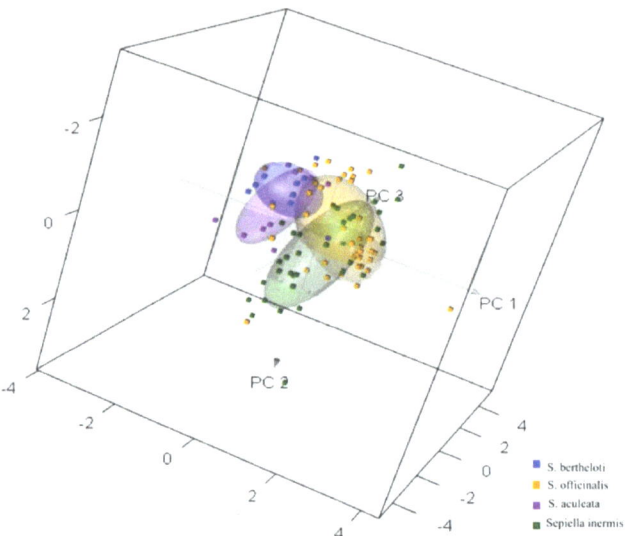

Figure 1. Principal component score plot for PC1, PC2, and PC3 of raw spectra.

The high variance explained by PC1 indicates that it effectively captures the significant and relevant characteristics inherent in the raw spectrum. This emphasizes the importance of PC1 in representing the primary sources of variation among the samples. This observation implies that species identification could potentially be facilitated by leveraging the distinct spectral attributes present in the samples. However, a partial separation among samples related to the different cuttlefish species was observed, suggesting that species identification could be possible due to the different spectral attributes of the samples associated with the characteristics of the species considered. Nonetheless, it is important to acknowledge that while PCA is valuable for dimensionality reduction and highlighting major sources of variance, it may not capture all intricacies related to species classification, thus explaining the partial overlapping among groups.

The findings align with the outcomes of previous studies conducted by Ottavian et al. [17] and Lv et al. [18], where PCA was used for classifying fish species. These studies demonstrated that PCA groups' segregation provided promising results for species classification; thus, the congruence between these studies and the current research suggests that PCA is a suitable method for exploring data trends in species differentiation.

Figure 2 illustrates the average raw spectra acquired from cuttlefish species within the specified range (900–1680 nm). The observed divergences between species can likely be attributed to variations in their physical and chemical properties, which, in turn, are influenced by differences in their habitats and diets [14]. These environmental factors play a crucial role in shaping the spectrum of each species showing a noticeable graphical divergence among the species.

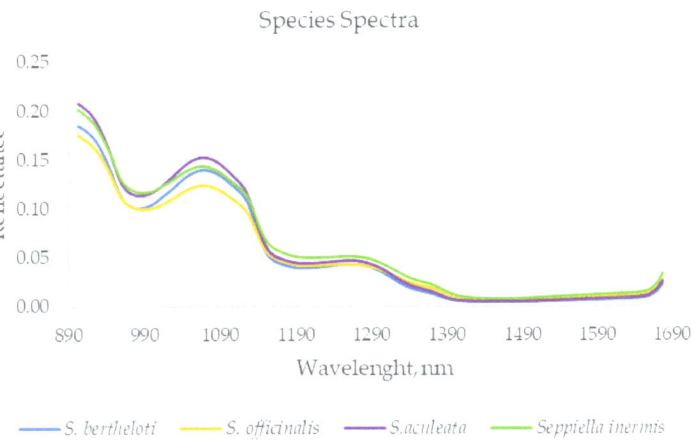

Figure 2. NIR spectra (mean) of cuttlefish species collected using the NIR portable device.

3.2. Classification by Species

In recent years, there has been an exploration of the application of NIRS to recognize different fishery species [16,19]. However, to date, research on species identification utilizing NIRS has predominantly focused on species within the Teleost infraclass. In detail, the study of Cavallini et al. [10] focused on differentiating between two closely resembling flatfish species, *Synaptura cadenati* (Guinean sole; $n = 50$) and *Pleuronectes platessa* (European plaice; $n = 50$). The fillets of these species were analyzed using portable NIRS devices operating at wavelengths of 740–1070 nm and 908–1676 nm, as well as a benchtop NIRS device operating at wavelengths of 800–2500 nm. The collected spectra were then subjected to chemometric analysis employing Partial Least Squares-Discriminant Analysis (PLS-DA) classification model. Such a study demonstrated an accuracy of 94.1% in species classification using the portable NIRS device and an accuracy of 90.1% using the benchtop device. In the study conducted by Ottavian et al. [17], fish minced samples were classified according to the species considered (*Sparus aurata*, $n = 106$; *Mullus barbatus*, $n = 106$; *Solea vulgaris*, $n = 88$; *Xiphias gladius*, $n = 175$) using a NIRS reflectance device and a PLS-DA classification model. The samples were categorized, obtaining a classification accuracy of 100% in validation.

The study of Lv et al. [18], using an NIRS reflectance device (1000–1799 nm) and chemometrics (PCA-Linear Discriminant Analysis) to distinguish among seven different carp species (*Hypophthalmichthys molitrix*, $n = 100$; *Mylopharyngodon piceus*, $n = 100$; *Aristichthys nobilis*, $n = 100$; *Ctenopharyngodon idellus*, $n = 100$; *Cyprinus carpio*, $n = 80$; *Carassius auratus*, $n = 100$; *Parabramis pekinensis*, $n = 70$), showed a complete classification capability (100%). Analog outcomes were noted in the investigation conducted by Alamprese et al. [20], wherein *Mullus surmuletus* (Red mullet) and *Pseudupeneus prayensis* (Atlantic mullet) were successfully identified using FT-NIR through the application of the Soft Independent Modelling of Class Analogies (SIMCA) technique. In contrast, the study conducted by Cozzolino et al. [21] demonstrated a lower classification capability compared to previous studies, probably because it was performed on by-products using an NIRS device (1100–2500 nm) to collect spectra. The classification accuracy (using Linear Discriminant Analysis) achieved using fish meals from *Salmon salar*, *Micromesistius poutassau*, and other species such as *Scomber scombrus* and *Clupea harengus* ranged from 70% to 90%. These studies demonstrate the potential of NIRS combined with chemometric analysis for species identification and classification in various fish species. The accuracy levels achieved vary across the studies, which can be influenced by factors such as the type of fish species, the specific NIRS device used, the wavelength range, and the analytical techniques employed.

However, to the best of our knowledge, there is a noticeable gap in studies that specifically explore cephalopod species identification.

Indeed, to address the existing research gap, the present study focuses on four distinct cuttlefish species, including *Sepia officinalis* and *Sepia bertheloti*, which have overlapping distributions in the Central and Eastern Atlantic (FAO fishing area 34). The study aimed to assess the Near-Infrared Spectroscopy (NIRS) classification capability in differentiating and recognizing these cuttlefish species. From the obtained confusion matrix (Table 2), the overall accuracy of the NIRS classification was found to be 93%.

Table 2. Performance of classification of Support Vector Machine model to discriminate cuttlefish according to the species in hold-out validation.

Predicted Species	Reference Species			
	S. bertheloti	S. officinalis	S. aculeata	Seppiella inermis
S. bertheloti	2	0	0	0
S. officinalis	0	12	2	0
S. aculeata	0	0	1	0
Seppiella inermis	0	0	0	10
Overall Accuracy (%)	93			
Balanced Accuracy (%)	100	93	66	100

The balanced accuracy, calculated for each class, demonstrated complete accuracy for the *S. bertheloti* and *Sepiella inermis* species. However, it was lower (93%) for *S. officinalis* and the lowest (67%) for *S. aculeata* species. Among the 27 samples in the test set, only 7% of cuttlefish were misclassified. The SVM linear classification model used in this study exhibited a perfect sensitivity (100%) in detecting positive cases for *S. bertheloti*, *S. officinalis*, and *Sepiella inermis*. This indicates that the model accurately identified all instances of these species in the dataset, reflecting a high level of accuracy in species detection. These results provide encouraging prospects for species identification and classification tasks using NIRS technology. However, the model showed lower sensitivity in identifying *S. aculeata* species, with two out of three samples being misclassified as *S. officinalis*. This misclassification affected the specificity of *S. officinalis* (86%). Nevertheless, the model demonstrated high specificity in correctly identifying negative cases for *S. bertheloti*, *S. aculeata*, and *Sepiella inermis* species. In the present study, there were four species considered, and two of them (*S. bertheloti* and *S. officinalis*) overlapped for the 34 FAO fishing area collections (Central Atlantic Oceans). However, this overlap did not have any negative impact on species identification. Similar to the study conducted by Varrà et al. [22], the present study confirmed that the samples exhibited different spectral attributes associated with the characteristics of each species. Indeed, despite sharing the same fishing area, the distinct spectral properties allowed for accurate identification and differentiation between *S. bertheloti* and *S. officinalis*. This finding emphasizes that even when species overlap spatially (habitat), their unique spectral attributes remain reliable markers for species identification and are more prominently identified through the supervised approach. In detail, with NIRS being an untargeted approach, the combination of essential molecular vibrations and overtones associated with specific functional chemical groups highlight the capability of NIRS to classify cuttlefish based on species as a qualitative trait. Specifically, this differentiation is attributed to the evaluation of the molecular phenotype derived from averaging the vibration modes of all molecules within the specimen. The molecular phenotype exhibits variations among species within the same genus, reflecting their distinct genome expression [23,24].

4. Conclusions

This study highlights the efficacy of NIRS classification in identifying the four species of cuttlefish examined. Despite an overall high accuracy of 93% in species identification, it is imperative to account for greater sample variability within each species to enhance the precision of the classification process. Nonetheless, the findings underscore the potential of rapid, eco-friendly, and easy-to-use NIRS devices for the online authentication of cuttlefish species, especially when morphological characteristics have been removed and the dichotomous keys employment are difficult to be considered (prepared product). However, the practical implications of these results are substantial; indeed, the ability to swiftly analyze a large number of samples not only strengthens consumer protection against adulteration and fraudulent claims but also empowers commercial stakeholders to verify the trustworthiness of their suppliers and ensure the integrity of received prepared products. Furthermore, this approach provides a legitimate means to investigate suspected fraudulent activities, enabling the evaluation and substantiation of such claims through more sophisticated analyses. This study contributes to highlighting the potential of NIRS-based species identification as a valuable tool for quality control and supply chain integrity in the context of fishery product authentication.

Author Contributions: Conceptualization, S.B., S.C. and L.F.; methodology, S.B., S.C. and L.F.; validation, S.C.; formal analysis, S.C.; investigation, S.C.; data curation, S.C.; writing—original draft preparation, S.C.; writing—review and editing, S.B., S.C., E.N. and L.F.; visualization, E.N.; project administration, L.F.; funding acquisition, L.F. All authors have read and agreed to the published version of the manuscript.

Funding: This research was funded by OIS-AIR project: Device for the on-line evaluation of shelf life, authenticity, and quality of seafood products (CUP C14I19001270007).

Institutional Review Board Statement: Not applicable.

Informed Consent Statement: Not applicable.

Data Availability Statement: Not applicable.

Acknowledgments: The authors would like to thank the Blu Pesca S.r.l. and Chioggiamar S.r.l. companies (Chioggia (VE), Italy) for their help with sample logistics.

Conflicts of Interest: The authors declare no conflict of interest.

References

1. Vargheese, S.; Basheer, V.S. Resolving the taxonomic ambiguity of Sepia ramani using integrative taxonomy. *Molluscan Res.* **2022**, *42*, 91–98. [CrossRef]
2. MIPAAF; FEAMP 2014–2020. Seppia, Analisi Economica e Prospettive di Consumo. Available online: https://ittico.bmti.it/CaricaPdfRegolamenti.do?doc=20 (accessed on 6 July 2023).
3. Hassoun, A.E.R.; Ujević, I.; Mahfouz, C.; Fakhri, M.; Roje-Busatto, R.; Jemaa, S.; Nazlić, N. Occurrence of domoic acid and cyclic imines in marine biota from Lebanon-Eastern Mediterranean Sea. *Sci. Total Environ.* **2021**, *755*, 142542. [CrossRef] [PubMed]
4. Drábková, M.; Jachníková, N.; Tyml, T.; Sehadová, H.; Ditrich, O.; Myšková, E.; Hypša, V.; Štefka, J. Population co-divergence in common cuttlefish (*Sepia officinalis*) and its dicyemid parasite in the Mediterranean Sea. *Sci. Rep.* **2019**, *9*, 14300. [CrossRef] [PubMed]
5. Jereb, P.; Roper, C.F. *Cephalopods of the World—An Annotated and Illustrated Catalogue of Cephalopod Species Know to Date*, 2nd ed.; FAO: Rome, Italy, 2010; Volume 2, ISBN 978-92-5-106720-8.
6. Neige, P.; Neige, P.; Life, M. Morphometrics of hard structures in cuttlefish. *Vie Milieu/Life Environ.* **2006**, *56*, 121–127.
7. Cermakova, E.; Lencova, S.; Mukherjee, S.; Horka, P.; Vobruba, S.; Demnerova, K.; Zdenkova, K. Identification of Fish Species and Targeted Genetic Modifications Based on DNA Analysis: State of the Art. *Foods* **2023**, *12*, 228. [CrossRef] [PubMed]
8. Currò, S.; Fasolato, L.; Serva, L.; Boffo, L.; Carlo, J.; Novelli, E.; Balzan, S. Use of a portable near-infrared tool for rapid on-site inspection of freezing and hydrogen peroxide treatment of cuttlefish (*Sepia officinalis*). *Food Control* **2022**, *132*, 108524. [CrossRef]
9. O'Brien, N.; Hulse, C.A.; Pfeifer, F.; Siesler, H.W. Near infrared spectroscopic authentication of seafood. *J. Near Infrared Spectrosc.* **2013**, *21*, 299–305. [CrossRef]
10. Cavallini, N.; Pennisi, F.; Giraudo, A.; Pezzolato, M.; Esposito, G.; Gavoci, G.; Magnani, L.; Pianezzola, A.; Geobaldo, F.; Savorani, F.; et al. Chemometric Differentiation of Sole and Plaice Fish Fillets Using Three Near-Infrared Instruments. *Foods* **2022**, *11*, 1643. [CrossRef] [PubMed]
11. O' Brien, N.A.; Hulse, C.A.; Siesler, H.W.; Hsiung, C. Spectroscopic Characterization of Seafood U.S. Patent No. US 9316628 B2, 19 April 2016.

12. European Commission. Commission Implementing Regulation (EU) 2022/2503 Amending and correcting Implementing Regulation (EU) 2019/627 as regards practical arrangements for the performance of official controls in live bivalve molluscs, fishery products, or related to UV-radiation. *Off. J. Eur. Union.* **2022**, *L325*, 58–61.
13. Chapela, M.J.; Sotelo, C.G.; Calo-Mata, P.; Pérez-Martín, R.I.; Rehbein, H.; Hold, G.L.; Quinteiro, J.; Rey-Méndez, M.; Rosa, C.; Santos, A.T. Identification of Cephalopod Species (Ommastrephidae and Loliginidae) in Seafood Products by Forensically Informative Nucleotide Sequencing (FINS). *J. Food Sci.* **2002**, *67*, 1672–1676. [CrossRef]
14. Currò, S.; Balzan, S.; Serva, L.; Boffo, L.; Ferlito, J.C.; Novelli, E.; Fasolato, L. Fast and green method to control frauds of geographical origin in traded cuttlefish using a portable infrared reflective instrument. *Foods* **2021**, *10*, 1678. [CrossRef] [PubMed]
15. Fox, M.; Mitchell, M.; Dean, M.; Elliott, C.; Campbell, K. The seafood supply chain from a fraudulent perspective. *Food Secur.* **2018**, *10*, 939–963. [CrossRef]
16. Ghidini, S.; Varrà, M.O.; Zanardi, E. Approaching authenticity issues in fish and seafood products by qualitative spectroscopy and chemometrics. *Molecules* **2019**, *24*, 1812. [CrossRef] [PubMed]
17. Ottavian, M.; Fasolato, L.; Facco, P.; Barolo, M. Foodstuff authentication from spectral data: Toward a species-independent discrimination between fresh and frozen-thawed fish samples. *J. Food Eng.* **2013**, *119*, 765–775. [CrossRef]
18. Lv, H.; Xu, W.; You, J.; Xiong, S. Classification of freshwater fish species by linear discriminant analysis based on near infrared reflectance spectroscopy. *J. Near Infrared Spectrosc.* **2017**, *25*, 54–62. [CrossRef]
19. Nieto-Ortega, S.; Lara, R.; Foti, G.; Melado-Herreros, Á.; Olabarrieta, I. Applications of near-infrared spectroscopy (NIRS) in fish value chain. In *Infrared Spectroscopy*; El-Azazy, M., Al-Saad, K., El-Shafie, A.S., Eds.; IntechOpen: Rijeka, Croatia, 2022; Chapter 5.
20. Alamprese, C.; Casiraghi, E. Application of FT-NIR and FT-IR spectroscopy to fish fillet authentication. *LWT Food Sci. Technol.* **2015**, *63*, 720–725. [CrossRef]
21. Cozzolino, D.; Chree, A.; Scaife, J.R.; Murray, I. Usefulness of Near-infrared reflectance (NIR) spectroscopy and chemometrics to discriminate fishmeal batches made with different fish species. *J. Agric. Food Chem.* **2005**, *53*, 4459–4463. [CrossRef] [PubMed]
22. Varrà, M.O.; Ghidini, S.; Fabrile, M.P.; Ianieri, A.; Zanardi, E. Country of origin label monitoring of musky and common octopuses (Eledone spp. and Octopus vulgaris) by means of a portable near-infrared spectroscopic device. *Food Control* **2022**, *138*, 109052. [CrossRef]
23. Rodríguez-Fernández, J.I.; De Carvalho, C.J.B.; Pasquini, C.; De Lima, K.M.G.; Moura, M.O.; Arízaga, G.G.C. Barcoding without DNA? Species identification using near infrared spectroscopy. *Zootaxa* **2011**, *2933*, 46–54. [CrossRef]
24. De Azevedo, R.A.; de Morais, J.W.; Lang, C.; de Sales Dambros, C. Discrimination of termite species using Near-Infrared Spectroscopy (NIRS). *Eur. J. Soil Biol.* **2019**, *93*, 103084. [CrossRef]

Disclaimer/Publisher's Note: The statements, opinions and data contained in all publications are solely those of the individual author(s) and contributor(s) and not of MDPI and/or the editor(s). MDPI and/or the editor(s) disclaim responsibility for any injury to people or property resulting from any ideas, methods, instructions or products referred to in the content.

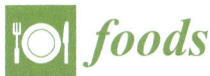

Review

Molecular Barcoding: A Tool to Guarantee Correct Seafood Labelling and Quality and Preserve the Conservation of Endangered Species

Laura Filonzi [1], Alessia Ardenghi [1,*], Pietro Maria Rontani [1], Andrea Voccia [1], Claudio Ferrari [1], Riccardo Papa [2], Nicolò Bellin [2] and Francesco Nonnis Marzano [1]

1. Department of Chemistry, Life Sciences and Environmental Sustainability, University of Parma, 43124 Parma, Italy; laura.filonzi@unipr.it (L.F.); pietromaria.rontani@unipr.it (P.M.R.); voccia.andrea@gmail.com (A.V.); claudio.ferrari1@unipr.it (C.F.); francesco.nonnismarzano@unipr.it (F.N.M.)
2. Department Biology, University of Puerto Rico, Rio Piedras, San Juan 00925, Puerto Rico; rpapa.lab@gmail.com (R.P.); nicolo.bellin@unipr.it (N.B.)
* Correspondence: aalessia.ardenghi@gmail.com

Abstract: The recent increase in international fish trade leads to the need for improving the traceability of fishery products. In relation to this, consistent monitoring of the production chain focusing on technological developments, handling, processing and distribution via global networks is necessary. Molecular barcoding has therefore been suggested as the gold standard in seafood species traceability and labelling. This review describes the DNA barcoding methodology for preventing food fraud and adulteration in fish. In particular, attention has been focused on the application of molecular techniques to determine the identity and authenticity of fish products, to discriminate the presence of different species in processed seafood and to characterize raw materials undergoing food industry processes. In this regard, we herein present a large number of studies performed in different countries, showing the most reliable DNA barcodes for species identification based on both mitochondrial (*COI*, *cytb*, *16S* rDNA and *12S* rDNA) and nuclear genes. Results are discussed considering the advantages and disadvantages of the different techniques in relation to different scientific issues. Special regard has been dedicated to a dual approach referring to both the consumer's health and the conservation of threatened species, with a special focus on the feasibility of the different genetic and genomic approaches in relation to both scientific objectives and permissible costs to obtain reliable traceability.

Keywords: molecular barcoding; fraud; mislabelling; species identification

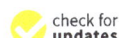

Citation: Filonzi, L.; Ardenghi, A.; Rontani, P.M.; Voccia, A.; Ferrari, C.; Papa, R.; Bellin, N.; Nonnis Marzano, F. Molecular Barcoding: A Tool to Guarantee Correct Seafood Labelling and Quality and Preserve the Conservation of Endangered Species. *Foods* **2023**, *12*, 2420. https://doi.org/10.3390/foods12122420

Academic Editor: Zhuohong Xie

Received: 4 May 2023
Revised: 14 June 2023
Accepted: 16 June 2023
Published: 20 June 2023

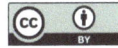

Copyright: © 2023 by the authors. Licensee MDPI, Basel, Switzerland. This article is an open access article distributed under the terms and conditions of the Creative Commons Attribution (CC BY) license (https://creativecommons.org/licenses/by/4.0/).

1. Seafood Commerce and Fraud

The global fish production industry plays a crucial role in national economies, supporting an estimated 59.5 million jobs in the primary sector of capture fisheries and aquaculture [1]. Dealing with the most valuable traded food commodity worldwide, seafood has also become a fundamental income product for developing countries with net exports valued more than sugar, tobacco, meat and rice combined [1,2]. Staggering numbers highlight a constant worldwide increase both in the sector of natural seafood capture and in aquaculture production. According to available data, global fish production has reached almost 300 million tonnes [3], also considering world aquaculture, which accounts for about one third of total fish production [1]. In 2018, aquaculture fish production was dominated by finfish (54.3 million tonnes—47 million tonnes from inland aquaculture and 7.3 million tonnes from marine and coastal aquaculture); molluscs, mainly bivalves (17.7 million tonnes) and crustaceans (9.4 million tonnes) [1].

However, if there is production, there is also consumption. In fact, according to the FAO [1], global food fish exploitation increased at an average annual rate of 3.1% from 1961 to 2017, a rate almost twice than the annual world population growth (1.6%) for the same period, and higher than all the other animal protein foods (meat, dairy, milk, etc.), which increased by 2.1% per year. At the individual level, global fish consumption rose by 122% from 1990 to 2018 [1]. The annual per capita seafood consumption of fisheries and aquaculture products approximately doubled in 2018 compared to the level in the 1960s. In particular, per capita fish consumption grew significantly from 9.0 kg in 1961 to 20.5 kg in 2018, by about 1.5% per year [1]. Europeans consume, on average, 24.4 kg per person of fishery products annually, 4 kg more than the world average [4]. Despite persistent differences in levels of fish consumption between regions and states, significant trends and trajectories were observed [5]. All the above cited data are graphically illustrated in Figure 1.

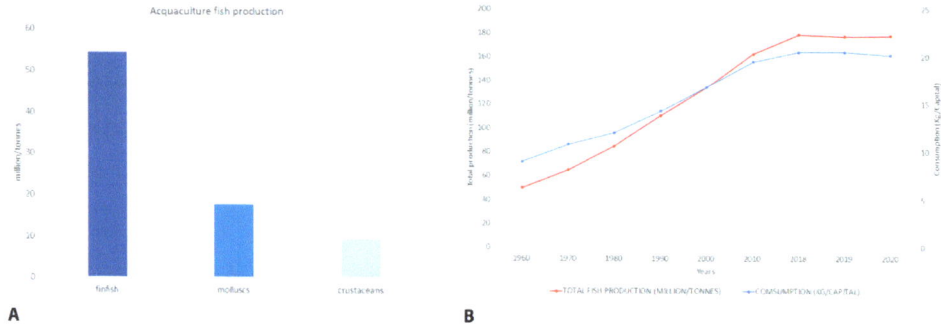

Figure 1. Aquaculture seafood production (million tonnes) in 2018 distributed among main production sectors (**A**); total fish production and consumption in the period 1961–2020 (**B**).

The rise of international fish trade leads to the need to improve the traceability of fishery products. In relation to this, innovation must be introduced at technological level to support the consistent production increase, with a special focus on the monitoring chain assessing product handling, processing and distribution via global networks [6]. A wide number of fish species are nowadays commercialized for human consumption on a world scale, most of which derive from aquaculture production and fishery activities [7]. On the other hand, cultural improvements and attention from the media has led consumers to demand more comprehensive and precise information on fish labelling. Therefore, issues concerning food quality and safety have recently become crucial points, also considering the still-frequent habit of fish species substitutions under certain conditions.

In fact, species substitution happens to expand profits; higher value species are replaced with other less precious, often cheaper, less well-known or even illegal and protected species [8,9]. Fish traceability is nowadays fundamental to avoid substitutions that may carry hidden risks for consumers; basic consequences may be health problems that occur primarily through the consumption of cryptic species coming from contaminated areas without any sanitary checks or able to trigger allergy problems [10,11]. It must be remarked that species substitution might even occur accidentally when taxa are difficult to recognize at a morphological level, and consequently the systematics of closely related species are trivial [4].

The European Union (EU), within the renewal plan of the Common Fisheries Policy and the Common Market Organization, has introduced new requirements for the labelling of fisheries and aquaculture products through the Cape IV of Regulation EU No. 1379/2013. Although this regulation requests appropriate species traceability and labelling (scientific binomial nomenclature based on genus and species collectively with the common name), the identification of processed species is frequently difficult to perform. Morphology-based identification methods may lead to incorrect species identification. Nowadays, more innovative methods and technologies are used to assess taxa determination and authenticity. Molecular diagnostic techniques have been developed to identify food fraud using different approaches, from the use of single proteins through enzyme-linked immunosorbent assay (ELISA) [12] or species-specific DNA sequences (DNA Barcode) [13] to near infrared spectroscopy [14] or modern genomic approaches [15].

In relation to the above cited issues, the aim of this review is to highlight the main barcoding approaches to identify the most reliable ones, which are able to allow affordable taxonomic identification of cryptic seafood species and limit commercial fraud that might threaten the consumer's health or the survival of endangered species.

The review has been prepared searching mainly in "ResearchGate", "Google Scholar", "PubMed", "Scopus" and "Web of Science". Considering that a high-quality search cannot rely on a single database, inclusion of different datasets is helpful to obtain more reliable literature. High-impact journals were preferred to avoid scarce quality of data and, above all, to have a wider audience.

2. DNA Barcoding and Seafood Mislabelling

In recent years, molecular barcoding (DNA barcoding) has been suggested as the gold standard in forensic taxonomy [16] and can be considered a further development of the previously applied technique proposed by Bartlett and Davidson [17]. About 30 years ago, these scientists presented an innovative methodology directed at cryptic food identification based on the use of short nucleotide regions for species authentication called Forensically Informative Nucleotide Sequence (FINS). This technique consists of a specific segment of DNA amplified using PCR and combines DNA sequencing and phylogenetic analysis to identify the most closely related taxon. Despite that, the modern concept of DNA barcoding was not established yet; the actual idea of DNA barcoding was developed in 2003 by Hebert et al. [18]. DNA barcoding is the analysis of variability in a specific genomic region, which is therefore designated the "DNA barcode", to be compared with specific databases of previously analysed sequences that become a priori reference DNA fragments determined for the species of interest [3]. The predominant precept driving DNA barcoding is the amplification of homologous genes by means of PCR and subsequent DNA sequencing. Sequences of interest are used as a "barcode" to determine the identity and authenticity of food products, for example, for DNA identification of various plant and animal species, to discriminate the presence of different taxa in processed food and to assess the presence of raw materials in food industry processes [19]. DNA barcodes consist of a standardized short sequence of DNA (in the range 400–800 bp) that, in theory, should be easily generated and characterized for all species [20]. The central notion of DNA barcoding asserts that a short sequence of DNA should display low variability within species and greater differentiation between species [20]. Kress and Erickson [21] proposed three criteria that have to be satisfied to consider a gene region as a DNA barcode: (i) contain significant species-level genetic variability and divergence, (ii) possess conserved flanking sites for developing universal PCR primers for wide taxonomic application and (iii) have a short sequence length to facilitate current capabilities of DNA extraction and amplification.

Nowadays, although both mitochondrial (mtDNA) and nuclear (nDNA) genes are involved in variegated approaches, the most reliable barcodes for the discrimination of different animal species are obtained using the mitochondrial gene coding for *cytochrome c oxidase 1* (*COI*) and *cytochrome b* (*cytb*) [18,22–25]. In particular, the most-used DNA barcode for seafood identification is a ~650 bp fragment of the mitochondrial gene *COI*. Many studies have shown the applicability of *COI* barcoding for accurate identification of a wide range of fish species and mislabelling detection [24,26–30].

It must be remarked that the use of mitochondrial markers for species' correct taxonomy displays several advantages with respect to nDNA (Table 1). In particular, mtDNA has a matrilinear inheritance and is not subjected to recombination. For this reason, nucleotide variation within the same taxon is at a minimum level while, in nDNA, great differentiation emerges among different species [3]. In fact, in spite of the high mutation rate of some mitochondrial regions, *COI* and *cytb* are conserved genes within each species.

Table 1. Comparison of advantages and disadvantages of mitochondrial and nuclear DNA.

	mtDNA	nDNA
Advantages	High number of copies of mtDNA	Useful when occur hybridization and introgression
	Matrilinear inheritance	
	Low variability within species and greater differentiation between	
Disadvantages	Nomenclature difficulties in differentiating closely related species	Subjected to recombination
		Single copy genes present in each cell

Another advantage can be referred to the high number of copies of mtDNA contained in the same specimen that allows a more reliable amplification in case of degraded samples such as those derived from processed seafood. It is noteworthy that DNA redundancy is generated by several contemporary copies of mtDNA within the same tissue; attention must be dedicated to the correct evaluation of data, and alternative analyses using nDNA might also be considered.

3. DNA Mini-Barcoding for Processed Seafood

Some of the processing and preservation techniques used with commercial seafood products might cause a limitation when full-length barcode regions (~650 bp) need to be analysed. In relation to the type of processing, the DNA may be degraded into fragments with sizes lower than 350 bp [31]. This is often the case with commercial fish, for which the correct preservation based on stable refrigerated conditions is a major issue along the entire production chain: fishing, transportation and distribution [32]. In addition, the quantity and quality of extracted DNA from processed seafood is affected by several additives, preservatives and flavours that these products contain [33]. In relation to this, a mini-barcoding approach has been suggested as valuable alternative to solve these problems and to obtain a reliable amplification of degraded DNA extracted from processed seafood. Precisely, the DNA mini-barcoding extrapolates reliable shorter DNA fragments (e.g., 100–200 bp) within the lost full length. DNA mini-barcoding is therefore a powerful method to recover DNA sequence information from specimens containing degraded DNA [23,32–38].

In particular, Shokralla et al. [33] developed an appropriate set of six mini-barcode primer pairs targeting short (127–314 bp) fragments of the cytochrome c oxidase I region. Results were successful after examining over 8000 DNA barcodes from species listed in the U.S. Food and Drug Administration (FDA) Seafood List. Authors obtained the greatest mini-barcoding success rate with the individual primer pair SH-E (226 bp). The success rate of targeting short primers reached a value of 88.6%, and it was higher than full-length DNA barcode primers that displayed a success rate of 20.5% [33]. In relation to this, Armani et al. [35] demonstrated that compared to full length *COI* barcode (655 bp), a mini barcode of 190 bp increased the success rate of PCR amplification from degraded DNA samples. In fact, 655 bp amplicon amplified from 91% (fresh) to 50% (cooked) and 81% (ethanol-preserved) samples, while the proposed 190 bp amplicon amplified 100% (cooked) and 94% (ethanol-preserved) samples. Chakraborty et al. [39] found that a 154-bp fragment from the transversion-rich domain of 1367 *COI* barcode sequences can successfully delimit species in the three most diverse orders of freshwater fishes (Cypriniformes, Siluriformes and Perciformes). Interestingly, variegated approaches can be applied according to the researcher experience and the type of product: Sultana et al. [38] proposed a novel mini barcode marker (295 bp) to discriminate fish species in both raw and processed states, while Pollack et al. [40] analysed in the same year the effects of cooking methods on DNA integrity using both full-length (655 bp) and mini-barcodes (208–226 bp). The highest overall success rate was found for one of the tested mini-barcodes (SH-E mini-barcode), regarding canned samples. Recently, Filonzi et al. [32] performed molecular analysis of

71 commercial fish samples based on mini-*COI* sequencing, testing two different primer sets. The first pair of universal primers called "Fish_mini" (295 bp) was the one proposed by Sultana et al. [38], while the second primer pair (SH-E, 226 bp) called "Fish_miniE" was tested following the protocol suggested by Shokralla et al. [33]. "Fish_miniE" successfully amplified 62 samples out of 71, reaching an amplification success rate of 87.3%, while "Fish_mini" displayed a positive result in 69 of 71 samples and a success rate of 97.2%.

It is noteworthy that the DNA mini-barcoding method might show loss of discriminatory power, especially for species that are closely related. Therefore, a key point to select a DNA barcode region is the presence of enough polymorphisms to allow discrimination among species in combination with high homology to design common primers [3]. From this point of view, the *COI* sequence of a small mini-barcode fragment ($\geq$100 bp) carries the information required for identification of individual species with more than 90% of resolution [33]. However, it must be remarked that when the barcode length is too short ($\leq$150 bp), further problems may emerge. In fact, despite the fact that the DNA region could be easily amplified, the correct species attribution might not be retrieved via direct comparison, and an erroneous identification could happen due to overlapping of closely related taxa [38].

4. The Impact of Seafood Frauds on Human Health

As mentioned above, a food fraud is committed when food is illegally placed on the market, most of the time for financial gain. Deliberate mislabelling and replacement of high-value species with cheaper ones is defined an Economically Motivated Adulteration (EMA) and is considered fraud [41]. In a specific document published in 2013 by the European Parliament, seafood was identified as the second most likely food item to be subject to fraud, following olive oil [42]. This voluntary or involuntary practice can also lead to unexpected events concerning different aspects of human health (from food allergies to poisoning and to multiorgan disfunctions). For example, roasted fillet products of codfish called Xue Yu (order Gadiformes) are largely consumed in China [43]. According to Xiong et al. [44], out of a total of 153 samples of roasted Xue Yu fillet products collected from 16 cities in China, only 42% of the samples were identified as belonging to Gadiformes, while the others were Scorpaeniformes, Tetraodontiformes and Lophiiformes. Moreover, the identification of poisonous *Lagocephalus* spp. from 37 samples highlighted the danger of mislabelling for human health. The consumption of this poisonous fish leads to several diseases: diarrhoea, body and organ (liver, kidney) weight loss, oxidative stress evidenced by an increase in lipid peroxidation (TBARS) and, conversely, a decrease in activities of such antioxidant enzymes as SOD, catalase and GSH-Px in different tissues (blood cells, liver, kidneys) as well as a decrease in alanine aminotransferase (ALT) and alkaline phosphatase (ALP) concentrations detected in blood plasma [45]. Furthermore, some species' flesh can be toxic if not treated properly. Lowenstein et al. [46] showed how several New York City sushi restaurants sold Escolar (*Lepidocybum flavorunneum*) as a variant of "white tuna". Escolar is a species banned for sale in Italian and Japanese markets due to high-risk health concerns. The large amount of wax esters in the lipidic fraction of its raw flesh is responsible for toxic activity over the gastroenteric apparatus [47]. Some species such as *Solea solea*, *Pleuronectes platessa* and *Merluccius merluccius* were mislabelled with less valuable species including *Pangasius hypophthalmus* in South Italy [48]. Pangasius farms were found contaminated by heavy metals in the Mekong River (Vietnam) with a potentially unhealthy status for human consumption [49].

5. Implications for the Conservation of Endangered Species

Another important aspect is that food fraud threatens the conservation of several endangered species. The International Union for the Conservation of Nature (IUCN) was founded in 1948 and was the first international organization to deal with environmental sustainability. It soon became the world's most comprehensive association dedicated to the global conservation of endangered animal, fungi and plant species. Among IUCN tools, the

Red List is a fundamental indicator of the conservation status of the world's biodiversity. Far more than a list of species, it is a strategic document to inform and define guidelines for species preservation, helpful for policy makers both at regional and global levels [50]. In particular, the "The IUCN Red List of Threatened Species" reports all living beings showing conservation issues, listed in different categories of severity: NE (not evaluated), DD (data deficient), LC (least concern), NT (near threatened), VU (vulnerable), EN (endangered), CR (critically endangered), EW (extinct in the wild), RE (regionally extinct), EX (globally extinct) [50].

One of the most common seafood frauds based on a species substitution occurs in the swordfish (*Xiphias gladius*, NT) trade [51]. *X. gladius* species substitution usually involves the taxon Selachimorpha. Currently, 153 shark species are classified as vulnerable (VU), endangered (EN) or critically endangered (CE) by the International Union for the Conservation of Nature [50]. Furthermore, 14 of them are listed in Appendix I, II or III by the Convention on International Trade in Endangered Species of Wild Fauna and Flora (CITES), which regulates their international commercial trade. The fact that the flesh of many fish species is similar in appearance, taste and texture [1] means that fraudulent practices could be unnoticed, especially in processed fish products. Ferrito et al. [51] reported the identification of the species *Prionace glauca* (Blue shark, NT), *Mustelus mustelus* (common smoothhound, EN) and *Oxynotus centrina* (angular roughshark, EN) in slices labelled as swordfish bought in fishmarkets in Southern Italy. Shehata et al. [52] reported a case of an individual of *Sphyrna lewini* (scalloped hammerhead, classified EN) mislabelled as *Prionace glauca* (blue shark, NT). A similar finding was previously reported by Willette et al. [53]. This fraudulent mislabelling of fish products is quite widespread and affects other endangered species. Juveniles of *Thunnus obesus* (VU), *T. alalunga* (LC), *T. albacares* (LC) and *T. thynnus* (LC) are sold as anchovy [54]. Although some of these species are considered LC on a global scale, most of their populations are seriously threatened at the regional level. This is particularly the case of the Mediterranean Sea. Anyway, Selachimorpha is one of the most mislabelled taxa. The shortfin mako *Isurus oxyrinchus*, which has recently been assessed in the "EN" category [50], is often sold, similarly to the Lamnidae, *Lamna nasus* (VU) (Porbeagle), as swordfish in some fish markets of Santiago (Chile); respectively, 2.13% of swordfish samples were shortfin mako and 6.39% were identified as porbeagle [55]. Interestingly, French and Wainwright [56] used DNA barcoding to identify the presence of shark DNA in pet food commercialized in Singapore. The most common identified sharks were the blue shark *Prionace glauca*, an overexploited species, and *Carcharinus falciformis* (silky shark), the latter listed in CITES Appendix II and "vulnerable" in the Red List [50]. In Filonzi et al. [32], a barcoding investigation was carried out in Italian fish markets over the last 10 years. Results have shown an improved situation compared to previously presented data from the same authors, witnessing a general improvement in the management and control of Italian fish markets [24]. Nevertheless, two samples labelled as *Katsowomus pelamis*, not directly involved in conservation issues, turned out to be either *Thunnus thynnus* (LC) or *Thunnus maccoyii* (EN). Similarly, *Lamna nasus* (VU) was *Isurus oxyrinchus* (EN), a more endangered species [32]. According to Lowenstein et al. [46], 19 out of 68 sushi products based on tuna purchased from 31 restaurants in Manhattan (New York City) and Denver (Colorado) were *T. thynnus* (LC) or the endangered southern bluefin tuna (*T. maccoyii*, EN), though 9 out of 31 restaurants that were involved did not list these species on their menus.

Interestingly, two bluefin tuna species, yellowfin and albacore, are no longer critically endangered, and the recent revision of IUCN classification has removed these species from the major risk categories [50]. The unexpectedly fast recovery bears witness to the effort dedicated over the past decade to end overfishing and limit unauthorized trading. On the other hand, researchers caution that, unlike tunas, many other marine species remain highly endangered. In fact, more than a third of the world's sharks and rays are still threatened to extinction due to overfishing, illegal commerce, habitat loss and climate change.

A further problem related to conservation of endangered species concerns the habit of using same/similar common names generating a sort of confusion over different taxa. For example, in the internal market of Brazil, which is an important country managing shark fisheries, besides being one of the largest importers of shark meat worldwide, several elasmobranch species are traded under the common popular name "caçao". In 2018, Almeròn Souza et al. [57] published a study about "caçao" fish, analysing 63 samples with DNA barcoding based on mitochondrial *COI* gene. As a result, they found DNA coming from 20 different species, 18 of which belonged to seven elasmobranch orders. It is noteworthy that some species belonged to such evolutionary distant taxa as *Xiphias gladius*. Considering IUCN criteria, 47% of the detected elasmobranch species were threatened at the global level, while 53% were threatened and 47% critically endangered in Brazil [57].

As shown in Table 2, seafood fraud is a common widespread practice all around the world. Sharks and unidentified local fish are the most involved species. In some cases, mislabelling also involves endangered species, frustrating fauna conservation measures. It must therefore be remarked that DNA barcoding is one of the most effective analysis tools to discover dangerous, unhealthy and unethical activities in commercial fisheries. The capability of mitochondrial and nuclear markers to allow fast identification processes has represented a turning point not only for food safety issues but also in the field of wildlife crime investigations. Interestingly, molecular tools not only support a fast taxonomic identification but may also define population genetic parameters.

Table 2. Examples of seafood mislabelling concerning species included in the IUCN "Red List" detected with DNA barcoding.

Reference	Collected Sample	Species Discovered	Global "Red List"	World Region
Almeròn-Souza F. et al., 2018 [57]	"Caçao" fish	*Carcharhinus brachyurus*	VU	Brazil
	"Caçao" fish	*Galeorhinus galeus*	CR	Brazil
	"Caçao" fish	*Gymnura altavela*	EN	Brazil
	"Caçao" fish	*Myliobatis goodei*	VU	Brazil
	"Caçao" fish	*Narcine brasiliensis*	NT	Brazil
	"Caçao" fish	*Prionace glauca*	NT	Brazil
	"Caçao" fish	*Pseudobatos horkelii*	CR	Brazil
	"Caçao" fish	*Rhizoprionodon lalandii*	VU	Brazil
	"Caçao" fish	*Rhizoprionodon porosus*	VU	Brazil
	"Caçao" fish	*Sphyrna lewini*	CR	Brazil
	"Caçao" fish	*Sphyrna zygaena*	VU	Brazil
	"Caçao" fish	*Squalus mitsukurii*	EN	Brazil
	"Caçao" fish	*Squatina occulta*	CR	Brazil
	"Caçao" fish	*Xiphias gladius*	NT	Brazil
	"Caçao" fish	*Zapteryx brevirostris*	EN	Brazil
	Engraulis encrasicolus	*Thunnus albacares*	LC	Europe
	Engraulis encrasicolus	*Thunnus alalunga*	LC	Europe
Blanco-Fernandez C. et al., 2021 [54]	*Thunnus alalunga*	*Thunnus thynnus*	LC	Africa
	Thunnus alalunga	*Thunnus obesus*	VU	Africa
	Merluccius capensis	*Gadus morhua*	VU	Africa
Filonzi L. et al., 2021 [32]	*Katsowomus pelamis*	*Thunnus thynnus*	LC	Italy
	Katsowomus pelamis	*Thunnus maccoyii*	EN	Italy
	Lamna nasus	*Isurus oxyrinchus*	EN	Italy
Lowenstein J.H. et al., 2009 [46]	*Thunnus* sp.	*Thunnus thynnus*	LC	USA
	Thunnus sp.	*Thunnus maccoyii*	EN	USA
Dufflocq P. et al., 2022 [55]	*Xiphias gladius*	*Isurus oxyrinchus*	EN	Chile
	Xiphias gladius	*Lamna nasus*	VU	Chile

Table 2. Cont.

Reference	Collected Sample	Species Discovered	Global "Red List"	World Region
Ferrito V. et al., 2019 [51]	Xiphias gladius	Mustelus mustelus	EN	Italy
	Xiphias gladius	Oxyntus centrina	EN	Italy
Staffen C.F. et al., 2017 [58]	Conger sp.	Micropogonias furnieri	LC	Brazil
	Salmo salar	Thunnus alalunga	NT	Brazil
	Thunnus sp.	Seriola zonata	LC	Brazil
	Thunnus sp.	Lepidocybium flavobrunneum	LC	Brazil
	Thunnus sp.	Salmo salar	LC	Brazil
	Thunnus sp.	Seriola lalandii	LC	Brazil
	"White fish"	Thunnus obesus	VU	Brazil
	"White fish"	Salmo salar	LC	Brazil
	Peprilus paru	Micropogonias furnieri	LC	Brazil
	Micropogonias undulatus	Prionace glauca	NT	Brazil
	Lepidocybium flavobrunneum	Ruvettus pretiosus	LC	Brazil
	Flounder gen.	Isopisthus parvipinnis	LC	Brazil
	Flounder gen.	Micropogonias furnieri	LC	Brazil
	Epinephelus sp.	Micropogonias furnieri	LC	Brazil
	Molva sp.	Micropogonias furnieri	LC	Brazil
	Pangasius pangasius	Micropogonias furnieri	LC	Brazil
	Salmo salar	Seriola zonata	LC	Brazil
	Salmo salar	Prionace glauca	NT	Brazil
	Salmo salar	Micropogonias furnieri	LC	Brazil
	Carcharias taurus	Prionace glauca	NT	Brazil
	Xiphias gladius	Trichiurus lepturus	LC	Brazil
	Cynoscion regalis	Isopisthus parvipinnis	LC	Brazil
Barbuto M. et al., 2010 [59]	Mustelus mustelus	Squalus acanthias	VU	Italy
	Mustelus mustelus	Prionace glauca	NT	Italy
	Mustelus mustelus	Galeorhinus galeus	CR	Italy
	Mustelus mustelus	Alopias superciliosus	VU	Italy
	Mustelus mustelus	Isurus oxyrinchus	EN	Italy

6. DNA Barcode Regions

6.1. Cytochrome c Oxidase I (COI) Gene

The *cytochrome c oxidase I (COI)* gene is the preferred sequence that serves as a "barcode" to identify and delineate the animal life form [22]. This DNA barcoding region is called the Folmer region and consists of a 648–655 bp long DNA segment near the 5' end of mitochondrial cytochrome c oxidase subunit 1. This region was first proposed by Folmer et al. [60] to identify metazoans and used in several studies on insects [38,61], mammals [62,63], amphibians [64], reptiles [65] and birds [18]. Considering birds, Hebert et al. [18] described a success rate of species identification from 98% to 100%. Ward et al. [26] proposed the *COI* mitochondrial gene as a barcode marker in fish. In particular, 207 species, mainly Australian marine fish, were sequenced for the 655 bp region of the mitochondrial cytochrome oxidase subunit I gene, demonstrating that cryptic fish species are revealed through the discovery of deep divergence of *COI* sequences within currently recognized species. However, to recover the variable segment flanking on both sides of the *COI* region, multiple rounds of PCR and multiple primer combinations were required [26]. Ivanova et al. [27] improved the *COI* barcoding protocol through identifying a primer set that could ensure wider use on more taxonomic groups, focusing on fishes. Primer cocktails were tested in 94 fish to identify the different *COI* sequences. Interestingly, the COI-2 primer cocktail was developed for mammalian barcode region amplification [63] but was proven to work in fish as well. Conversely, the COI-3 cocktail developed for fish was very effective in mammals, amphibians and reptiles. Together, these cocktails amplified the barcode region for every tested species [27]. The mitochondrial *COI* gene has been implemented as the preferred barcode region for the animal kingdom because it provides regular resolution at the species level and it is a region present in a large number of species [34,66]. For this reason, in the following years, *COI* barcoding became a standard method for the identification of fish specimens and products, Ref. [59] due to the need of finding adequate tools to confirm species authenticity and product labelling to avoid commercial fraud [59,67,68]. Seafood authentication and food safety became a wide scientific interest all over the world. In this regard, Filonzi et al. [24] developed molecular barcoding using 650 bp of *COI* gene to identify seafood frauds in Italy. A special focus was put on Italian commercial markets during 2008 when the results were obtained in 69 processed fish products belonging to 27 teleost species. DNA barcoding using Sanger's sequencing revealed incorrect labelling in 22 samples (32%). Among the replaced species, 18 (26%) were severe frauds from both economic and nutritional perspectives [24]. Armani et al. [35] dedicated further attention to ethnic seafood sold in the Italian market. Sixty-eight variously processed ethnic seafood products were collected from the Italian market and full cytochrome c oxidase DNA barcode (FDB, ~655 bp) or a mini-*COI* barcode (MDB, ~139 bp) were performed. Discrepancies between labelling and molecular identification were revealed in 48.5% of all products. In particular, two samples were labelled as squid but identified as *Lagocephalus* spp., which is a poisonous puffer fish species banned from the EU market. This result confirmed the importance of DNA barcoding as a golden tool for protecting consumers' health and economic interests [35].

During recent decades, using the analysis of the *cytochrome c-oxidase I* gene sequence, seafood mislabelling was identified in different countries of Europe such as Germany [37], Italy [32,69], United Kingdom [8,70], France [71], Spain [72], Greece [73], Portugal [74] and Northern Europe [75]. The work proposed by Tinacci et al. [76] underlined the urgency to review and update the Bulgarian official seafood list. Ninety-seven labelled seafood products collected from Bulgarian wholesalers were analysed using COI barcoding and revealed a species substitution rate of 17.7%. The analysis of the official seafood denomination label highlighted the presence of commercial and scientific names not included within the official list (59.2%), the lack of a scientific name (34.1%), the incomplete reference to the catching area (85.2%) and the absence of the fishing gear (55.2%). Pardo et al. [77] focused their studies on fish mislabelling rate in the mass caterer (HoReCa) sector across Europe. A total of 283 samples were collected in 180 mass cafeterias inside commercial outlets in 23 European countries. Molecular analysis based on the *COI* gene sequence revealed that 26% of the samples were mislabelled.

Several studies were performed in different places such as South America [28,78], Asia [79–81], the US [53,82,83], Africa [84,85] and Australia [86,87]. In relation to this, Cawthorn et al. [88] estimated the prevalence of species substitution and fraud prevailing in commercial fish in the South African market. The region of the *COI* gene was sequenced from 248 fish samples collected in seafood wholesalers and retail outlets. DNA barcoding was able to provide unambiguous species-level identifications, and 9% of samples from wholesalers and 31% from retailers were identified as different species from the ones indicated. Munguia-Vega et al. [89] conducted a DNA barcoding study in three cities within Mexico and sequenced the *COI* gene in 376 fish samples sold as 48 distinct commercial names at fish markets, grocery stores and restaurants. Overall, the study mislabelling rate was 30.8%. Dissimilar mislabelling rates [3,90] have been shown depending on countries, species groups, the dealer, strict regulation of government, the processing of fish and the year. In Europe, for example, Bénard-Capelle et al. [71] detected only 14 mislabelling cases (3.7%) among the 371 samples collected in France. On the contrary, the average seafood mislabelling in Belgium was 31.1%, while the substitution of bluefin tuna was up to 95% [75]. A similar scenario characterizes the rest of the world; indeed, high rates of mislabelling, using the *COI* gene, were observed in North America, respectively, 47% in the USA [53] and 41.2% in Canada [91]. In contrast, in South Korea, one of the biggest seafood markets in the world with strict laws of the Korean Government, a low mislabelling rate was found by Do et al. [92]. This study used the *COI* gene to investigate mislabelling of 157 seafood samples;

12 mislabelling cases were found with a mislabelling rate of 7.6%. A wide variety of fish products have been studied using DNA barcoding, but little investigation of sushi, poke and ceviche dishes sold at restaurants has been performed. In relation to this, Kitch and colleagues [93] dedicated their research to this type of product based on raw fish, analysing 105 samples collected in Orange County (CA). Among these, 103 samples were positively identified using DNA barcoding and a species substitution rate of 23.3% was evidenced. On the other hand, non-congruent labelling was found in 45.6% of samples, while 63.1% of samples had some form of mislabelling. When the assessment was stratified in relation to the product category, ceviche had the highest overall mislabelling rate with 85.3%, followed by poke with 61.8% and sushi with 42.9%. Some authors [72,93] hypothesized that a general lower rate occurred in specimens obtained from local grocery stores in comparison with larger supermarkets, wholesalers or restaurants.

At last, the suitability of the *COI* gene for species identification using the mini-barcode version must be remarked. The proposal of a wide set of primers [33] allows the application of this approach to detect short informative fragments useful for analysing particularly degraded samples (see dedicated Section 3 in this review).

6.2. Cytochrome b (cytb) Gene

In 1989, Kocher et al. [94] identified the cytochrome b region as a possible genetic marker for species identification. A standard set of primers headed for conserved mtDNA regions was amplified and sequenced in more than 100 animal species, among which were mammals, amphibians, birds, some invertebrates and fishes. The results of this study showed different genetic variability between different species of the same biological class. This unexpected taxonomic utility of cytochrome b (*cytb*) primers provided opportunities for phylogenetic and population research [94]. Several studies proposed mtDNA for species identification, considering this particular genome one of the most useful for phylogenetic work [95–98]. At the beginning of the twenty-first century, the mitochondrial *cytb* gene was probably the best-known mitochondrial gene in terms of the structure and function of its protein product [99,100]. Parson et al. [101] attempted to identify DNA from 44 different animal species covering the five major vertebrate groups (15 mammals, 22 birds, 1 amphibian, 2 reptiles, and 4 fish species). The *cytb* fragment was amplified, sequenced and compared to the database's homologous 300 bp fragment sequence. Similarly to Ivanova et al. [27], who defined the best primer set to assess the correct taxonomic groups using *COI* sequences (see previous chapter), Sevilla et al. [102] tried to improve the *cytb* barcoding protocol for fish. A set of 21 PCR primers and amplification conditions were developed to barcode any teleost fish species according to their mitochondrial cytochrome b gene sequences. Overall, the above procedure yielded > 99.9% successful amplifications [102]. In fish, *cytb* has also proved to be a useful marker for the identification of seafood species and/or resolving species phylogenies [25,103–106]. In particular, mt *cytb* has been used to identify flatfish, gadoids, anchovies, eels, scombroids and many other species [107–112]. *Cytb* barcoding as a molecular method involving DNA sequencing can be successfully used for fish species identification, giving a key contribution to the correct labeling of fish products [6,24,113,114]. For instance, using *cytb* sequences, Marko et al. [6] showed that 70% of 22 red snapper samples (*Lutjanus campechanus*) from US markets were less-valuable species of Lutjanidae.

Armani et al. [115] analysed the genera *Neosalanx* and *Protosalanx* belonging to the *Salangidae* fish family, also known as icefish or silverfish, which is imported processed from China to Italy. Direct gene sequencing was carried out to taxonomically classify the correct species in 10 specimens of *Neosalanx taihuensis* directly collected from Lake Taihu. In addition, 200 specimens of icefish whose indirect origin was attributed to 40 markets (27 from Italy and 13 from China) were analysed with the same technique. The main purpose of the taxonomic approach was to investigate any potential mislabelling. Obtained *cytb* sequences identified 90% of market samples as *N. taihuensis*. The data rose to 93% when only products collected in Italy were considered. Interestingly, 15% of samples coming from Italian markets were mislabelled, thus confirming the existence of commercial fraud at an international level. In similar research, Ha et al. [116] carried out an analysis of 10 processed fillets collected from department stores in Hanoi (Vietnam). Only four of these products matched common and corresponding scientific names after the appropriate barcoding evaluation. The other six samples exhibited inappropriate labelling, switching from *P. hypophthalmus* into *P. boucourti*. Although no real commercial fraud was found in these products, the correct scientific names of fish species should always be considered for elaborated products as they are publicly available in supermarkets where people have no specific consciousness of this problem [116]. Meanwhile, Cutarelli et al. [117] analysed 60 samples of canned fish belonging to three genera and five species collected by Italian Health authorities: PIF (Border Inspection Posts), NAS (Anti-Sophistication Police) and ASL (Local Health Authority). The species declared were confirmed in all samples except two, which were labelled as *Thunnus alalunga* instead of *Thunnus thynnus*. All other samples were correctly labelled as *Thunnus albacares*, *Thunnus obesus*, *Sardina pilchardus* and *Engraulis encrasicolus* [117]. Gomes et al. [118] evaluated the authenticity of 107 frozen fillets tagged as Gurijuba (*Sciades parkeri*) and Uritinga (*Sciades proops*) bought from local markets located on the northern Amazon coast. About 16% of fillets initially attributed to *S. parkeri* were substituted with *S. proops*. Forensic analysis using mtDNA markers proved to be highly efficient in the discrimination of processed seafood, providing unequivocal taxonomy. In fact, commercial fraud pertaining to Gurijuba fillets was discovered using *cytb* sequences as a barcode in fish [118]. The same markers were adopted by Souza et al. [119] to estimate the mislabelling prevalence of seafood displayed in street markets, fishmongers, supermarkets and restaurants of Rio de Janeiro (Brazil). Analyses were carried out between 2012 ($n = 77$) and 2020 ($n = 183$). Nearly 50% (130/260) of the analysed products had no correspondence. It is noteworthy that the frequency of mislabelling varied across the commercialization chain. Once again, a split evaluation displayed higher mislabelling values detected in street markets (61%) and restaurants (82%) compared to fishmongers (38%) and supermarkets (22%). The most commonly exploited species as substitutes were *Pangasianodon hypophthalmus* (75%) and *Xystreurys rasile* (17%). Substitute taxa were usually lower priced, supporting an economic motivation as the general idea formulated for mislabelling. These results reinforce the need for updated and consistent regulations addressed to a more stringent control of sales of a wide variety of species in street markets and restaurants [119].

6.3. 16S rDNA and 12S rDNA

The two ribosomal RNAs, *12S* rRNA (819 to 975 bp in vertebrates) and *16S* rRNA (1571 to 1640 bp in vertebrates) genes, similarly to other mitochondrial genes, have numerous nucleotide substitutions, suggesting their use as a tool for species identification [120]. In relation to this, the mitochondrial *12S* rRNA and/or *16S* rRNA genes have been used as molecular markers to identify mammals, birds, shrimp and other species [121–127].

In particular, the mitochondrial gene coding for *12S* rRNA has been reported to be an excellent tool for the authentication of fish and seafood due to its mutation rate, acceptable length and availability of sequence information in databases [128]. Meanwhile, there is evidence that the *16S* rDNA is adequate for discriminating some *Epinephelus* and *Mycteroperca* species from non-target species [129]. Various studies were carried out to investigate and implement the use of these rRNA genes as molecular markers for species identification. Variants belonging to *12S* and *16S* molecular markers have been used to identify a wide variety of flatfish, eel, cardinalfish, cephalopods, mackerel, hairtail species, crab and several others [39,128,130,131]. Worldwide, *12S* and *16S* rDNAs have become valuable barcoding tools to assess seafood fraud verification cases. Their application to high-value fish has been demonstrated by Von der Heyden et al. [132], who tested several widely available and generally expensive fish in South African high-priced markets utilizing mtDNA *16S* rRNA sequencing. Interestingly, half of 178 tested samples revealed mislabelling with a special focus on kob. In fact, 84% of kob fillets, *Argyrosomus* spp, provided an attribution to other species, such as mackerel, croaker and warehou. Phylogenetic analyses supported the general idea of frequent species substitution among barracuda, wahoo and king mackerel. Genetic analyses gave the opportunity to reveal that red snapper fillets included those of river snapper *Lutjanus argentimaculatus*, which is a prohibited species for sale in South African markets. From preliminary population genetic comparisons, some 30% of kingklip samples probably had their origin in New Zealand rather than southern Africa. A similar mislabelling rate was found in seafood products sold in South America. In northern Brazil, an investigation was carried out for critically endangered species' (*Pristis perotteti*, largetooth sawfish) commercialization in fish markets, typically labelled as "sharks". Based on partial DNA sequences of the mitochondrial *16S*, 55% of samples were unequivocally identified as *P. perotteti*, while the others (45%) belonged to the families Carcharhinidae and Ginglymostomatidae [133]. Considering one of most exploited species in Caribbean regions, also including part of South America, Lee-Charris et al. [134] focused their attention on the common snook *Centropomus undecimalis*, realizing that populations drastically decreased in that marine sector due to overfishing and environmental degradation. Thus, there is a market imbalance between the availability of snook products and their demand by consumers, which generates such fraudulent actions as species substitution. Therefore, to investigate the existence of mislabelling in common snook products, 15 fresh snook fillets from six of the main fish markets and 44 frozen snook fillets from the five commercial brands available in Santa Marta (Colombia) were identified through molecular barcodes (*16S* rDNA and *COI*). A sort of discrepancy emerged between department stores and local shops. In fact, an astonishing 98% of processed fillets were found to be fraudulent in the commercial markets in comparison to a much lower involvement of fish shops, where only a single case was registered. The species used to substitute snook included the Pacific bearded brotula *Brotula clarkae* (38 samples), the Nile perch *Lates niloticus* (4 samples) and the acoupa weakfish *Cynoscion acoupa* (1 sample) [134]. To contribute to the current knowledge on mislabelling rates in Europe, some studies have been performed on seafood products in Spain [135,136]. Horreo et al. [135] tested 77 fish dishes from 53 different restaurants located in nine districts of Madrid (Spain). A short fragment of the *16S* rDNA was sequenced and compared with sequences in databases to verify that seven species or genera and almost 30% of the samples were mislabelled. Mislabelling was present in 37% of the sampled restaurants and 71% of the sampled districts.

In more recent years, several researchers have verified the presence of seafood fraud in Asia [137–139]. Hossain et al. [137] experimented with a pair of universal primers with the aim to target a 198 bp fragment of the mitochondrial *16S* rDNA to assess species identification in partially degraded samples. The *16S* rRNA gene was tested on 24 processed fish products commonly consumed in Malaysia. The newly developed marker successfully identified 92% of the tested commercial fish products based on 96–100% sequence similarities. Five out of 24 (20.8%) fish products revealed a considerable degree of species mislabelling. According to its limited fragment length, the new molecular marker developed in Hossain et al. [137] is a reliable tool to identify fish species even in highly processed products. Results were particularly helpful to detect species substitutions with the objective to protect both consumers' health and economic interests [137]. Xing et al. [138] compared the results obtained using the shorter sequence of the mitochondrial region of *16S* rDNA (~220 bp) with a region of *COI* gene to test a variety of sold animal-derived food products in the Chinese market. More precisely, 52 samples, quite variegated and including meat, poultry and fish purchased from retail companies and online sources, were assessed. Approximately 94% of the samples generated barcode sequences. On the opposite, the failure rate for barcodes based on the entire *COI* region was 44%. Despite this, they obtained valuable data using the *16S* rDNA mini-barcode from 87% of the *COI*-failed cases. Overall, the survey revealed that 23% of animal-derived products were mislabelled and, in most cases, contained undeclared species [138].

A higher mislabelling rate was also found in canned tuna sold in Taiwan. Chang et al. [139] sequenced two mitochondrial regions, *16S* and the control region (D-Loop), to assess 90 canned tuna products, also including 25 animal food items. Results revealed that *Sarda orientalis*, *Euthynnus affinis*, *Auxis rochei* and *Auxis thazard* are commonly exploited as substitutes in place of declared tuna products. Specifically, only 63.33% of investigated samples are true canned tuna, i.e., containing *Thunnus* species or skipjack tuna [139]. On the other hand, a low mislabelling rate was found in the study of Helgoe et al. [140], in which Atlantic cod (*Gadus morhua*) samples (n = 546) were collected from local markets, supermarkets and restaurants from eight cities across Spain. DNA barcoding was performed used PCR-based assays of the mitochondrial cytochrome oxidase-I (*COI*) and *16S* rRNA loci. A 6.2% mislabelling rate was discovered. Although no evidence emerged for possible distinct geographic patterns of mislabelling, biologic samples obtained from restaurants were more likely to be mislabelled than those sampled in department stores. In relation to sample preparation, such processed products as elaborated or salted/smoked fish were more likely to be mislabelled than fresh or frozen products. Common ling (*Molva molva*), haddock (*Melanogrammus aeglefinus*), saithe (*Pollachius virens*) and Alaska pollock (*Gadus chalcogrammus*) were the most common substitutes, while Nile perch (*Lates niloticus*) and striped catfish (*Pangasianodon hypophthalmus*) were the most taxonomically dissimilar to Atlantic cod.

6.4. Nuclear DNA

Despite the advantages of using mtDNA for species identification, some nDNA targets have also established to be successful in the recognition of fish and seafood species. Frequently, nuclear genes have been used in combination with mitochondrial genes to improve the efficiency and robustness of the analysis. In fact, to overcome limitations connected to mtDNA in defining closely related taxa, different regions of nDNA have been proposed as helpful markers to reach a reliable identification. In particular, nuclear regions are fundamental to solve issues related to hybridization and introgression [3]. The most common is the nuclear *5S* rRNA gene (*5S* rDNA), which consists of a small 120 bp conserved region coding for *5S* rRNA and a variable region of noncoding DNA, termed the non-transcribed spacer (NTS), that has a species-specific length and sequence [141–143]. In particular, the *5S* rRNA gene has been used to identify gadoids, salmonids, sharks, mackerel and others [143–146]. Perez and Garcia-Vazquez [147], using PCR amplification and sequencing of the nuclear *5S* rDNA, demonstrated that hake products commercialized in southern European (Spanish and Greek) market chains presented more than 30% of incorrect species labelling. DNA analysis showed that tails and fillets were more mislabelled than other products, and African species were substitute species for products labelled as American and European taxa [147]. Triantafyllidis et al. [148] used the *5S* rRNA gene as molecular marker for detecting and quantifying allergenic fish species contained in Greek commercial seafood labelled with generic and unspecific names. Almost 85% of the analysed products contained highly allergenic hake or grenadier species and only 15% contained less histaminergic species such as cod and haddock [148]. Frigerio et al. [149] performed a new set of primers on the *5S* rDNA and non-transcribed spacer (*NTS*) on 27 processed and unprocessed products collected at the Milan fish market and across different Italian supermarkets. In their research, a new DNA mini-barcoding region suitable for species identification was identified [149].

Another important nDNA region which has been used for species identification is the intronless nuclear rhodopsin gene (*RHO*) [150], which has been proposed for recognizing teleost fishes by Sevilla et al. [102]. Under certain circumstances, such as hybridization and introgression that are frequent in fish populations, the intronless nuclear rhodopsin gene results to be a useful additional marker for fish species identification in combination with mtDNA targets [91,151]. In particular, Abdullah and Rehbein [152,153] demonstrated the usefulness of the rhodopsin gene as nuclear marker for fish species differentiation, particularly tuna food products from Indonesian markets.

Variations in the gene coding for *18S* rDNAs allowed the identification of four species of abalone in Thailand, *Haliotis asinina, H. ovina* and *H. varia* [154]. Several authors used the *18S* rDNA for fish identification [155–157]. *18S* rDNA-barcode possesses several advantages: the complete *18S* rRNA gene sequence displays different variability levels [158]; a well-developed *18S* rDNA-sequence library, including a wide spectrum of taxa, is available on Genbank and facilitates the identification of variable and conserved regions; the presence of multiple nuclear copies [159] increases the probability of amplifying degraded prey DNA from predator faeces and, thus, increases the sensitivity of the method [160].

Finally, the myosin heavy chain 6 cardiac muscle alpha gene (*MYH6*) has been used to identify genetic diversity between species [161,162]. In particular, Ramirez et al. [161] proposed this gene to highlight the phylogenetic relationships among the *Laemolyta* genus. Twenty-four samples of four valid nominal *Laemolyta* species were investigated using barcoding analysis.

7. DNA Barcoding Databases

The organization and storage of sequences in several comprehensive and consistent barcode databases is one of the major strengths of the DNA barcode-based technologies related to species identification, authentication and phylogenetic analysis [163–165].

In most cases, each database contains an organized set of information concerning species name, voucher data, collection records, specimen identifiers and genetic sequences [164]. The computation of nucleotide variation, using evolutionary models such as the Kimura2-parameter distance method [166], allows to assess the correct match between the target and reference sequences. To ensure the correct identification, the database must contain reference sequences representing that species; this implies the accuracy of the association between the loaded sequences and the referred species, and this may be a problem especially in seafood cases due to many morphological similarities between different species and taxa [167].

DNA barcoding is successfully applied to seafood for many reasons: (1) in comparison to other animal sources (e.g., cattle, sheep, goat, horse) where taxonomic discrimination must be carried out at race level, the assessment of seafood is mainly performed on a high number of species and the effectiveness of this technique is therefore enhanced; (2) classical identification approaches are not useful in many cases, particularly with processed food; (3) in seafood more than in other living groups, molecular identification can go further than the species level, allowing in several cases the identification of varieties that belong to local natural resources and hence the identification of the geographical origin of a certain product [163].

The support of bioinformatics associated with the laboratory approach is therefore fundamental. One of the most popular public databases is GenBank, which is part of the NCBI (International Nucleotide Sequence Database Collaboration) that also includes the DNA DataBank of Japan (DDBJ) and the European Nucleotide Archive (ENA). Conceived in 1982, at this time, there are more than 200 million sequences (release Aug 2022: 239,915,786 sequences). From 1982 to the present, the number of bases in GenBank has approximately doubled every 18 months [168]. GenBank also has a useful tool that provides a rapid sequence comparison to identify unknown species. This software, called BLAST (Basic Local Alignment Search Tool), directly approximates alignments that optimize a measure of local similarity between sequences and calculates the statistical significance of matches [169]. This database is also widely used in food safety to perform correct specimen identification due to the many available sequences. Despite this, it has been criticized as being susceptible to problems such as incorrect species identification and missing information [170], especially with fish and seafood [171].

It must be remarked that despite the large number of sequences so far deposited in GenBank, the database is not appropriately dedicated to seafood and, therefore, a lack of information or unreliable taxonomy may complicate correct species attribution [3]. For this reason, more specific databases dedicated to barcoding or fish species are more helpful for the solution of traceability issues.

Alternatively to GenBank, the Barcode of Life Database (BOLD) is a cloud-based data storage and shared platform that supports the assembly and use of DNA barcode data. It has been created by the organization iBOL, which has the main purpose of developing a globally accessible DNA-based system for the discovery and identification of all multicellular life [172]. Currently, BOLD consists of more than 11 million sequences belonging to 243,000 animal species. All the stored barcodes have been deposited after identification by expert taxonomists. Moreover, BOLD has a useful component called BOLD-IDS, an identification engine tool that provides, whenever possible, a match between the target barcode sequence and the referred one, allowing a taxonomic assignment.

Both BOLD and Genbank concern all species and, in food safety, they are widely used for specimen identification of many products, from raw to processed food [163], but also for the detection of parasite and pathogens in human and animal food [173,174]. BOLD identification normally achieves higher acceptability and scientific merit since it is based on verified sequences and tagged specimens. However, BOLD records suffer from some shortcomings such as a low number of species, and it usually depends on GenBank sequences. Some pitfalls were documented, such as mistakes in private submission or records gleaned from the GenBank database that can create incorrect identification when BOLD-IDS are used [38,175].

With the aim to collect and assemble standardized DNA barcode sequences within a well-organized reference library to aid the molecular identification of all fish species, the Fish Barcode of Life Initiative (FISH-BOL) is a concerted global research project launched in 2005 [164,176]. FISH-BOL currently has DNA barcode records in place for nearly 8000 species. So far, several studies have shown a high success rate of DNA barcoding for species identification [177] using FISH-BOL, with 93% of freshwater species and 98% of marine species tested with unambiguous taxa differentiation [167].

Fish-Trace is a public European database which has been created to compile and deliver accessible data and material needed for the genetic identification of marine fish species in Europe. Fish-Trace consists of 220 species belonging to 75 different families [178]. To minimize the risk of incorrect association between the loaded sequence and the referred species, all the fish specimens have been identified by taxonomists and stored in natural history museums [179]. Every sequence loaded contains metadata information of both sampling and geographic origin. The Fish-Trace catalogue is based on two genes, one mitochondrial (*cytb*) and one nuclear (*rhodopsin*), used in analysis validation and quality control. Although Fish-Trace is specifically dedicated to fish species, its data are limited to European species based only on two genes, not on *COI*, which nowadays represents the most reliable one.

Further, Aquagene is a free-access database of genetic information of marine species. This database now consists of 603 species referenced by 1093 individuals and 1383 barcodes. All species are characterized by multiple gene sequences including the standard COI barcoding gene together with *cytb*, *MYH6* and *RHO*, therefore facilitating unambiguous species determination even for closely related species or those with high intraspecific diversity. Moreover, it is possible to find data concerning the sampled specimen, such as digital images, voucher number and geographic origin [180].

It is noteworthy that one of the strengths of this technology is the availability of many sequences stored in multiple databases. Although this may allow reliable comparisons, it can also generate a certain degree of complexity in species identification due to different variations on the information sources. This usually occurs more often in seafood identification due to many morphological similarities in closely related groups [167]. As shown in Table 3, expert-verified databases present a lower number of species, while NCBI Genbank, despite a large number of species and sequences, suffers from the absence of data validation and a lack of sample information [179]. In this regard, in some cases, the same barcode produces different results in those databases [32,38]. For this reason, integration of different databanks coupled to an expert based judgment is fundamental for reaching a reliable specific attribution, integrating the result provided from the databases and the sampling information [32].

Table 3. DNA barcoding principal database specifications.

Database	Molecular Markers	Taxa	N° of Sequences	World Region
GenBank	All	All	239 milions	All
BOLD	COI, ITS, rbcL, matK	Animal, Plants, Fungi, Protists	11 milions	All
FISH-BOL	COI	Freshwater and Marine Species	Not Available	All
Fish-Trace	cytb, rhodopsin	Marine Species	Not Available	Europe
Aquagene	COI, cytb, MYH6, rhodopsin	Marine Species	1383	Central Eastern Atlantic

8. Evolution of Seafood Barcoding through the Genomic Era

New genomic technologies (NGTs) have been developed over the last two decades. NGTs may lead to several and variegated advantages in the fields of food safety, agriculture, industry and pharmaceutics. A connection between genomics and food issues is also considered in "The Farm to Fork Strategy", which is a focal point of the European Green Deal with the intent to make food systems fair, healthy and environmentally friendly. Among different approaches, DNA sequencing is still fundamental to trace elaborated foods that gather a mixture of sources within a single product. Although the traditional Sanger sequencing technology is still the gold standard for species identification, innovative approaches are emerging to analyse processed seafood samples that may contain more than one species [15]. According to the above-mentioned concepts, in the last decade, genomics techniques have become more common and exploited in all fields in science and have consequently led to technological improvements and a decrease in costs.

Alternative next-generation DNA barcodes have been proposed, starting from innovative approaches in taxonomy and population genetics [181]. In particular, Restriction Site Associated DNA (RAD) sequencing has been proposed to distinguish closely related species. This technique is very efficient at generating sequence data from many thousands of nuclear loci; however, taxon-specific optimization is requested and precludes the application of RAD sequencing as a universal barcoding approach. Approaches based on genome skim are mostly used for floristic species and will therefore not be considered in this manuscript, while a more common method is based on the use of capture probes. Probe sets are being developed for both mitochondrial and nuclear markers, and they may offer powerful extended barcodes. However, the need to develop probes having wide phylogenetic coverage is still a limiting step.

On the other hand, Next Generation Sequencing (NGS) has been proposed as the most valuable substitute to the classical Sanger approach. The major difference between Sanger technology and NGS is the capacity of the latter technique to identify up to 15 or more different fish species potentially present in a single highly processed product [182]. The progress of NGS has recently spread out as no other technique has done before. Its ability to sequence millions of small DNA fragments in parallel has revolutionized the genomic research. In fact, the simultaneous identification of animal and plant species in food products is one of the main goals to reach a reliable food safety using high-throughput sequencing formats [183,184].

Most of literature in this field has been increasing exponentially since the last 5 years, and the majority of approaches are nowadays managed through the Ion Torrent™ and Illumina™ technologies. Kappel et al. [185] exploited metabarcoding using the Illumina MiSeq platform, targeting two short *cytb* fragments useful for tuna species identification in mixtures containing one to four species. Results provided precise sequence recoveries, allowing the identification of a minimum percentage of *Katsuwonus pelamis* (around 1% w/w) mixed inside major quantities of *Thunnus alalunga* within the same canned product. In the same year, Carvalho et al. [186] explored barcoding with the Ion torrent PGM method for the identification of fish species in highly processed codfish products, reporting a mislabelling rate of 41%. Giusti et al. [187] analysed surimi products, applying the same technology, using *16S* rDNA barcodes from a wide range of fish and cephalopod species. The authors verified that 37.5% of the products were mislabelled, 25% declared a species different from those identified and 25% did not label the presence of molluscs. Wang et al. [15] tested the feasibility of next-generation sequencing in identifying mixed salmon products sold in Shanghai. Salmon samples containing up to eight species were amplified using *16S* rDNA mini-barcode primers and sequenced on an Illumina HiSeq2500 platform. All species were accurately identified, and mixtures as low as 1% (w/w) could be detected. Both Sanger and NGS techniques were used to compare species identification, and a final cross-validation was obtained with real-time PCR to verify the accuracy of the DNA metabarcoding technology. DNA barcoding and metabarcoding of commercial salmon food products revealed the presence of mislabelling in 16 of 32 (50%) samples. The characterization of novel nuclear targets functional to flatfish samples identification was performed by Paracchini et al. [188] in silico study and NGS. Samples of various species of the Pleuronectidae family were analysed using short candidate nuclear regions. The advantages of these novel targets over the mitochondrial ones were demonstrated particularly for the capability to identify hybrid individuals, as well as multiple fish species in complex mixtures. More precisely, the ring finger protein 41 gene, also known as *Nrdp1*, showed the highest level of species differentiation, followed by the genes encoding the homeobox C13a/C13b proteins and midline 2 [188]. Two years later, the same research group [189] proposed additional nuclear genes and four non-coding regions assessed on raw or mildly treated commercial products. Using the NGS technique, gadoid species were successfully identified in complex mixtures and processed samples.

Interestingly, the NGS method can recover complete or near-complete barcodes under challenging experimental conditions, even in century-old samples where DNA is highly degraded [190]. Nevertheless, NGS represents a valuable tool to detect bacterial contamination in seafood with the aim of avoiding food-borne diseases [191], which represent an additional threat to consumers in addition to species substitution, particularly in popular tourist destinations [58].

It must be remarked that the application of NGS in food science is quite a recent acquisition and therefore under continuous development. The constant search for the best approach in terms of time, costs, quality and efficiency to obtain entire mitogenome sequences is leading to new advances both in terms of laboratory activities and bioinformatics tools for data analysis. Continued improvements in sequencing platforms and analysis tools will make this approach even more reliable and cost effective very shortly [192].

9. Conclusions

To protect consumers from food frauds and health hazards and to improve the monitoring of species endangered by overfishing and illegal commercial activities, reliable molecular tools to perform barcoding DNA analysis were developed. In this review, we explored and presented a wide number of barcoding approaches with a special focus on fish species traceability both in terms of taxonomic identification and labelling. The proposed methods can identify with high accuracy the different species (or even lower taxa) in a wide range of raw and processed seafood products. For each method, a plethora of different studies has been discussed highlighting the main advantages and pitfalls.

Considering the overall evaluation and the highlighted differences between more classical markers and novel nuclear and mitochondrial barcoding regions, it is noteworthy that the choice for the best approach must still consider variegated aspects that have to be evaluated under an expert-based judgement. As a matter of fact, the combination of different methods to improve the accuracy scores of correct identifications seems the best practical way to reach a reliable species validation. Nevertheless, independent or integrated data-sharing platforms are nowadays available to align, validate and classify the generated barcoding sequences.

The recent description and application of novel powerful genomics technologies open new perspectives. Innovative approaches based on NGS may generate millions of sequence reads in parallel, also under challenging experimental conditions, such as sample degradation due to bad preservation within the commercial pathway. Its power will have to be fully implemented in the future to reach constant improvements in terms of time, costs, quality and efficiency with the aim of increasing the application of DNA barcoding as one of most effective tools to discover unethical activities in seafood consumption. On the other hand, it must be remarked that constant technological improvements in the fields of molecular genetics and genomics make biotechnological approaches more reliable. Adaptation of protocols starting from DNA extraction coupled to enrichment techniques [192] up to bioinformatic elaboration of millions of available sequences [181] allows the presentation of barcoding as an affordable strategy becoming more and more popular, also considering the continuous fall of costs.

Author Contributions: L.F. was involved in the conceptualisation, supervision, writing and editing of the original draft. A.A. was involved in references, data collection and writing of the original draft. P.M.R., A.V. and C.F. were involved in writing original draft. R.P. contributed through supervision and final manuscript editing. N.B. was involved in the editing of the manuscript's final version. F.N.M. contributed through conceptualisation, supervision, project administration and writing—review and editing. All authors have read and agreed to the published version of the manuscript.

Funding: This research was partly developed with local funding by the University of Parma—Grant FIL2022—and with the financial support of Spin Off Gen-Tech S.r.l.

Data Availability Statement: Data is contained within the article.

Acknowledgments: This work has benefited from the equipment and framework of the COMP-R Initiative, funded by the 'Departments of Excellence' program of the Italian Ministry for University and Research (MUR, 2023–2027).

Conflicts of Interest: The authors declare no conflict of interest.

References

1. The State of World Fisheries and Aquaculture 2020 | FAO. Available online: https://www.fao.org/family-farming/detail/en/c/1279714/ (accessed on 25 March 2023).
2. Lofstedt, A.; de Roos, B.; Fernandes, P.G. Less than Half of the European Dietary Recommendations for Fish Consumption Are Satisfied by National Seafood Supplies. *Eur. J. Nutr.* **2021**, *60*, 4219–4228. [CrossRef] [PubMed]
3. Fernandes, T.J.R.; Amaral, J.S.; Mafra, I. DNA Barcode Markers Applied to Seafood Authentication: An Updated Review. *Crit. Rev. Food Sci. Nutr.* **2021**, *61*, 3904–3935. [CrossRef] [PubMed]
4. Vindigni, G.; Pulvirenti, A.; Alaimo, S.; Monaco, C.; Spina, D.; Peri, I. Bioinformatics Approach to Mitigate Mislabelling in EU Seafood Market and Protect Consumer Health. *Int. J. Environ. Res. Public. Health* **2021**, *18*, 7497. [CrossRef] [PubMed]
5. Costello, C.; Cao, L.; Gelcich, S.; Cisneros-Mata, M.; Free, C.M.; Froehlich, H.E.; Golden, C.D.; Ishimura, G.; Maier, J.; Macadam-Somer, I.; et al. The Future of Food from the Sea. *Nature* **2020**, *588*, 95–100. [CrossRef] [PubMed]
6. Marko, P.B.; Lee, S.C.; Rice, A.M.; Gramling, J.M.; Fitzhenry, T.M.; McAlister, J.S.; Harper, G.R.; Moran, A.L. Fisheries: Mislabelling of a Depleted Reef Fish. *Nature* **2004**, *430*, 309–310. [CrossRef] [PubMed]
7. Naylor, R.L.; Hardy, R.W.; Buschmann, A.H.; Bush, S.R.; Cao, L.; Klinger, D.H.; Little, D.C.; Lubchenco, J.; Shumway, S.E.; Troell, M. A 20-Year Retrospective Review of Global Aquaculture. *Nature* **2021**, *591*, 551–563. [CrossRef]
8. Helyar, S.J.; Lloyd, H.A.D.; De Bruyn, M.; Leake, J.; Bennett, N.; Carvalho, G.R. Fish Product Mislabelling: Failings of Traceability in the Production Chain and Implications for Illegal, Unreported and Unregulated (IUU) Fishing. *PLoS ONE* **2014**, *9*, e98691. [CrossRef]
9. Acutis, P.L.; Cambiotti, V.; Riina, M.V.; Meistro, S.; Maurella, C.; Massaro, M.; Stacchini, P.; Gili, S.; Malandra, R.; Pezzolato, M.; et al. Detection of Fish Species Substitution Frauds in Italy: A Targeted National Monitoring Plan. *Food Control* **2019**, *101*, 151–155. [CrossRef]
10. Van Leeuwen, S.P.J.; Van Velzen, M.J.M.; Swart, C.P.; Van Der Veen, I.; Traag, W.A.; De Boer, J. Halogenated Contaminants in Farmed Salmon, Trout, Tilapia, Pangasius, and Shrimp. *Environ. Sci. Technol.* **2009**, *43*, 4009–4015. [CrossRef]

11. D'Amico, P.; Armani, A.; Gianfaldoni, D.; Guidi, A. New Provisions for the Labelling of Fishery and Aquaculture Products: Difficulties in the Implementation of Regulation (EU) n. 1379/2013. *Mar. Policy* **2016**, *71*, 147–156. [CrossRef]
12. Asensio, L.; González, I.; García, T.; Martín, R. Determination of Food Authenticity by Enzyme-Linked Immunosorbent Assay (ELISA). *Food Control* **2008**, *19*, 1–8. [CrossRef]
13. Woolfe, M.; Primrose, S. Food Forensics: Using DNA Technology to Combat Misdescription and Fraud. *Trends Biotechnol.* **2004**, *22*, 222–226. [CrossRef]
14. Osborne, B.G. Near-Infrared Spectroscopy in Food Analysis. *Encycl. Anal. Chem.* **2006**, 1–14. [CrossRef]
15. Wang, N.; Xing, R.R.; Zhou, M.Y.; Sun, R.X.; Han, J.X.; Zhang, J.K.; Zheng, W.J.; Chen, Y. Application of DNA Barcoding and Metabarcoding for Species Identification in Salmon Products. *Food Addit. Contam. Part. A Chem. Anal. Control. Expo. Risk Assess.* **2021**, *38*, 754–768. [CrossRef]
16. Dawnay, N.; Ogden, R.; McEwing, R.; Carvalho, G.R.; Thorpe, R.S. Validation of the Barcoding Gene COI for Use in Forensic Genetic Species Identification. *Forensic Sci. Int.* **2007**, *173*, 1–6. [CrossRef]
17. Bartlett, S.E.; Davidson, W. FINS (Forensically Informative Nucleotide Sequencing): A Procedure for Identifying the Animal Origin of Biological Specimens. *Biotechniques* **1992**, *12*, 408–411.
18. Hebert, P.D.N.; Cywinska, A.; Ball, S.L.; DeWaard, J.R. Biological Identifications through DNA Barcodes. *Proc. Biol. Sci.* **2003**, *270*, 313–321. [CrossRef]
19. Nehal, N.; Choudhary, B.; Nagpure, A.; Gupta, R.K. DNA Barcoding: A Modern Age Tool for Detection of Adulteration in Food. *Crit. Rev. Biotechnol.* **2021**, *41*, 767–791. [CrossRef]
20. Savolainen, V.; Cowan, R.S.; Vogler, A.P.; Roderick, G.K.; Lane, R. Towards Writing the Encyclopedia of Life: An Introduction to DNA Barcoding. *Philos. Trans. R. Soc. Lond. B Biol. Sci.* **2005**, *360*, 1805–1811. [CrossRef]
21. Kress, W.J.; Erickson, D.L. DNA Barcodes: Genes, Genomics, and Bioinformatics. *Proc. Natl. Acad. Sci. USA* **2008**, *105*, 2761–2762. [CrossRef]
22. Roe, A.D.; Sperling, F.A.H. Patterns of Evolution of Mitochondrial Cytochrome c Oxidase I and II DNA and Implications for DNA Barcoding. *Mol. Phylogenet. Evol.* **2007**, *44*, 325–345. [CrossRef] [PubMed]
23. Hajibabaei, M.; Smith, M.A.; Janzen, D.H.; Rodriguez, J.J.; Whitfield, J.B.; Hebert, P.D.N. A Minimalist Barcode Can Identify a Specimen Whose DNA Is Degraded. *Mol. Ecol. Notes* **2006**, *6*, 959–964. [CrossRef]
24. Filonzi, L.; Chiesa, S.; Vaghi, M.; Nonnis Marzano, F. Molecular barcoding reveals mislabelling of commercial fish products in Italy. *Food Res. Int.* **2010**, *43*, 1383–1388. [CrossRef]
25. Imoto, J.M.; Saitoh, K.; Sasaki, T.; Yonezawa, T.; Adachi, J.; Kartavtsev, Y.P.; Miya, M.; Nishida, M.; Hanzawa, N. Phylogeny and Biogeography of Highly Diverged Freshwater Fish Species (Leuciscinae, Cyprinidae, Teleostei) Inferred from Mitochondrial Genome Analysis. *Gene* **2013**, *514*, 112–124. [CrossRef] [PubMed]
26. Ward, R.D.; Zemlak, T.S.; Innes, B.H.; Last, P.R.; Hebert, P.D.N. DNA Barcoding Australia's Fish Species. *Philos. Trans. R. Soc. Lond. B Biol. Sci.* **2005**, *360*, 1847–1857. [CrossRef]
27. Ivanova, N.V.; Zemlak, T.S.; Hanner, R.H.; Hebert, P.D.N. Universal Primer Cocktails for Fish DNA Barcoding. *Mol. Ecol. Notes* **2007**, *7*, 544–548. [CrossRef]
28. Carvalho, D.C.; Neto, D.A.P.; Brasil, B.S.A.F.; Oliveira, D.A.A. DNA Barcoding Unveils a High Rate of Mislabelling in a Commercial Freshwater Catfish from Brazil. *Mitochondrial DNA* **2011**, *22* (Suppl. S1), 97–105. [CrossRef]
29. Cline, E. Marketplace Substitution of Atlantic Salmon for Pacific Salmon in Washington State Detected by DNA Barcoding. *Food Res. Int.* **2012**, *45*, 388–393. [CrossRef]
30. Pappalardo, A.M.; Ferrito, V. DNA Barcoding Species Identification Unveils Mislabelling of Processed Flatfish Products in Southern Italy Markets. *Fish. Res.* **2015**, *164*, 153–158. [CrossRef]
31. Naaum, A.M.; Hanner, R.H. An Introduction to DNA-Based Tools for Seafood Identification. In *Seafood Authenticity and Traceability*; Academic Press: Cambridge, MA, USA, 2016; pp. 99–111. [CrossRef]
32. Filonzi, L.; Vaghi, M.; Ardenghi, A.; Rontani, P.M.; Voccia, A.; Nonnis Marzano, F. Efficiency of DNA Mini-Barcoding to Assess Mislabelling in Commercial Fish Products in Italy: An Overview of the Last Decade. *Foods* **2021**, *10*, 1449. [CrossRef]
33. Shokralla, S.; Hellberg, R.S.; Handy, S.M.; King, I.; Hajibabaei, M. A DNA Mini-barcoding system for authentication of processed fish products. *Sci. Rep.* **2015**, *5*, 15894. [CrossRef]
34. Meusnier, I.; Singer, G.A.C.; Landry, J.F.; Hickey, D.A.; Hebert, P.D.N.; Hajibabaei, M. A Universal DNA Mini-Barcode for Biodiversity Analysis. *BMC Genom.* **2008**, *9*, 214. [CrossRef]
35. Armani, A.; Guardone, L.; La Castellana, R.; Gianfaldoni, D.; Guidi, A.; Castigliego, L. DNA Barcoding Reveals Commercial and Health Issues in Ethnic Seafood Sold on the Italian Market. *Food Control* **2015**, *55*, 206–214. [CrossRef]
36. Chin, T.C.; Adibah, A.B.; Danial Hariz, Z.A.; Siti Azizah, M.N. Detection of Mislabelled Seafood Products in Malaysia by DNA Barcoding: Improving Transparency in Food Market. *Food Control* **2016**, *64*, 247–256. [CrossRef]
37. Günther, B.; Raupach, M.J.; Knebelsberger, T. Full-Length and Mini-Length DNA Barcoding for the Identification of Seafood Commercially Traded in Germany. *Food Control* **2017**, *73*, 922–929. [CrossRef]
38. Sultana, S.; Ali, M.E.; Hossain, M.A.M.; Asing; Naquiah, N.; Zaidul, I.S.M. Universal Mini COI Barcode for the Identification of Fish Species in Processed Products. *Food Res. Int.* **2018**, *105*, 19–28. [CrossRef]
39. Chakraborty, M.; Dhar, B.; Ghosh, S.K. Design of Character-Based DNA Barcode Motif for Species Identification: A Computational Approach and Its Validation in Fishes. *Mol. Ecol. Resour.* **2017**, *17*, 1359–1370. [CrossRef]

40. Pollack, S.J.; Kawalek, M.D.; Williams-Hill, D.M.; Hellberg, R.S. Evaluation of DNA Barcoding Methodologies for the Identification of Fish Species in Cooked Products. *Food Control* **2018**, *84*, 297–304. [CrossRef]
41. Spink, J.; Moyer, D.C. Defining the Public Health Threat of Food Fraud. *J. Food Sci.* **2011**, *76*, 157–163. [CrossRef]
42. Committee on the Environment. Draft report on the food crisis, fraud in the food chain and the control thereof. In *Public Health and Food Safety from European Parliament, 2091*; EU Parliament Publisher: Strasbourg, France, 2013; pp. 1–9.
43. Xiong, X.; D'Amico, P.; Guardone, L.; Castigliego, L.; Guidi, A.; Gianfaldoni, D.; Armani, A. The Uncertainty of Seafood Labeling in China: A Case Study on Cod, Salmon and Tuna. *Mar. Policy* **2016**, *68*, 123–135. [CrossRef]
44. Xiong, X.; Yao, L.; Ying, X.; Lu, L.; Guardone, L.; Armani, A.; Guidi, A.; Xiong, X. Multiple Fish Species Identified from China's Roasted Xue Yu Fillet Products Using DNA and Mini-DNA Barcoding: Implications on Human Health and Marine Sustainability. *Food Control* **2018**, *88*, 123–130. [CrossRef]
45. Saoudi, M.; Abdelmouleh, A.; Kammoun, W.; Ellouze, F.; Jamoussi, K.; El Feki, A. Toxicity Assessment of the Puffer Fish Lagocephalus Lagocephalus from the Tunisian Coast. *Comptes Rendus Biol.* **2008**, *331*, 611–616. [CrossRef] [PubMed]
46. Lowenstein, J.H.; Amato, G.; Kolokotronis, S.O. The Real Maccoyii: Identifying Tuna Sushi with DNA Barcodes—Contrasting Characteristic Attributes and Genetic Distances. *PLoS ONE* **2009**, *4*, e7866. [CrossRef] [PubMed]
47. Zarza, M.C.P.; Gutiérrez, V.R.; Bravo, L. Lipid Composition of Two Purgative Fish: Ruvettus Pretiosus and Lepidocybium Flavobrunneum. *Grasas Aceites* **1993**, *44*, 47–52. [CrossRef]
48. Tantillo, G.; Marchetti, P.; Mottola, A.; Terio, V.; Bottaro, M.; Bonerba, E.; Bozzo, G.; Di Pinto, A. Occurrence of mislabelling in prepared fishery products in Southern Italy. *Ital. J. Food Saf.* **2015**, *4*, 5358. [CrossRef]
49. Duarte, G.S.C.; Takemoto, R.M.; Yamaguchi, M.U.; de Matos, L.S.; Pavanelli, G.C. Evaluation of the Concentration of Heavy Metals in Fillets of Pangasius Hypophthalmus (Sauvage, 1878), Panga, Imported from Vietnam. *Int. J. Dev. Res.* **2019**, *9*, 30181–30186.
50. IUCN. The IUCN Red List of Threatened Species. Version 2022-2. 2022. Available online: https://www.iucnredlist.org (accessed on 30 March 2023).
51. Ferrito, V.; Raffa, A.; Rossitto, L.; Federico, C.; Saccone, S.; Pappalardo, A.M. Swordfish or Shark Slice? A Rapid Response by COIBar–RFLP. *Foods* **2019**, *8*, 537. [CrossRef]
52. Shehata, H.R.; Naaum, A.M.; Garduño, R.A.; Hanner, R. DNA Barcoding as a Regulatory Tool for Seafood Authentication in Canada. *Food Control* **2018**, *92*, 147–153. [CrossRef]
53. Willette, D.A.; Simmonds, S.E.; Cheng, S.H.; Esteves, S.; Kane, T.L.; Nuetzel, H.; Pilaud, N.; Rachmawati, R.; Barber, P.H. Using DNA Barcoding to Track Seafood Mislabeling in Los Angeles Restaurants. *Conserv. Biol.* **2017**, *31*, 1076–1085. [CrossRef]
54. Blanco-Fernandez, C.; Ardura, A.; Masiá, P.; Rodriguez, N.; Voces, L.; Fernandez-Raigoso, M.; Roca, A.; Machado-Schiaffino, G.; Dopico, E.; Garcia-Vazquez, E. Fraud in Highly Appreciated Fish Detected from DNA in Europe May Undermine the Development Goal of Sustainable Fishing in Africa. *Sci. Rep.* **2021**, *11*, 11423. [CrossRef]
55. Dufflocq, P.; Larraín, M.A.; Araneda, C. Species Substitution and Mislabelling in the Swordfish (*Xiphias gladius*) Market in Santiago, Chile: Implications in Shark Conservation. *Food Control* **2022**, *133*, 108607. [CrossRef]
56. French, I.; Wainwright, B.J. DNA Barcoding Identifies Endangered Sharks in Pet Food Sold in Singapore. *Front. Mar. Sci.* **2022**, *9*. [CrossRef]
57. Almerón-Souza, F.; Sperb, C.; Castilho, C.L.; Figueiredo, P.I.C.C.; Gonçalves, L.T.; Machado, R.; Oliveira, L.R.; Valiati, V.H.; Fagundes, N.J.R. Molecular Identification of Shark Meat from Local Markets in Southern Brazil Based on DNA Barcoding: Evidence for Mislabelling and Trade of Endangered Species. *Front. Genet.* **2018**, *9*, 138. [CrossRef]
58. Staffen, C.F.; Staffen, M.D.; Becker, M.L.; Löfgren, S.E.; Muniz, Y.C.N.; de Freitas, R.H.A.; Marrero, A.R. DNA Barcoding Reveals the Mislabelling of Fish in a Popular Tourist Destination in Brazil. *PeerJ* **2017**, *5*, e4006. [CrossRef]
59. Barbuto, M.; Galimberti, A.; Ferri, E.; Labra, M.; Malandra, R.; Galli, P.; Casiraghi, M. DNA barcoding reveals fraudulent substitutions in shark seafood products: The Italian case of "palombo" (*Mustelus* spp.). *Food Res. Int.* **2010**, *43*, 376–381. [CrossRef]
60. Folmer, O.; Black, M.; Hoeh, W.; Lutz, R.; Vrijenhoek, R. DNA primers for amplification of mitochondrial cytochrome c oxidase subunit I from diverse metazoan invertebrates. *Mol. Mar. Biol. Biotechnol.* **1994**, *3*, 294–299.
61. Ball, S.L.J.; Hebert, P.D.N.; Burian, S.K.; Webb, M. Biological Identifications of Mayflies (Ephemeroptera) Using DNA Barcodes. *J. N. Am. Benthol. Soc.* **2005**, *24*, 508–524. [CrossRef]
62. Hajibabaei, M.; Singer, G.A.C.; Hebert, P.D.N.; Hickey, D.A. DNA Barcoding: How It Complements Taxonomy, Molecular Phylogenetics and Population Genetics. *Trends Genet.* **2007**, *23*, 167–172. [CrossRef]
63. Clare, E.L.; Lim, B.K.; Engstrom, M.D.; Eger, J.L.; Hebert, P.D.N. DNA Barcoding of Neotropical Bats: Species Identification and Discovery within Guyana. *Mol. Ecol. Notes* **2007**, *7*, 184–190. [CrossRef]
64. Vences, M.; Thomas, M.; Bonett, R.M.; Vieites, D.R. Deciphering Amphibian Diversity through DNA Barcoding: Chances and Challenges. *Philos. Trans. R. Soc. B Biol. Sci.* **2005**, *360*, 1859–1868. [CrossRef]
65. Supikamolseni, A.; Ngaoburanawit, N.; Sumontha, M.; Chanhome, L.; Suntrarachun, S.; Peyachoknagul, S.; Srikulnath, K. Molecular Barcoding of Venomous Snakes and Species-Specific Multiplex PCR Assay to Identify Snake Groups for Which Antivenom Is Available in Thailand. *Genet. Mol. Res.* **2015**, *14*, 13981–13997. [CrossRef] [PubMed]
66. Rock, J.; Costa, F.O.; Walker, D.I.; North, A.W.; Hutchinson, W.F.; Carvalho, G.R. DNA Barcodes of Fish of the Scotia Sea, Antarctica Indicate Priority Groups for Taxonomic and Systematics Focus. *Antarct. Sci.* **2008**, *20*, 253–262. [CrossRef]
67. Wong, E.H.K.; Shivji, M.S.; Hanner, R.H. Identifying Sharks with DNA Barcodes: Assessing the Utility of a Nucleotide Diagnostic Approach. *Mol. Ecol. Resour.* **2009**, *9* (Suppl. S1), 243–256. [CrossRef] [PubMed]

68. Wallace, L.J.; Boilard, S.M.A.L.; Eagle, S.H.C.; Spall, J.L.; Shokralla, S.; Hajibabaei, M. DNA Barcodes for Everyday Life: Routine Authentication of Natural Health Products. *Food Res. Int.* **2012**, *49*, 446–452. [CrossRef]
69. Pappalardo, A.M.; Raffa, A.; Calogero, G.S.; Ferrito, V. Geographic Pattern of Sushi Product Misdescription in Italy-A Crosstalk between Citizen Science and DNA Barcoding. *Foods* **2021**, *10*, 756. [CrossRef]
70. Miller, D.; Jessel, A.; Mariani, S. Seafood Mislabelling: Comparisons of Two Western European Case Studies Assist in Defining Influencing Factors, Mechanisms and Motives. *Fish. Fish.* **2012**, *13*, 345–358. [CrossRef]
71. Bénard-Capelle, J.; Guillonneau, V.; Nouvian, C.; Fournier, N.; Loët, K.L.; Dettai, A. Fish Mislabelling in France: Substitution Rates and Retail Types. *PeerJ* **2015**, *2*, e714. [CrossRef]
72. Muñoz-Colmenero, M.; Blanco, O.; Arias, V.; Martinez, J.L.; Garcia-Vazquez, E. DNA Authentication of Fish Products Reveals Mislabelling Associated with Seafood Processing. *Fisheries* **2016**, *41*, 128–138. [CrossRef]
73. Minoudi, S.; Karaiskou, N.; Avgeris, M.; Gkagkavouzis, K.; Tarantili, P.; Triantafyllidou, D.; Palilis, L.; Avramopoulou, V.; Tsikliras, A.; Barmperis, K.; et al. Seafood Mislabelling in Greek Market Using DNA Barcoding. *Food Control* **2020**, *113*, 107213. [CrossRef]
74. Harris, D.J.; Rosado, D.; Xavier, R. DNA Barcoding Reveals Extensive Mislabelling in Seafood Sold in Portuguese Supermarkets. *J. Aquat. Food Prod. Technol.* **2016**, *25*, 1375–1380. [CrossRef]
75. Christiansen, H.; Fournier, N.; Hellemans, B.; Volckaert, F.A.M. Seafood Substitution and Mislabelling in Brussels' Restaurants and Canteens. *Food Control* **2018**, *85*, 66–75. [CrossRef]
76. Tinacci, L.; Guidi, A.; Toto, A.; Guardone, L.; Giusti, A.; D'Amico, P.; Armani, A. DNA Barcoding for the Verification of Supplier's Compliance in the Seafood Chain: How the Lab Can Support Companies in Ensuring Traceability. *Ital. J. Food Saf.* **2018**, *7*, 83–88. [CrossRef]
77. Pardo, M.Á.; Jiménez, E.; Viðarsson, J.R.; Ólafsson, K.; Ólafsdóttir, G.; Daníelsdóttir, A.K.; Pérez-Villareal, B. DNA Barcoding Revealing Mislabelling of Seafood in European Mass Caterings. *Food Control* **2018**, *92*, 7–16. [CrossRef]
78. Barbosa, A.J.; Sampaio, I.; Santos, S. Re-visiting the occurrence of mislabelling in frozen "pescada-branca" (*Cynoscion leiarchus* and *Plagioscion squamosissimus*–Sciaenidae) sold in Brazil using DNA barcoding and octaplex PCR assay. *Food Res. Int.* **2021**, *143*, 110308. [CrossRef]
79. Nagalakshmi, K.; Annam, P.K.; Venkateshwarlu, G.; Pathakota, G.B.; Lakra, W.S. Mislabelling in Indian Seafood: An Investigation Using DNA Barcoding. *Food Control* **2016**, *59*, 196–200. [CrossRef]
80. Wen, J.; Tinacci, L.; Acutis, P.L.; Riina, M.V.; Xu, Y.; Zeng, L.; Ying, X.; Chen, Z.; Guardone, L.; Chen, D.; et al. An Insight into the Chinese Traditional Seafood Market: Species Characterization of Cephalopod Products by DNA Barcoding and Phylogenetic Analysis Using COI and 16SrRNA Genes. *Food Control* **2017**, *82*, 333–342. [CrossRef]
81. Neo, S.; Kibat, C.; Wainwright, B.J. Seafood Mislabelling in Singapore. *Food Control* **2022**, *135*, 108821. [CrossRef]
82. Khaksar, R.; Carlson, T.; Schaffner, D.W.; Ghorashi, M.; Best, D.; Jandhyala, S.; Traverso, J.; Amini, S. Unmasking Seafood Mislabelling in U.S. Markets: DNA Barcoding as a Unique Technology for Food Authentication and Quality Control. *Food Control* **2015**, *56*, 71–76. [CrossRef]
83. Vandamme, S.G.; Griffiths, A.M.; Taylor, S.A.; Di Muri, C.; Hankard, E.A.; Towne, J.A.; Watson, M.; Mariani, S. Sushi Barcoding in the UK: Another Kettle of Fish. *PeerJ* **2016**, *4*, e1891. [CrossRef]
84. Galal-Khallaf, A.; Ardura, A.; Mohammed-Geba, K.; Borrell, Y.J.; Garcia-Vazquez, E. DNA Barcoding Reveals a High Level of Mislabelling in Egyptian Fish Fillets. *Food Control* **2014**, *46*, 441–445. [CrossRef]
85. Cawthorn, D.M.; Duncan, J.; Kastern, C.; Francis, J.; Hoffman, L.C. Fish Species Substitution and Misnaming in South Africa: An Economic, Safety and Sustainability Conundrum Revisited. *Food Chem.* **2015**, *185*, 165–181. [CrossRef] [PubMed]
86. Lamendin, R.; Miller, K.; Ward, R.D. Labelling Accuracy in Tasmanian Seafood: An Investigation Using DNA Barcoding. *Food Control* **2015**, *47*, 436–443. [CrossRef]
87. Mitchell, A.; Rothbart, A.; Frankham, G.; Johnson, R.N.; Neaves, L.E. Could Do Better! A High School Market Survey of Fish Labelling in Sydney, Australia, Using DNA Barcodes. *PeerJ* **2019**, *7*, e7138. [CrossRef] [PubMed]
88. Cawthorn, D.M.; Steinman, H.A.; Witthuhn, R.C. DNA Barcoding Reveals a High Incidence of Fish Species Misrepresentation and Substitution on the South African Market. *Food Res. Int.* **2012**, *46*, 30–40. [CrossRef]
89. Munguia-Vega, A.; Terrazas-Tapia, R.; Dominguez-Contreras, J.F.; Reyna-Fabian, M.; Zapata-Morales, P. DNA Barcoding Reveals Global and Local Influences on Patterns of Mislabelling and Substitution in the Trade of Fish in Mexico. *PLoS ONE* **2022**, *17*, e0265960. [CrossRef] [PubMed]
90. Mariani, S.; Griffiths, A.M.; Velasco, A.; Kappel, K.; Jerome, M.; Perez-Martin, R.I.; Schroder, U.; Verrez-Bagnis, V.; Silva, H.; Vandamme, S.G.; et al. Low Mislabelling Rates Indicate Marked Improvements in European Seafood Market Operations. *Front. Ecol. Environ.* **2015**, *13*, 536–540. [CrossRef]
91. Hanner, R.; Floyd, R.; Bernard, A.; Collette, B.B.; Shivji, M. DNA Barcoding of Billfishes. *Mitochondrial DNA* **2011**, *22*, 27–36. [CrossRef]
92. Do, T.D.; Choi, T.J.; Kim, J.; An, H.E.; Park, Y.J.; Karagozlu, M.Z.; Kim, C.B. Assessment of Marine Fish Mislabelling in South Korea's Markets by DNA Barcoding. *Food Control* **2019**, *100*, 53–57. [CrossRef]
93. Kitch, C.J.; Tabb, A.M.; Marquis, G.E.; Hellberg, R.S. Species Substitution and Mislabelling of Ceviche, Poke, and Sushi Dishes Sold in Orange County, California. *Food Control* **2022**, *146*, 109525. [CrossRef]

94. Kocher, T.D.; Thomas, W.K.; Meyer, A.; Edwards, S.V.; Paabo, S.; Villablanca, F.X.; Wilson, A.C. Dynamics of Mitochondrial DNA Evolution in Animals: Amplification and Sequencing with Conserved Primers. *Proc. Natl. Acad. Sci. USA* **1989**, *86*, 6196–6200. [CrossRef]
95. Avise, J.C.; Ankney, C.D.; Nelson, W.S. Mitochondrial gene trees and the evolutionary relationship of mallard and black ducks. *Evolution* **1990**, *44*, 1109–1119. [CrossRef]
96. Hedges, S.B. Molecular Evidence for the Origin of Birds. *Proc. Natl. Acad. Sci. USA* **1994**, *91*, 2621–2624. [CrossRef]
97. Moore, W.S. Inferring phylogenies from MtDNA variation: Mitochondrial-gene trees versus nuclear-gene trees. *Evolution* **1995**, *49*, 718–726. [CrossRef]
98. Mindell, D.P.; Sorenson, M.D.; Huddleston, C.J.; Miranda, H.C.; Knight, A.; Sawchuk, S.J.; Yuri, T. Phylogenetic Relationships among and within Select Avian Orders Based on Mitochondrial DNA. *Avian Mol. Evol. Syst.* **1997**, 213–247. [CrossRef]
99. Esposti, M.D.; De Vries, S.; Crimi, M.; Ghelli, A.; Patarnello, T.; Meyer, A. Mitochondrial Cytochrome b: Evolution and Structure of the Protein. *Biochim. Biophys. Acta* **1993**, *1143*, 243–271. [CrossRef]
100. Lau, C.H.; Drinkwater, R.D.; Yusoff, K.; Tan, S.G.; Hetzel, D.J.S.; Barker, J.S.F. Genetic Diversity of Asian Water Buffalo (*Bubalus bubalis*): Mitochondrial DNA D-Loop and Cytochrome b Sequence Variation. *Anim. Genet.* **1998**, *29*, 253–264. [CrossRef]
101. Parson, W.; Pegoraro, K.; Niederstätter, H.; Föger, M.; Steinlechner, M. Species Identification by Means of the Cytochrome b Gene. *Int. J. Legal. Med.* **2000**, *114*, 23–28. [CrossRef]
102. Sevilla, R.G.; Diez, A.; Norén, M.; Mouchel, O.; Jérôme, M.; Verrez-Bagnis, V.; Van Pelt, H.; Favre-Krey, L.; Krey, G.; Bautista, J.M. Primers and Polymerase Chain Reaction Conditions for DNA Barcoding Teleost Fish Based on the Mitochondrial Cytochrome b and Nuclear Rhodopsin Genes. *Mol. Ecol. Notes* **2007**, *7*, 730–734. [CrossRef]
103. Kartavtsev, Y.P.; Jung, S.O.; Lee, Y.M.; Byeon, H.K.; Lee, J.S. Complete Mitochondrial Genome of the Bullhead Torrent Catfish, Liobagrus Obesus (Siluriformes, Amblycipididae): Genome Description and Phylogenetic Considerations Inferred from the Cyt b and 16S RRNA Genes. *Gene* **2007**, *396*, 13–27. [CrossRef]
104. Kartavtsev, Y.P.; Park, T.J.; Vinnikov, K.A.; Ivankov, V.N.; Sharina, S.N.; Lee, J.S. Cytochrome b (Cyt-b) Gene Sequence Analysis in Six Flatfish Species (Teleostei, Pleuronectidae), with Phylogenetic and Taxonomic Insights. *Mar. Biol.* **2007**, *152*, 757–773. [CrossRef]
105. Ward, R.D.; Holmes, B.H.; Yearsley, G.K. DNA Barcoding Reveals a Likely Second Species of Asian Sea Bass (Barramundi) (*Lates calcarifer*). *J. Fish. Biol.* **2008**, *72*, 458–463. [CrossRef]
106. Chiesa, S.; Filonzi, L.; Vaghi, M.; Papa, R.; Marzano, F.N. Molecular Barcoding of an Atypical Cyprinid Population Assessed by Cytochrome B Gene Sequencing. *Zoolog Sci.* **2013**, *30*, 408–413. [CrossRef] [PubMed]
107. Sotelo, C.G.; Calo-Mata, P.; Chapela, M.J.; Pérez-Martín, R.I.; Rehbein, H.; Hold, G.L.; Russell, V.J.; Pryde, S.; Quinteiro, J.; Izquierdo, M.; et al. Identification of Flatfish (*Pleuronectiforme*) Species Using DNA-Based Techniques. *J. Agric. Food Chem.* **2001**, *49*, 4562–4569. [CrossRef] [PubMed]
108. Calo-Mata, P.; Sotelo, C.G.; Perez-Martin, R.I.; Rehbein, H.; Hold, G.L.; Russell, V.J.; Pryde, S.; Quinteiro, J.; Rey-Mendez, M.; Rosa, C.; et al. Identification of Gadoid Fish Species Using DNA-Based Techniques. *Eur. Food Res. Technol.* **2003**, *217*, 259–264. [CrossRef]
109. Chow, S.; Nohara, K.; Tanabe, T.; Itoh, T.; Tsuji, S.; Nishikawa, Y.; Uyeyanagi, S.; Uchikawa, K. Genetic and Morphological Identification of Larval and Small Juvenile Tunas (Pisces: Scombridae) Caught by a Midwater Trawl in the Western Pacific. *Bull. Fish. Res. Agen.* **2003**, *8*, 1–14.
110. Pepe, T.; Trotta, M.; Marco, I.D.I.; Cennamo, P.; Anastasio, A.; Cortesi, M.L. Mitochondrial Cytochrome b DNA Sequence Variations: An Approach to Fish Species Identification in Processed Fish Products. *J. Food Prot.* **2005**, *68*, 421–425. [CrossRef]
111. Teletchea, F.; Maudet, C.; Hänni, C. Food and Forensic Molecular Identification: Update and Challenges. *Trends Biotechnol.* **2005**, *23*, 359–366. [CrossRef]
112. Santaclara, F.J.; Espiñeira, M.; Cabado, A.G.; Aldasoro, A.; Gonzalez-Lavín, N.; Vieites, J.M. Development of a Method for the Genetic Identification of Mussel Species Belonging to Mytilus, Perna, Aulacomya, and Other Genera. *J. Agric. Food Chem.* **2006**, *54*, 8461–8470. [CrossRef]
113. Michelini, E.; Cevenini, L.; Mezzanotte, L.; Simoni, P.; Baraldini, M.; De Laude, L.; Roda, A. One-Step Triplex-Polymerase Chain Reaction Assay for the Authentication of Yellowfin (*Thunnus albacares*), Bigeye (*Thunnus obesus*), and Skipjack (*Katsuwonus pelamis*) Tuna DNA from Fresh, Frozen, and Canned Tuna Samples. *J. Agric. Food Chem.* **2007**, *55*, 7638–7647. [CrossRef]
114. Cutarelli, A.; Amoroso, M.G.; De Roma, A.; Girardi, S.; Galiero, G.; Guarino, A.; Corrado, F. Italian Market Fish Species Identification and Commercial Frauds Revealing by DNA Sequencing. *Food Control* **2014**, *37*, 46–50. [CrossRef]
115. Armani, A.; Castigliego, L.; Tinacci, L.; Gianfaldoni, D.; Guidi, A. Molecular Characterization of Icefish, (Salangidae Family), Using Direct Sequencing of Mitochondrial Cytochrome b Gene. *Food Control* **2011**, *22*, 888–895. [CrossRef]
116. Ha, T.T.T.; Huong, N.T.; Hung, N.P.; Guiguen, Y. Species Identification Using DNA Barcoding on Processed Panga Catfish Products in Viet Nam Revealed Important Mislabelling. *Turk. J. Fish. Aquat. Sci.* **2018**, *18*, 457–462. [CrossRef]
117. Cutarelli, A.; Galiero, G.; Capuano, F.; Corrado, F. Species Identification by Means of Mitochondrial Cytochrome b DNA Sequencing in Processed Anchovy, Sardine and Tuna Products. *Food Nutr. Sci.* **2018**, *09*, 369–375. [CrossRef]
118. Gomes, G.; Correa, R.; Veneza, I.; da Silva, R.; da Silva, D.; Miranda, J.; Sampaio, I. Forensic Analysis Reveals Fraud in Fillets from the "Gurijuba" Sciades Parkeri (Ariidae—Siluriformes): A Vulnerable Fish in Brazilian Coastal Amazon. *Mitochondrial DNA Part A* **2019**, *30*, 721–729. [CrossRef]

119. Souza, D.S.; Clemente, W.R.; Henning, F.; Solé-Cava, A.M. From Fish-Markets to Restaurants: Substitution Prevalence along the Flatfish Commercialization Chain in Brazil. *Fish. Res* **2021**, *243*, 106095. [CrossRef]
120. Yang, L.; Tan, Z.; Wang, D.; Xue, L.; Guan, M.X.; Huang, T.; Li, R. Species Identification through Mitochondrial RRNA Genetic Analysis. *Sci. Rep.* **2014**, *4*, 4089. [CrossRef]
121. Simons, A.M.; Mayden, R.L. Phylogenetic Relationships of the Western North American Phoxinins (Actinopterygii: Cyprinidae) as Inferred from Mitochondrial *12S* and *16S* Ribosomal RNA Sequences. *Mol. Phylogenet Evol.* **1998**, *9*, 308–329. [CrossRef] [PubMed]
122. Saini, M.; Das, D.K.; Dhara, A.; Swarup, D.; Yadav, M.P.; Gupta, P.K. Characterisation of Peacock (*Pavo cristatus*) Mitochondrial *12S* RRNA Sequence and Its Use in Differentiation from Closely Related Poultry Species. *Br. Poult. Sci.* **2007**, *48*, 162–166. [CrossRef]
123. Kitano, T.; Umetsu, K.; Tian, W.; Osawa, M. Two Universal Primer Sets for Species Identification among Vertebrates. *Int. J. Legal. Med.* **2007**, *121*, 423–427. [CrossRef]
124. Gupta, A.R.; Patra, R.C.; Das, D.K.; Gupta, P.K.; Swarup, D.; Saini, M. Sequence Characterization and Polymerase Chain Reaction-Restriction Fragment Length Polymorphism of the Mitochondrial DNA *12S* RRNA Gene Provides a Method for Species Identification of Indian Deer. *Mitochondrial DNA* **2008**, *19*, 394–400. [CrossRef]
125. Pascoal, A.; Barros-Velázquez, J.; Cepeda, A.; Gallardo, J.M.; Calo-Mata, P. A Polymerase Chain Reaction-Restriction Fragment Length Polymorphism Method Based on the Analysis of a *16S* RRNA/TRNA(Val) Mitochondrial Region for Species Identification of Commercial Penaeid Shrimps (Crustacea: Decapoda: Penaeoidea) of Food Interest. *Electrophoresis* **2008**, *29*, 499–509. [CrossRef]
126. Wang, B.; Jiang, J.; Xie, F.; Chen, X.; Dubois, A.; Liang, G.; Wagner, S. Molecular Phylogeny and Genetic Identification of Populations of Two Species of Feirana Frogs (Amphibia: Anura, Ranidae, Dicroglossinae, Paini) Endemic to China. *Zoolog Sci.* **2009**, *26*, 500–509. [CrossRef]
127. Sarri, C.; Stamatis, C.; Sarafidou, T.; Galara, I.; Godosopoulos, V.; Kolovos, M.; Liakou, C.; Tastsoglou, S.; Mamuris, Z. A New Set of *16S* RRNA Universal Primers for Identification of Animal Species. *Food Control* **2014**, *43*, 35–41. [CrossRef]
128. Céspedes, A.; García, T.; Carrera, E.; González, I.; Fernández, A.; Asensio, L.; Hernández, P.E.; Martín, R. Genetic differentiation between sole (*Solea solea*) and Greenland halibut (*Reinhardtius hippoglossoides*) by PCR–RFLP analysis of a *12S* rRNA gene fragment. *J. Sci. Food Agric.* **2000**, *80*, 29–32. [CrossRef]
129. Trotta, M.; Schönhuth, S.; Pepe, T.; Cortesi, M.L.; Puyet, A.; Bautista, J.M. Multiplex PCR method for use in real-time PCR for identification of fish fillets from grouper (*Epinephelus* and *Mycteroperca* species) and common substitute species. *J. Agric. Food Chem.* **2005**, *53*, 2039–2045. [CrossRef]
130. Gharrett, A.J.; Gray, A.K.; Heifetz, J. Identification of Rockfish (*Sebastes* spp.) by Restriction Site Analysis of the Mitochondrial ND-3/ND-4 and *12S/16S* RRNA Gene Regions. *Fish. Bull.* **2001**, *99*, 49–62.
131. Applewhite, L.; Rasmussen, R.; Morrissey, M. *Species Identification of Seafood. The Seafood Industry: Species, Products, Processing, and Safety*, 2nd ed.; Wiley-Blackwell: Hoboken, NJ, USA, 2012; pp. 193–219. [CrossRef]
132. Von Der Heyden, S.; Barendse, J.; Seebregts, A.J.; Matthee, C.A. Misleading the Masses: Detection of Mislabelled and Substituted Frozen Fish Products in South Africa. *ICES J. Mar. Sci.* **2010**, *67*, 176–185. [CrossRef]
133. Melo Palmeira, C.A.; da Silva Rodrigues-Filho, L.F.; de Luna Sales, J.B.; Vallinoto, M.; Schneider, H.; Sampaio, I. Commercialization of a Critically Endangered Species (*Largetooth sawfish*, *Pristis perotetti*) in Fish Markets of Northern Brazil: Authenticity by DNA Analysis. *Food Control* **2013**, *34*, 249–252. [CrossRef]
134. Lea-Charris, E.; Castro, L.R.; Villamizar, N. DNA Barcoding Reveals Fraud in Commercial Common Snook (*Centropomus undecimalis*) Products in Santa Marta, Colombia. *Heliyon* **2021**, *7*, e07095. [CrossRef]
135. Horreo, J.L.; Fitze, P.S.; Jiménez-Valverde, A.; Noriega, J.A.; Pelaez, M.L. Amplification of *16S* RDna Reveals Important Fish Mislabelling in Madrid Restaurants. *Food Control* **2019**, *96*, 146–150. [CrossRef]
136. Parrondo, M.; López, S.; Aparicio-Valencia, A.; Fueyo, A.; Quintanilla-García, P.; Arias, A.; Borrell, Y.J. Almost Never You Get What You Pay for: Widespread Mislabelling of Commercial "Zamburiñas" in Northern Spain. *Food Control* **2021**, *120*, 107541. [CrossRef]
137. Hossain, M.M.; Uddin, S.M.K.; Chowdhury, Z.Z.; Sultana, S.; Johan, M.R.; Rohman, A.; Ali, M.E. Universal Mitochondrial *16S* RRNA Biomarker for Mini-Barcode to Identify Fish Species in Malaysian Fish Products. *Food Addit. Contam. Part A* **2019**, *36*, 493–506. [CrossRef] [PubMed]
138. Xing, R.R.; Hu, R.R.; Han, J.X.; Deng, T.T.; Chen, Y. DNA barcoding and mini-barcoding in authenticating processed animal-derived food: A case study involving the Chinese market. *Food Chem.* **2020**, *309*, 125653. [CrossRef] [PubMed]
139. Chang, C.H.; Kao, Y.T.; Huang, T.T.; Wang, Y.C. Product Authentication Using Two Mitochondrial Markers Reveals Inconsistent Labeling and Substitution of Canned Tuna Products in the Taiwanese Market. *Foods* **2021**, *10*, 2655. [CrossRef] [PubMed]
140. Helgoe, J.; Oswald, K.J.; Quattro, J.M. A Comprehensive Analysis of the Mislabelling of Atlantic Cod (*Gadus morhua*) Products in Spain. *Fish. Res.* **2020**, *222*, 105400. [CrossRef]
141. Suzuki, H.; Sakurai, S.; Matsuda, Y. Rat *5S* rDNA spacer sequences and chromosomal assignment of the genes to the extreme terminal region of chromosome 19. *Cytogenet. Genome Res.* **1996**, *72*, 1–4. [CrossRef]
142. Rodríguez, M.A.; García, T.; González, I.; Asensio, L.; Fernández, A.; Lobo, E.; Hernández, P.E.; Martín, R. Identification of goose (*Anser anser*) and mule duck (*Anas platyrhynchos* × *Cairina moschata*) foie gras by multiplex polymerase chain reaction amplification of the *5S* RDNA gene. *J. Agric. Food Chem.* **2001**, *49*, 2717–2721. [CrossRef]

143. Aranishi, F. Rapid PCR-RFLP Method for Discrimination of Imported and Domestic Mackerel. *Mar. Biotechnol.* **2005**, *7*, 571–575. [CrossRef]
144. Carrera, E.; García, T.; Céspedes, A.; González, I.; Fernández, A.; Asensio, L.M.; Hernández, P.E.; Martín, R. Differentiation of Smoked Salmo Salar, Oncorhynchus Mykiss and Brama Raii Using the Nuclear Marker 5S RDNA. *Int. J. Food Sci. Technol.* **2000**, *35*, 401–406. [CrossRef]
145. Clarke, S.C.; Magnussen, J.E.; Abercrombie, D.L.; McAllister, M.K.; Shivji, M.S. Identification of Shark Species Composition and Proportion in the Hong Kong Shark Fin Market Based on Molecular Genetics and Trade Records. *Conserv. Biol.* **2006**, *20*, 201–211. [CrossRef]
146. Morán, P.; Garcia-Vazquez, E. Identification of Highly Prized Commercial Fish Using a PCR-Based Methodology. *Biochem. Mol. Biol. Educ.* **2006**, *34*, 121–124. [CrossRef]
147. Perez, J.; Garcia-Vazquez, E. Genetic identification of nine hake species for detection of commercial fraud. *J. Food Prot.* **2004**, *67*, 2792–2796. [CrossRef]
148. Triantafyllidis, A.; Karaiskou, N.; Perez, J.; Martinez, J.L.; Roca, A.; Lopez, B.; Garcia-Vazquez, E. Fish Allergy Risk Derived from Ambiguous Vernacular Fish Names: Forensic DNA-Based Detection in Greek Markets. *Food Res. Int.* **2010**, *43*, 2214–2216. [CrossRef]
149. Frigerio, J.; Gorini, T.; Palumbo, C.; De Mattia, F.; Labra, M.; Mezzasalma, V. A Fast and Simple DNA Mini-Barcoding and RPA Assay Coupled with Lateral Flow Assay for Fresh and Canned Mackerel Authentication. *Food Anal. Methods* **2022**, *16*, 426–435. [CrossRef]
150. Venkatesh, B.; Ning, Y.; Brenner, S. Late Changes in Spliceosomal Introns Define Clades in Vertebrate Evolution. *Proc. Natl. Acad. Sci. USA* **1999**, *96*, 10267–10271. [CrossRef]
151. Abdullah, A.; Rehbein, H. DNA Barcoding for the Species Identification of Commercially Important Fishery Products in Indonesian Markets. *Int. J. Food Sci. Technol.* **2017**, *52*, 266–274. [CrossRef]
152. Abdullah, A.; Rehbein, H. Authentication of Raw and Processed Tuna from Indonesian Markets Using DNA Barcoding, Nuclear Gene and Character-Based Approach. *Eur. Food Res. Technol.* **2014**, *239*, 695–706. [CrossRef]
153. Abdullah, A.; Rehbein, H. The Differentiation of Tuna (Family: Scombridae) Products through the PCR-Based Analysis of the Cytochrome b Gene and Parvalbumin Introns. *J. Sci. Food Agric.* **2016**, *96*, 456–464. [CrossRef]
154. Klinbunga, S.; Pripue, P.; Khamnamtong, N.; Puanglarp, N.; Tassanakajon, A.; Jarayabhand, P.; Aoki, T.; Menasveta, P. Genetic diversity and molecular markers of the tropical abalone (*Haliotis asinina*) in Thailand. *Mar. Biotechnol.* **2003**, *5*, 505–517. [CrossRef]
155. Meistertzheim, A.L.; Héritier, L.; Lejart, M. High-Resolution Melting of 18S RDNA (18S-HRM) for Discrimination of Bivalve's Species at Early Juvenile Stage: Application to a Spat Survey. *Mar. Biol.* **2017**, *164*, 133. [CrossRef]
156. Zhang, J.; Hanner, R. Molecular Approach to the Identification of Fish in the South China Sea. *PLoS ONE* **2012**, *7*, e30621. [CrossRef] [PubMed]
157. Novotny, A.; Jan, K.M.G.; Dierking, J.; Winder, M. Niche Partitioning between Planktivorous Fish in the Pelagic Baltic Sea Assessed by DNA Metabarcoding, QPCR and Microscopy. *Sci. Rep.* **2022**, *12*, 10952. [CrossRef] [PubMed]
158. Van de Peer, Y.; Caers, A.; De Rijk, P.; De Wachter, R. Database on the Structure of Small Ribosomal Subunit RNA. *Nucleic Acids Res.* **1998**, *26*, 179–182. [CrossRef] [PubMed]
159. Beebee, T.; Rowe, G. *An Introduction to Molecular Ecology*; Oxford University Press: New York, NY, USA, 2004.
160. Corse, E.; Costedoat, C.; Chappaz, R.; Pech, N.; Martin, J.F.; Gilles, A. A PCR-Based Method for Diet Analysis in Freshwater Organisms Using 18S RDNA Barcoding on Faeces. *Mol. Ecol. Resour.* **2010**, *10*, 96–108. [CrossRef]
161. Ramirez, J.L.; Galetti, P.M. DNA Barcode and Evolutionary Relationship within Laemolyta Cope 1872 (Characiformes: Anostomidae) through Molecular Analyses. *Mol. Phylogenet. Evol.* **2015**, *93*, 77–82. [CrossRef]
162. Qu, M.; Tang, W.; Liu, Q.; Wang, D.; Ding, S. Genetic Diversity within Grouper Species and a Method for Interspecific Hybrid Identification Using DNA Barcoding and RYR3 Marker. *Mol. Phylogenet. Evol.* **2018**, *121*, 46–51. [CrossRef]
163. Galimberti, A.; De Mattia, F.; Losa, A.; Bruni, I.; Federici, S.; Casiraghi, M.; Martellos, S.; Labra, M. DNA Barcoding as a New Tool for Food Traceability. *Food Res. Int.* **2013**, *50*, 55–63. [CrossRef]
164. Clark, L.F. The Current Status of DNA Barcoding Technology for Species Identification in Fish Value Chains. *Food Policy* **2015**, *54*, 85–94. [CrossRef]
165. Bhattacharya, M.; Sharma, A.R.; Patra, B.C.; Sharma, G.; Seo, E.M.; Nam, J.S.; Chakraborty, C.; Lee, S.S. DNA Barcoding to Fishes: Current Status and Future Directions. *Mitochondrial DNA A DNA Mapp. Seq. Anal.* **2016**, *27*, 2744–2752. [CrossRef]
166. Kimura, M. A Simple Method for Estimating Evolutionary Rates of Base Substitutions through Comparative Studies of Nucleotide Sequences. *J. Mol. Evol.* **1980**, *16*, 111–120. [CrossRef]
167. Hellberg, R.S.; Morrissey, M.T. Advances in DNA-Based Techniques for the Detection of Seafood Species Substitution on the Commercial Market. *J. Lab. Autom.* **2011**, *16*, 308–321. [CrossRef]
168. Benson, D.A.; Cavanaugh, M.; Clark, K.; Karsch-Mizrachi, I.; Lipman, D.J.; Ostell, J.; Sayers, E.W. GenBank. *Nucleic Acids Res.* **2017**, *45*, D37–D42. [CrossRef]
169. Altschul, S.F.; Gish, W.; Miller, W.; Myers, E.W.; Lipman, D.J. Basic Local Alignment Search Tool. *J. Mol. Biol.* **1990**, *215*, 403–410. [CrossRef]
170. Bidartondo, M.I.; Bruns, T.D.; Blackwell, M.; Edwards, I.; Taylor, A.F.S.; Bianchinotti, M.V.; Padamsee, M.; Callac, P.; Lima, N.; White, M.M.; et al. Preserving Accuracy in GenBank. *Science* **2018**, *319*, 1616. [CrossRef]

171. Li, X.; Shen, X.; Chen, X.; Xiang, D.; Murphy, R.W.; Shen, Y. Detection of Potential Problematic Cytb Gene Sequences of Fishes in GenBank. *Front. Genet.* **2018**, *9*. [CrossRef]
172. Ratnasingham, S.; Hebert, P.D.N. Bold: The Barcode of Life Data System (http://www.barcodinglife.org). *Mol. Ecol. Notes* **2007**, *7*, 355–364. [CrossRef]
173. Cipriani, P.; Smaldone, G.; Acerra, V.; D'Angelo, L.; Anastasio, A.; Bellisario, B.; Palma, G.; Nascetti, G.; Mattiucci, S. Genetic Identification and Distribution of the Parasitic Larvae of *Anisakis pegreffii* and *Anisakis simplex* (s. s.) in European Hake Merluccius Merluccius from the Tyrrhenian Sea and Spanish Atlantic Coast: Implications for Food Safety. *Int. J. Food Microbiol.* **2015**, *198*, 1–8. [CrossRef]
174. Leonard, S.R.; Mammel, M.K.; Lacher, D.W.; Elkins, C.A. Application of Metagenomic Sequencing to Food Safety: Detection of Shiga Toxin-Producing Escherichia Coli on Fresh Bagged Spinach. *Appl. Environ. Microbiol.* **2015**, *81*, 8183–8191. [CrossRef]
175. Wong, L.L.; Peatman, E.; Lu, J.; Kucuktas, H.; He, S.; Zhou, C.; Na-nakorn, U.; Liu, Z. DNA Barcoding of Catfish: Species Authentication and Phylogenetic Assessment. *PLoS ONE* **2011**, *6*, e17812. [CrossRef]
176. Becker, S.; Hanner, R.; Steinke, D. Five Years of FISH-BOL: Brief Status Report. *Mitochondrial DNA* **2011**, *22*, 3–9. [CrossRef]
177. International Barcode of Life—Illuminate Biodiversity. Available online: https://ibol.org/ (accessed on 26 March 2023).
178. FishTrace–Home—European Commission. Available online: https://fishtrace.jrc.ec.europa.eu/ (accessed on 26 March 2023).
179. Zanzi, A.; Martinsohn, J.T. FishTrace: A Genetic Catalogue of European Fishes. *Database* **2017**, *2017*, bax075. [CrossRef] [PubMed]
180. AquaGene. Available online: https://www.aquagene.org/ (accessed on 26 March 2023).
181. Coissac, E.; Hollingsworth, P.M.; Lavergne, S.; Taberlet, P. From barcodes to genomes: Extending the concept of DNA barcoding. *Mol. Ecol.* **2016**, *25*, 1423–1428. [CrossRef] [PubMed]
182. Franco, C.M.; Ambrosio, R.L.; Cepeda, A.; Anastasio, A. Fish Intended for Human Consumption: From DNA Barcoding to a next-Generation Sequencing (NGS)-Based Approach. *Curr. Opin. Food Sci.* **2021**, *42*, 86–92. [CrossRef]
183. Haynes, E.; Jimenez, E.; Pardo, M.A.; Helyar, S.J. The Future of NGS (Next Generation Sequencing) Analysis in Testing Food Authenticity. *Food Control* **2019**, *101*, 134–143. [CrossRef]
184. Noh, E.S.; Lee, M.N.; Kim, E.M.; Nam, B.H.; Noh, J.K.; Park, J.Y.; Kim, K.H.; Kang, J.H. Discrimination of Raw Material Species in Mixed Seafood Products (Surimi) Using the next Generation Sequencing Method. *Food Biosci.* **2021**, *41*, 100786. [CrossRef]
185. Kappel, K.; Haase, I.; Käppel, C.; Sotelo, C.G.; Schröder, U. Species Identification in Mixed Tuna Samples with Next-Generation Sequencing Targeting Two Short Cytochrome b Gene Fragments. *Food Chem.* **2017**, *234*, 212–219. [CrossRef]
186. Carvalho, D.C.; Palhares, R.M.; Drummond, M.G.; Gadanho, M. Food Metagenomics: Next Generation Sequencing Identifies Species Mixtures and Mislabelling within Highly Processed Cod Products. *Food Control* **2017**, *80*, 183–186. [CrossRef]
187. Giusti, A.; Armani, A.; Sotelo, C.G. Advances in the Analysis of Complex Food Matrices: Species Identification in Surimi-Based Products Using Next Generation Sequencing Technologies. *PLoS ONE* **2017**, *12*, e0185586. [CrossRef]
188. Paracchini, V.; Petrillo, M.; Lievens, A.; Puertas Gallardo, A.; Martinsohn, J.T.; Hofherr, J.; Maquet, A.; Silva, A.P.B.; Kagkli, D.M.; Querci, M.; et al. Novel Nuclear Barcode Regions for the Identification of Flatfish Species. *Food Control* **2017**, *79*, 297–308. [CrossRef]
189. Paracchini, V.; Petrillo, M.; Lievens, A.; Kagkli, D.M.; Angers-Loustau, A. Nuclear DNA Barcodes for Cod Identification in Mildly-Treated and Processed Food Products. *Food Addit. Contam. Part. A Chem. Anal. Control. Expo. Risk Assess.* **2019**, *36*, 1–14. [CrossRef]
190. Prosser, S.W.J.; Dewaard, J.R.; Miller, S.E.; Hebert, P.D.N. DNA Barcodes from Century-Old Type Specimens Using next-Generation Sequencing. *Mol. Ecol. Resour.* **2016**, *16*, 487–497. [CrossRef] [PubMed]
191. Serra, C.R.; Oliva-Teles, A.; Tavares, F. Gut Microbiota Dynamics in Carnivorous European Seabass (*Dicentrarchus labrax*) Fed Plant-based Diets. *Sci. Rep.* **2021**, *11*, 447–460. [CrossRef] [PubMed]
192. Mascolo, C.; Ceruso, M.; Sordino, P.; Palma, G.; Anastasio, A.; Pepe, T. Comparison of Mitochondrial DNA Enrichment and Sequencing Methods from Fish Tissue. *Food Chem.* **2019**, *294*, 333–338. [CrossRef] [PubMed]

Disclaimer/Publisher's Note: The statements, opinions and data contained in all publications are solely those of the individual author(s) and contributor(s) and not of MDPI and/or the editor(s). MDPI and/or the editor(s) disclaim responsibility for any injury to people or property resulting from any ideas, methods, instructions or products referred to in the content.

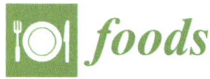 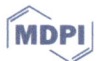

Article

Effects of Light Shading, Fertilization, and Cultivar Type on the Stable Isotope Distribution of Hybrid Rice

Syed Abdul Wadood [1,3,4,†], Yunzhu Jiang [1,3,†], Jing Nie [1,3], Chunlin Li [1,3], Karyne M. Rogers [1,3,5], Hongyan Liu [6], Yongzhi Zhang [3], Weixing Zhang [2,*] and Yuwei Yuan [1,3,*]

[1] State Key Laboratory for Managing Biotic and Chemical Threats to the Quality and Safety of Agro-Products, Hangzhou 310021, China; abwadood.fn@uhe.edu.pk (S.A.W.)
[2] China National Rice Research Institute, Hangzhou 310006, China
[3] Institute of Agro-Product Safety and Nutrition, Zhejiang Academy of Agricultural Sciences, Key Laboratory of Information Traceability for Agricultural Products, Ministry of Agriculture and Rural Affairs of China, Hangzhou 310021, China
[4] Department of Food Science, University of Home Economics Lahore, Lahore 54700, Pakistan
[5] National Isotope Centre, GNS Science, 30 Gracefield Road, Lower Hutt 5040, New Zealand
[6] Research Center for Plants and Human Health, Institute of Urban Agriculture, Chinese Academy of Agricultural Sciences, Chengdu 610213, China
* Correspondence: zhangwxcnrri@163.com (W.Z.); ywytea@163.com (Y.Y.); Tel.: +86-571-8640-6862 (Y.Y.); Fax: +86-571-8640-1834 (Y.Y.)
† These authors contributed equally to this work.

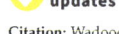

Citation: Wadood, S.A.; Yunzhu, J.; Nie, J.; Li, C.; Rogers, K.M.; Liu, H.; Zhang, Y.; Zhang, W.; Yuan, Y. Effects of Light Shading, Fertilization, and Cultivar Type on the Stable Isotope Distribution of Hybrid Rice. *Foods* **2023**, *12*, 1832. https://doi.org/10.3390/foods12091832

Academic Editor: Maria Castro-Puyana

Received: 10 March 2023
Revised: 10 April 2023
Accepted: 24 April 2023
Published: 28 April 2023

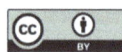

Copyright: © 2023 by the authors. Licensee MDPI, Basel, Switzerland. This article is an open access article distributed under the terms and conditions of the Creative Commons Attribution (CC BY) license (https://creativecommons.org/licenses/by/4.0/).

Abstract: The effect of fertilizer supply and light intensity on the distribution of elemental contents (%C and %N) and light stable isotopes (C, N, H, and O) in different rice fractions (rice husk, brown rice, and polished rice) of two hybrid rice cultivars (maintainer lines You-1B and Zhong-9B) were investigated. Significant variations were observed for δ^{13}C (−31.3 to −28.3‰), δ^{15}N (2.4 to 2.7‰), δ^{2}H (−125.7 to −84.7‰), and δ^{18}O (15.1‰ to 23.7‰) values in different rice fractions among different cultivars. Fertilizer treatments showed a strong association with %N, δ^{15}N, δ^{2}H, and δ^{18}O values while it did not impart any significant variation for the %C and δ^{13}C values. Light intensity levels also showed a significant influence on the isotopic values of different rice fractions. The δ^{13}C values showed a positive correlation with irradiance. The δ^{2}H and δ^{15}N values decreased with an increase in the irradiance. The light intensity levels did not show any significant change for δ^{18}O values in rice fractions. Multivariate ANOVA showed a significant interaction effect of different factors (light intensity, fertilizer concentration, and rice variety) on the isotopic composition of rice fractions. It is concluded that all environmental and cultivation factors mentioned above significantly influenced the isotopic values and should be considered when addressing the authenticity and origin of rice. Furthermore, care should be taken when selecting rice fractions for traceability and authenticity studies since isotopic signatures vary considerably among different rice fractions.

Keywords: light intensity; fertilizer treatment; stable isotopes; hybrid rice; cultivar; fractionation mechanism

1. Introduction

Rice (*Oryza sativa* L.) is a major cereal crop consumed by half of the global population and widely planted in Asia, Africa, and parts of America. In 2020, the total area under rice cultivation exceeded 195 million hectares. The quality characteristics of rice are mainly associated with its growing conditions, and recently the traceability of rice back to its growing origins has gained increasing interest from consumers, producers, and related industries since it is vulnerable to economic fraud [1]. Many methods have been developed to address the authenticity of rice, including multi-element, spectroscopic, omic, and DNA-based analysis [2–5]. Most recently, stable isotope analysis (SIA) has been widely employed to authenticate organic rice, determine its geographic origin, and identify rice cultivars [6,7].

However, there may be unknown stable isotope effects on rice, caused by cultivar type, light intensity, environmental factors, and fertilizer treatments which may reduce the accurate determination of its geographical origin, especially when it is procured from nearby or adjoining localities. Therefore, identifying the range of stable isotope compositions (δ^{13}C, δ^{15}N, δ^2H, and δ^{18}O) in different rice fractions according to the differences in light intensity level, fertilizer type and concentration, and cultivar/variety would improve the validity of traceability methods for rice and its products.

Different factors such as plant physiology, photosynthetic processes, climatic factors (temperature, sunshine, humidity, precipitation), and cultivation practices have been shown to induce stable isotope fractionation in plants [8]. Generally, the δ^{13}C values of plants reflect plant photosynthetic processes and water use efficiency. Carbon found in mature rice grains originates from the assimilation of CO_2 during the grain filling period [9]. Solar irradiance is the main factor that affects the net CO_2 assimilation rate and high temperature is also associated with stomatal closure and a reduction in CO_2 assimilation. Conversely, if the temperature is below the optimum range, the net CO_2 assimilation rate will become light-limited and lead to reduced photosynthetic productivity [10]. In addition, plant photosynthesis is also affected internally by photozymes, hydrolase C3 reductase, and CO_2 fixation enzymes [11]. This internal physiological response is referred as the physiological index which mainly reflects stomatal conductance, transpiration rates, net photosynthetic rate, and intercellular CO_2 concentration. Plant δ^2H and δ^{18}O values reflect physical factors such as rainfall and evapotranspiration, and are also associated with plant physiological parameters such as transpiration and stomatal conductance [12]. Nitrogen isotopes are mostly associated with farming practices, crop types, and soil characteristics and also reflect significant correlations between plant growth, photosynthetic capacity, and respiration rate [8,12].

Many studies have reported the limitation of stable isotopes in addressing the authenticity of agro-products when the samples are procured from close geographical locations or from a region where the same agricultural practices (fertilizer, etc.) are adopted [13]. Therefore, it is very important to understand the effects of different factors (light intensity, fertilizer type and concentration, and cultivar type) on the composition of rice stable isotopes. To explore these effects, we conducted two field experiments with a split plot design using two commonly used Chinese hybrid rice cultivars (maintainer lines) Zhong-9B and You-1B. The objective of this study was to investigate the variability of %C, %N, δ^{13}C, δ^{15}N, δ^2H, and δ^{18}O values in different rice fractions (husk, polished rice, and brown rice) in response to different fertilizer regimes and light intensity levels, and to identify how light shading and fertilizer application control isotopic ratios in rice. The results from this study will contribute more insight into the localized climatic, environmental, and farming effects on the isotopic composition of rice and will allow us to better predict rice origin and authenticity using stable isotope-based traceability models.

2. Material and Methods

2.1. Field Experiment

Field trials were carried out in 2018 at an experimental field at the China National Rice Research Institute (CNRRI) in Fuyang, Zhejiang province. Two commonly used hybrid rice maintainer lines (Zhong9B and You1B, which are the most popular cultivars in China provided by CNRRI), were studied. In total, three nitrogen treatments (N0, N6, and N12) with three light intensities (shading; 50% and 75%, and non-shading; ambient light) were arranged in a split plot design. The size of each plot was 10 m^2 with 3 replicates for each treatment. Nitrogenous fertilizer was applied as 0 kg/ha (N0), 90 kg/ha (N6), and 180 kg/ha (N12), respectively, at different growing stages including basal planting, tillering, and heading stages which accounted for 50%, 30%, and 20% of the application, respectively. Phosphate fertilizers were used only as basal fertilizer, whereas potash was used as both basal and tillering fertilizers and the fertilizer proportion was N:P:K = 1:0.5:0.5, respectively.

In the case of N0, urea was not applied during the entire production period. In total, 450 kg/ha of super phosphate was applied as basal fertilizer and 150 kg/ha of potash as basal (75 kg/ha) and tillering stage (75 kg/ha), respectively. For N6 treatment, 195 kg/ha of urea was applied, including 97.5 kg/ha as basal fertilizer, 58.5 kg/ha as tillering fertilizer (7 to 9 days after transplanting), and 39 kg/ha as heading fertilizer (30 days after transplanting), respectively. In the case of N12 treatment, a total of 390 kg/ha of urea was applied, of which 195 kg/ha was basal fertilizer, 117 kg/ha was tillering fertilizer, and 78 kg/ha was applied as heading fertilizer. The application rate of phosphate and potash fertilizers for both N6 and N12 treatments were the same as N0.

For the light intensity investigation, natural sunlight treatment, LS-0 (0% shading, no shading), and shaded treatments, LS-50 (50% shading) and LS-75 (75% shading) were applied. In the shaded treatments, plants were shaded with a shading screen/net. For LS-50, one layer was used and for LS-75 two layers of shading screen were applied over the top of the rice plants.

2.2. Elemental Content and Isotope Ratio Measurements

Rice grains (2 kg) from each plot were harvested at maturity and subsequently threshed by a hulling machine equipped with a rice polisher (PY-200, Hubei Pinyang Technology Co., Ltd., Xiaogan, China) to obtain different fractions including brown rice (BR), polished rice (PR), and rice husk (RH). All fractions were air-dried, then ground into a fine powder, and finally dried at 50 ± 2 °C for 24 h. The samples were stored in desiccators until further analysis. For the determination of elemental contents (% C, % N) and isotopes (δ^{13}C and δ^{15}N), dried powdered samples were weighed (4.5 to 5.5 mg) and packed into tin capsules (3 mm × 5 mm). The samples were combusted in an elemental analyzer (Vario Pyro Cube, Elementar, Hanau, Germany) and the combustion gases were analyzed using an isotope ratio mass spectrometer (IRMS) (IsoPrime100, Isoprime Ltd., Manchester, UK). Sample combustion was carried out in a combustion furnace at 1150 °C and reduction in the N_2O_x gases to N_2 over copper wire occurred at 850 °C. An inert gas (He) with a flow rate of 230 mL/min was passed through a CentrION prior to mass spectrometry. Acetanilide (Puriss. p.a., Sigma-Aldrich) was used to calibrate elemental % C and % N. For δ^{13}C and δ^{15}N analysis, multipoint calibration was applied using reference standard materials including B2155 (protein, δ^{13}C = −27.0‰, δ^{15}N = +6.0‰), IAEA-CH-6 (sucrose, δ^{13}C = −10.4‰), USGS40 (L-glutamic acid, δ^{13}C = −26.4‰, δ^{15}N = −4.5‰), USGS64 (glycine, δ^{13}C = −40.8‰, δ^{15}N = +1.8‰), and IAEA-N-2 (ammonium sulfate, δ^{15}N = +20.3‰). The δ^{13}C and δ^{15}N values were measured relative to V-PDB and AIR, respectively.

For δ^2H and δ^{18}O isotopes, around 1.0 mg powdered sample of each fraction was weighed into silver capsules (6 mm × 4 mm) and analyzed using EA (Vario Pyro Cube, Elementar, Hanau, Germany) IRMS (IsoPrime100, Isoprime Ltd., Manchester, England). Reference materials USGS54 (Canadian lodgepole pine, δ^2H = −150.4‰, δ^{18}O = +17.8‰) and USGS55 (Mexican ziricote, δ^2H = −28.2‰, δ^{18}O = +19.1‰) were used to calibrate the δ^2H and δ^{18}O measurements. Samples and reference materials were freeze-dried at −60 °C for three days to remove all adsorbed water and subsequently equilibrated for five days in the laboratory and exposed to local atmospheric conditions prior to H and O analysis. Pyrolysis was performed at 1450 °C to convert organic H and O to gaseous H_2 and CO, respectively, and finally the analytes were transferred into the IRMS for isotope determination. The δ^2H and δ^{18}O values were measured relative to Vienna Standard Mean Ocean Water (V-SMOW). All the samples were analyzed in triplicate. Reference materials were sourced from the International Atomic Energy Agency (IAEA, Vienna, Austria) and the United States Geological Survey (USGS, Reston, Virginia, United States). B2155 was supplied by Elemental Microanalysis (Okehampton, United Kingdom). The analytical precision for δ^{13}C, δ^{15}N, δ^2H, and δ^{18}O was less than ±0.1‰, ±0.2‰, ±2‰, and 0.5‰, respectively. The delta values (δ) were calculated as follows:

$$\delta E = \left(R_{sample} / R_{standard} \right) - 1 \qquad (1)$$

where δE represents $\delta^{13}C$, $\delta^{15}N$, δ^2H, and $\delta^{18}O$ whereas R_{sample} and $R_{standard}$ represent the $^{13}C/^{12}C$, $^{15}N/^{14}N$, $^2H/^1H$, or $^{18}O/^{16}O$ ratios in samples and reference materials, respectively.

2.3. Data Analysis

The effect of light intensity, fertilizer type and concentration, cultivars, and their interaction were studied using %C, %N, $\delta^{13}C$, $\delta^{15}N$, δ^2H, and $\delta^{18}O$ of different rice fractions with multivariate analysis of variance. Light shading level, fertilizer type and concentration, and cultivars were considered as fixed variables. Differences among the treatments were evaluated using Duncan's test at a significance level of 0.05. All analyses were performed using R software (version 3.0.3).

3. Results and Discussion

3.1. Multivariate ANOVA for Elemental Content and Isotope Ratios

Multivariate analysis of variance was applied to evaluate the effect of different factors such as variety (vty), shading level, and fertilizer (nitrogen) concentration on the carbon (%C), nitrogen (%N), $\delta^{13}C$, $\delta^{15}N$, δ^2H, and $\delta^{18}O$ values of different rice fractions, including polished rice (PR), brown rice (BR), and rice husk (RH). The results are summarized in Table 1 and shown in Figure 1. The results showed that the carbon content (%C) in different rice fractions was not affected by vty, light shading, fertilizer, or their interactions. For %N, light shading showed a significant influence on the total nitrogen content of PR and BR; however, no significant difference was observed in RH under different light shading levels. Moreover, an interaction (vty × light shading) effect was also observed for PR (Figure 1a). In the case of $\delta^{13}C$, light shading and variety significantly contributed to all rice fractions. The interaction (vty × fertilizer)/(vty × light shading) effect also showed significant influence for PR and (vty × light shading) for RH. No interaction effect was observed for BR (Figure 1b–d).

Table 1. A combined analysis of variance for different influencing factors on the stable carbon ($\delta^{13}C$), nitrogen ($\delta^{15}N$), oxygen ($\delta^{18}O$), and hydrogen (δ^2H) values among different rice fractions.

		Pr (>F)					
	Factor	%C	%N	$\delta^{13}C$ (‰)	$\delta^{15}N$ (‰)	δ^2H (‰)	$\delta^{18}O$ (‰)
Polished Rice	Fertilizer (N)	0.300	0.168	0.241	0.007 **	0.003 **	0.903
	Light shading (LS)	0.624	0.000 ***	0.000 ***	0.001 **	0.000 ***	0.408
	Variety (vty)	0.960	0.011 *	0.000 ***	0.541	0.222	0.004 **
	N × LS	0.945	0.528	0.291	0.061	0.190	0.893
	Vty × N	0.289	0.072	0.007 **	0.043 *	0.028 *	0.367
	Vty × LS	0.889	0.033 *	0.016 *	0.000 ***	0.030 *	0.456
Brown Rice	Fertilizer (N)	0.061	0.007 **	0.775	0.014 *	0.005 **	0.848
	Light shading (LS)	0.208	0.000 ***	0.000 ***	0.001 **	0.000 ***	0.920
	Variety (vty)	0.398	0.339	0.000 ***	0.338	0.029 *	0.683
	N × LS	0.432	0.630	0.087	0.073	0.273	0.954
	Vty × N	0.662	0.354	0.439	0.583	0.187	0.287
	Vty × LS	0.876	0.602	0.258	0.000 ***	0.114	0.403
Rice Husk	Fertilizer (N)	0.326	0.165	0.344	0.002 *	0.974	0.000 ***
	Light shading (LS)	0.081	0.053	0.000 ***	0.002 **	0.829	0.008 **
	Variety (vty)	0.833	0.000 ***	0.000 ***	0.004 **	0.000 ***	0.000 ***
	N × LS	0.208	0.581	0.153	0.015 *	0.541	0.283
	Vty × N	0.476	0.217	0.279	0.695	0.253	0.000 ***
	Vty × LS	0.586	0.363	0.025 *	0.000 ***	0.708	0.000 ***

Note: *** Indicates highly significant at $p < 0.001$, ** $p < 0.01$, and * $p < 0.05$.

The $\delta^{15}N$ values in RH, PR, and BR were significantly affected by fertilizer concentration, shading level, and interaction (vty × shading level) effects (Figure 1e–g). Significant interaction effects (vty × fertilizer) on $\delta^{15}N$ were also observed for PR (Figure 1h) and (fertilizer × light) for RH (Figure 1i). The fertilizer concentration and shading levels were the major factors that contributed significant variation among all rice fractions. In the case of δ^2H, the fertilizer concentration and shading level showed a significant difference for PR and BR, whereas no significant difference was observed for RH. The interaction (vty × fertilizer)/(vty × light shading) effect was only observed for PR (Figure 1j,k). Only cultivar imparted a significant variation for the δ^2H values in RH. In the case of δ^{18}O, different trends were observed. Almost all factors contributed to a significant variation for RH but no significant differences were observed for BR and PR. The interaction (vty × fertilizer)/(vty × light shading) effects for δ^{18}O are shown in Figure 1l,m, respectively.

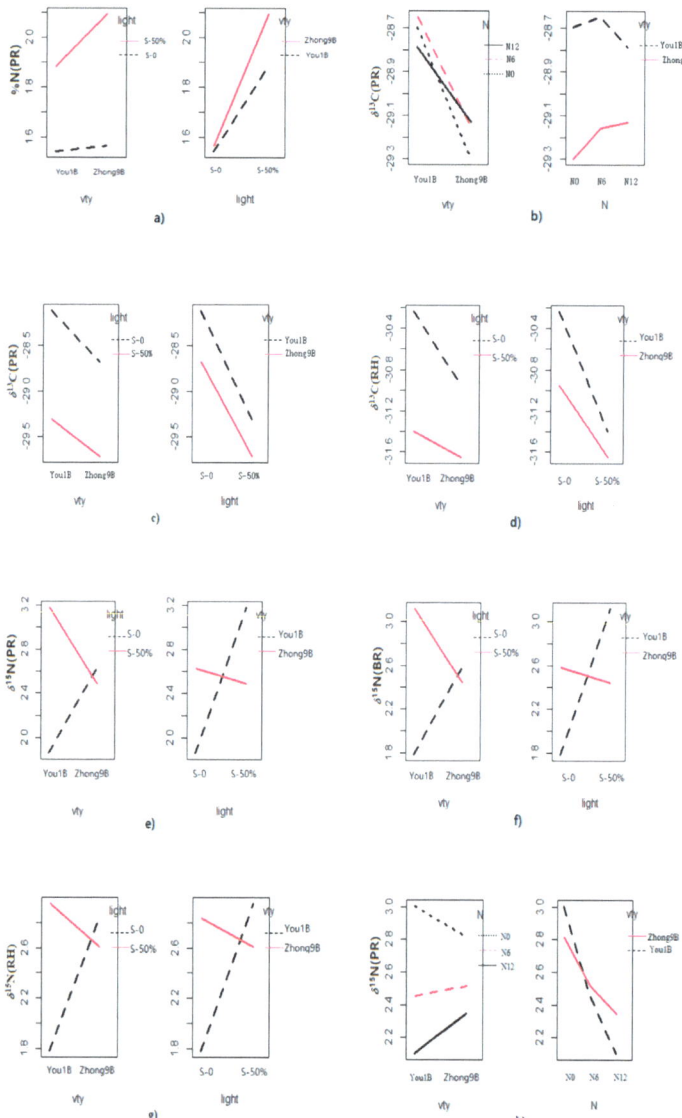

Figure 1. Cont.

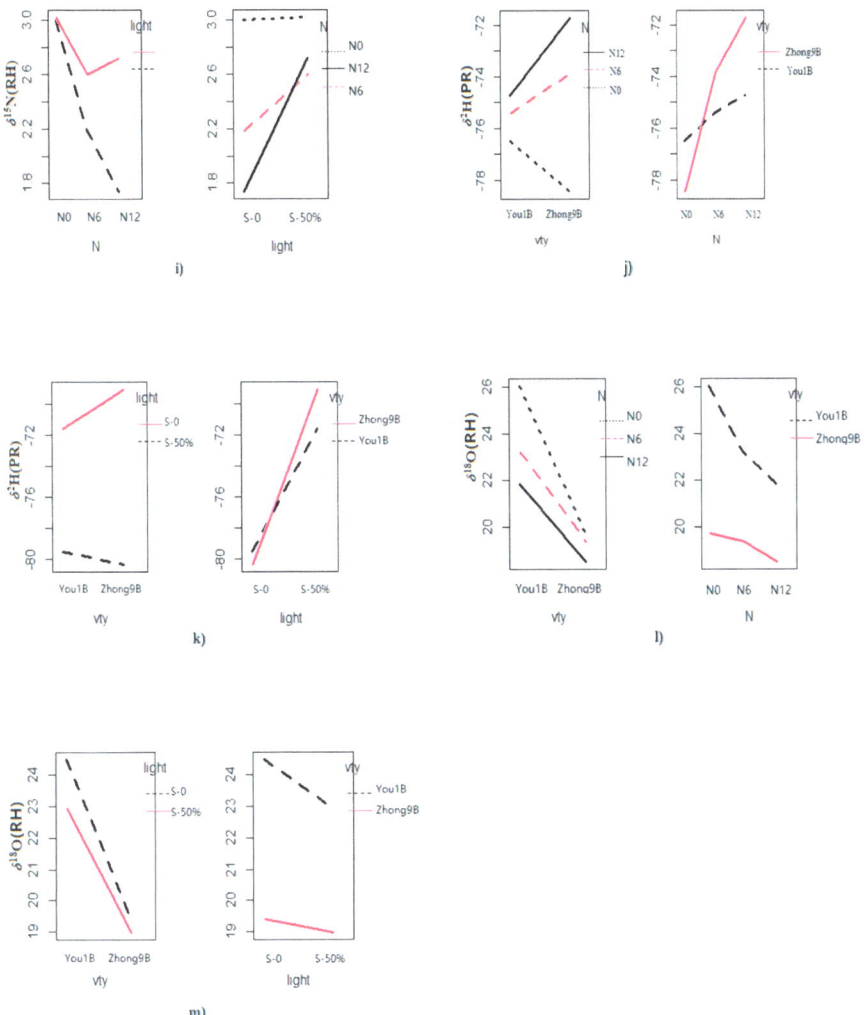

Figure 1. Interaction effects for the δ^{13}C, δ^{15}N, δ^2H, and δ^{18}O values among rice varieties (vty), fertilizer concentration (N), and light intensity of different rice fractions. (**a**) vty × light (PR, %N); (**b**) vty × N (PR, δ^{13}C); (**c**) vty × light (PR, δ^{13}C); (**d**) vty × light (RH, δ^{13}C); (**e**) vty × light (PR, δ^{15}N); (**f**) vty × light (BR, δ^{15}N); (**g**) vty × light (RH, δ^{15}N); (**h**) vty × N (PR, δ^{15}N); (**i**) N × light (RH, δ^{15}N); (**j**) vty × N (PR, δ^2H); (**k**) vty × light (PR, δ^2H); (**l**) vty × N (RH, δ^{18}O); (**m**) vty × light (RH, δ^{18}O).

3.2. Elemental and Isotope Differences between the Rice Varieties

Differences in the %C, %N, δ^{13}C, δ^{15}N, δ^2H, and δ^{18}O values among the different rice cultivar fractions under different fertilizer concentrations and light intensities were determined. The results showed significant differences for all the analyzed parameters except for %C. Multiple comparisons were made between %N, δ^{13}C, δ^{15}N, δ^2H, and δ^{18}O values (Figure 2). The %N in RH showed a strong significant difference between the two rice varieties. The total %N of You-1B rice (1.8 ± 0.2%) was significantly higher than Zhong-9B rice (1.5 ± 0.4%). Similarly, the δ^{13}C values of You-1B RH (−30.8‰), PR (−28.3‰), and BR (−29.1‰) were significantly higher than Zhong-9B (−31.3‰, −29.2‰, and −29.7‰), respectively. The lower δ^{13}C values of Zhong-9B rice suggest higher water use efficiency. Different factors are responsible for genetic variations in the δ^{13}C values, including diffusive conductance, water use efficiency, stomatal activity, etc. [14]. For the δ^{18}O values, the two varieties also showed significant differences for PR and RH. Higher δ^{18}O values of You-1B RH (23.7‰) indicate higher transpiration rates. Our results are consistent with previous findings where a similar trend was observed for δ^{18}O variations among different rice cultivars [15]. Differences in the δ^{18}O values are mainly due to the vegetative cycle of water [16].

A different pattern was observed for the δ^2H values. You-1B BR (−88.6‰) and RH (−125.7‰) were significantly lower than Zhong-9B BR and RH (−84.7‰ and −117.0‰), respectively. This difference suggests that less water fractionation occurred in Zhong-9B rice. A previous study also reported a significant difference in the δ^2H values among different rice cultivars [17].

The δ^{15}N values also followed the same trend where Zhong-9B rice values were higher than You-1B, although the difference in traits between rice varieties was primarily reflected in RH. δ^{15}N values of PR, BR, and RH in Zhong-9B and You-1B rice was (2.6‰, 2.5‰, 2.7‰) and (2.5‰, 2.4‰, and 2.4‰), respectively. Our results are consistent with previous findings where significant differences in the δ^{15}N values among different rice cultivars were reported [18].

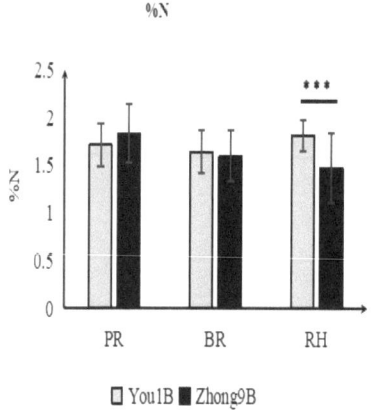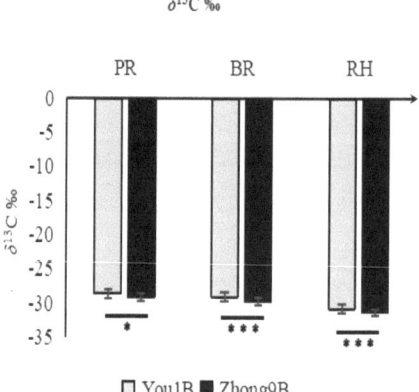

Figure 2. *Cont.*

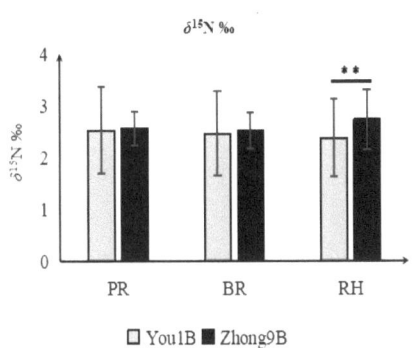
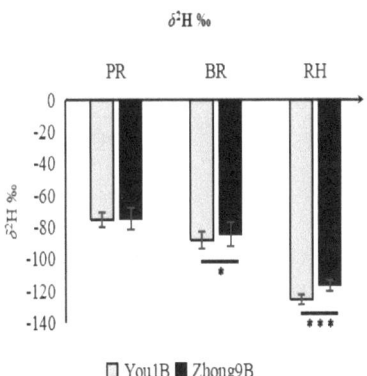
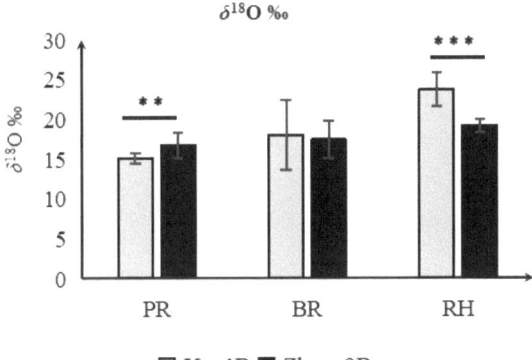

Figure 2. Variation of %N, δ^{13}C, δ^{15}N, δ^{2}H, and δ^{18}O values in the polished rice (PR), brown rice (BR), and rice husk (RH) between two rice varieties. *** Indicates high significance at $p < 0.001$, ** $p < 0.01$, and * $p < 0.05$ (Duncan's test).

3.3. Effect of Fertilizer Regimes on Elemental and Isotope Values of Rice Fractions

The effect of different fertilizer treatments on the %C, %N, δ^{13}C, δ^{15}N, δ^{2}H, and δ^{18}O values was measured and the results are shown in Figure 3. %N did not show any significant effect among the rice fractions and the only interaction effect (variety × nitrogen) was detected in PR rice (Table 1). The %N and δ^{15}N values among different rice fractions were significantly affected by nitrogen fertilizer application levels. The %N and δ^{15}N values of different rice fractions under different fertilizer concentrations (N0, N6, and N12) followed different patterns of accumulation. Figure 3 shows that the %N of rice grains was higher when subjected to higher nitrogen application levels. The %N for BR (1.8 ± 0.2%) grown under N12 conditions was significantly higher than N6 (1.6 ± 0.26%) and N0 (1.6 ± 0.2%), respectively. However, the δ^{15}N value for N0 was significantly higher than N6 and N12 indicating that the synthetic urea fertilizer application level was negatively correlated with the δ^{15}N values in different rice fractions (Figure 3).

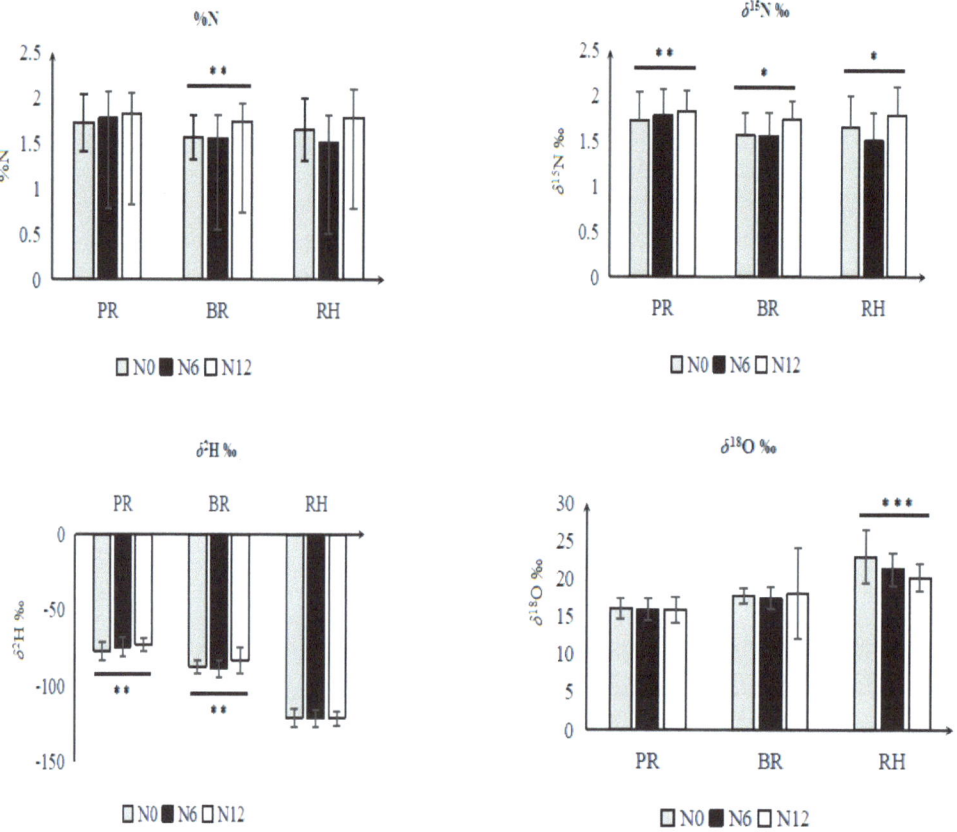

Figure 3. The value of %N, δ^{15}N, δ^2H, and δ^{18}O stable isotopes in rice husk (RH), polished (PR), and brown rice (BR) under different nitrogen fertilization levels. *** Indicates high significance at $p < 0.001$, ** $p < 0.01$, and * $p < 0.05$ (Duncan's test).

These results appear consistent with previous findings which suggest conventionally fertilized rice has lower δ^{15}N values compared to control samples (without fertilizer) [19]. The interpretation of δ^{15}N signatures in plant tissues is generally complex since it can differ from the nutrient source as ^{15}N fractionation occurs during plant physiological processes, mainly during nitrogen uptake, nitrate assimilation, and reduction, as well as during remobilization to the rice grain [20,21]. Lower δ^{15}N values in the fertilized plant fractions during pre-anthesis reflect the direct N availability from the fertilizer applied. Discrimination against ^{15}N occurs during the assimilation of inorganic nitrogen within the plant, and the enzymes responsible for this isotope discrimination include nitrate reductase and glutamine synthase [22].

Higher N assimilation rates in fertilized plants enhance the uptake of inorganic fertilizer which results in the reduction in ^{15}N in fertilized plants compared to non-fertilized plants [22]. In addition, the isotopic discrimination against ^{15}N is marginal in non-fertilized rice ears (glumes, awns, grains) as compared to fertilized rice ears, probably because N limitation prevents discrimination and promotes a higher efficiency for N remobilization [23]. The higher amount of N carried over into the grain results in a higher ^{15}N discrimination. This fact suggests a decrease in the δ^{15}N values for the rice grain in fertilized plants compared to non-fertilized plants. Discrimination within the plant is lower in the non-fertilized grains (N0; lacking nitrogen fertilizer) because the ratio between the plant demand vs. available N is high [24].

Nitrogen fertilizer application had a significant effect on the δ^2H values in PR and BR. The highest δ^2H values in PR ($-73.2‰$) and BR ($-83.2‰$) were observed for the N12 treatment which indicates that the δ^2H values increased with N fertilizer level. There is limited literature on this topic, which restricts the discussion of this mechanism, although a similar trend was observed for the δ^2H values in a previous study, where it was reported that BS-fertilized (biogas slurry) rice had higher δ^2H values than a control rice (without fertilizer) [19]. The effects of nitrogen application levels on the δ^{18}O values contrasted with δ^2H values. There was no significant effect in the PR and BR grains, probably due to a weak or no effect on grain morphological parameters, and a lack of N effect on stomatal conductance and transpiration rates [25].

A significant difference was observed in the δ^{18}O values in RH. The mean δ^{18}O values for N6 (21.3‰) and N12 (20.2‰) treatments were significantly lower than N0 treatments (22.9‰) suggesting that the δ^{18}O values in RH decreased with increasing nitrogen fertilization. Lower δ^{18}O values in RH than the rice grain may be associated with progressive enrichment in plant components from the root, to the stem, to the leaf, and finally to the grain, as well as physiological factors such as dehydration and plant tissue degradation that occurs during husk development [26].

3.4. Elemental and Isotopic Variations among Different Light Shading Treatments

Different shading treatments including LS-0, LS-50, and LS-75 were applied and the effect was observed on the %N, %C, δ^{13}C, δ^{15}N, δ^2H, and δ^{18}O values of different rice fractions. The experiment was performed using two shading treatments (LS-0 and LS-50) for rice plants grown with fertilizer treatment N0 and N6, respectively (Figure 4a), and three shading treatments (LS-0, LS-50, and LS-75) for rice plants cultivated using N12 fertilizer treatment (Figure 4b). The shading effect on the %N, %C, δ^{13}C, δ^{15}N, δ^2H, and δ^{18}O values of rice grown under different fertilizer treatments followed the same pattern. The light shading treatment showed a significant effect on the %N, δ^{15}N, δ^{13}C, and δ^2H values in different rice fractions. The values of %N were significantly lower at LS-0 than that of LS-50 and LS-75 in all three rice grain fractions. In the case of PR, the highest %N value was observed LS-75 (2.3 ± 0.2%) followed by LS-50 (2.0 ± 0.2%) and the lowest was observed in LS-0 (1.6 ± 0.1%), respectively. The δ^{15}N values followed a unique pattern. It can be seen in Figure 4b that the δ^{15}N signature among different rice fractions was significantly higher in LS-50 compared to LS-0 (non-shaded), but it decreased in LS-75. No significant difference was found in the δ^{15}N values for LS-0 and LS-75. Further investigation is required to explore this mechanism since no literature was found that explained this phenomenon in rice. However, previous research has shown that the effect of maize kernel shading (40%) on %N at different stages showed a decrease in the %N content (up to 60%) compared to the control (ambient sunlight), which is not consistent with our study [27]. This crop difference suggests that plant physiological characteristics can impart significant crop variation for N uptake, retention, utilization, and isotopic fractionation.

The δ^{13}C values among different rice fractions also showed significant variations for different shading treatments. The %C values of LS-0 in different rice fractions including PR ($-28.3‰$), BR ($-28.8‰$), and RH ($-30.5‰$) were significantly higher than those of LS-50 (29.5‰, $-30.0‰$, $-31.6‰$), and LS-75 ($-29.7‰$, $-30.1‰$, $-31.5‰$), respectively, indicating that at greater light intensity, the ^{13}C isotopic fractionation is higher. In previous studies, a similar trend in δ^{13}C values for citrus, grapefruit, and banana plants were reported under different shading treatments [10,28,29]. The δ^{13}C values are positively correlated with irradiance and a similar trend of increasing δ^{13}C values with increasing irradiance has been found in banana plants [28]. The δ^{13}C values have been shown to be negatively correlated to internal CO_2 concentration in plants during carbon uptake, so a decrease in δ^{13}C values under shaded treatments indicates increased conductance during the time that the CO_2 was fixed and/or a decreased photosynthetic rate [10]. Another study argued that lower $\delta^{13}C$ values in shaded treatments clearly indicated that shading disrupted the photosynthate metabolism, reducing the photosynthate accumulation in grains [30].

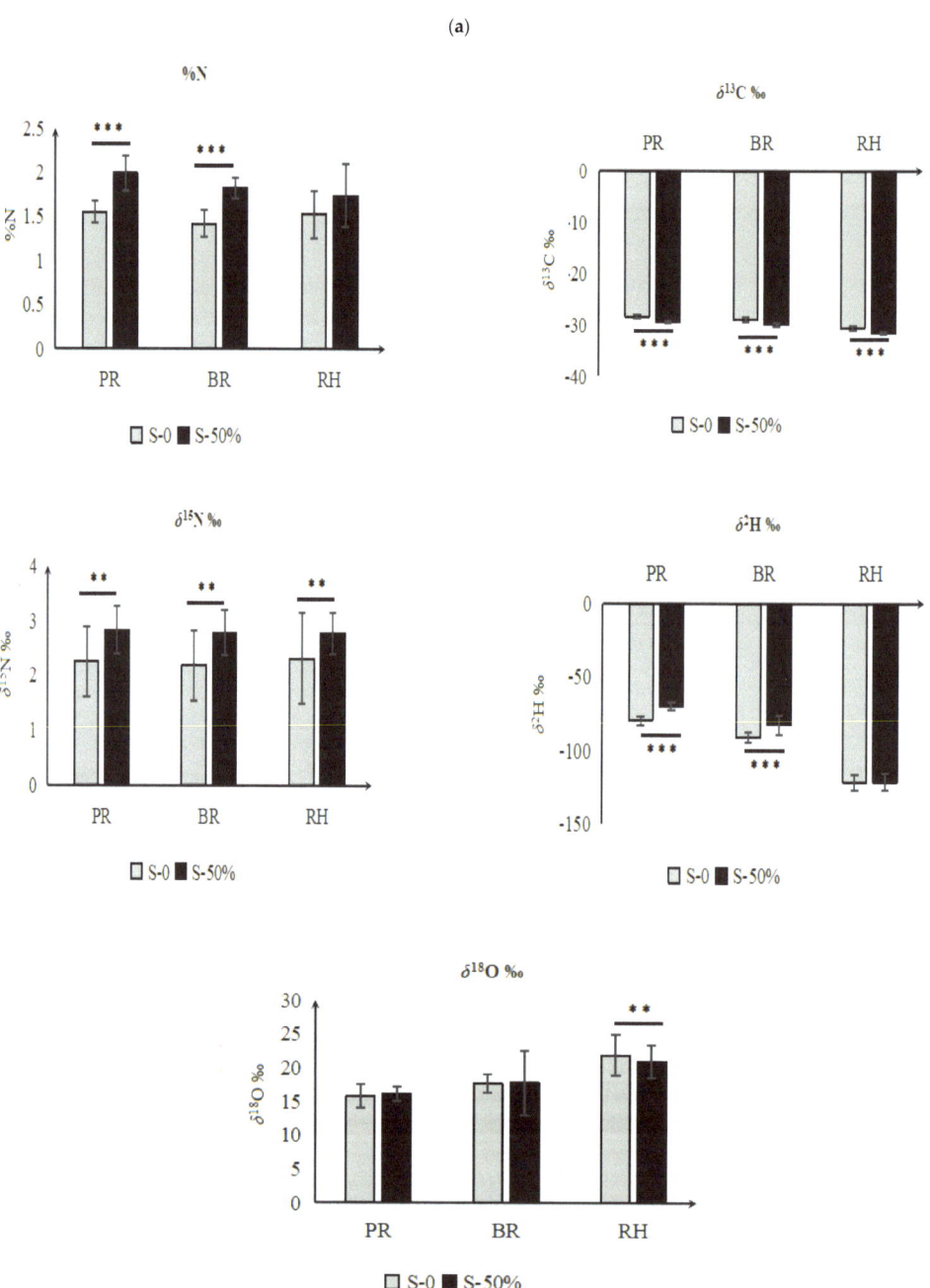

Figure 4. *Cont.*

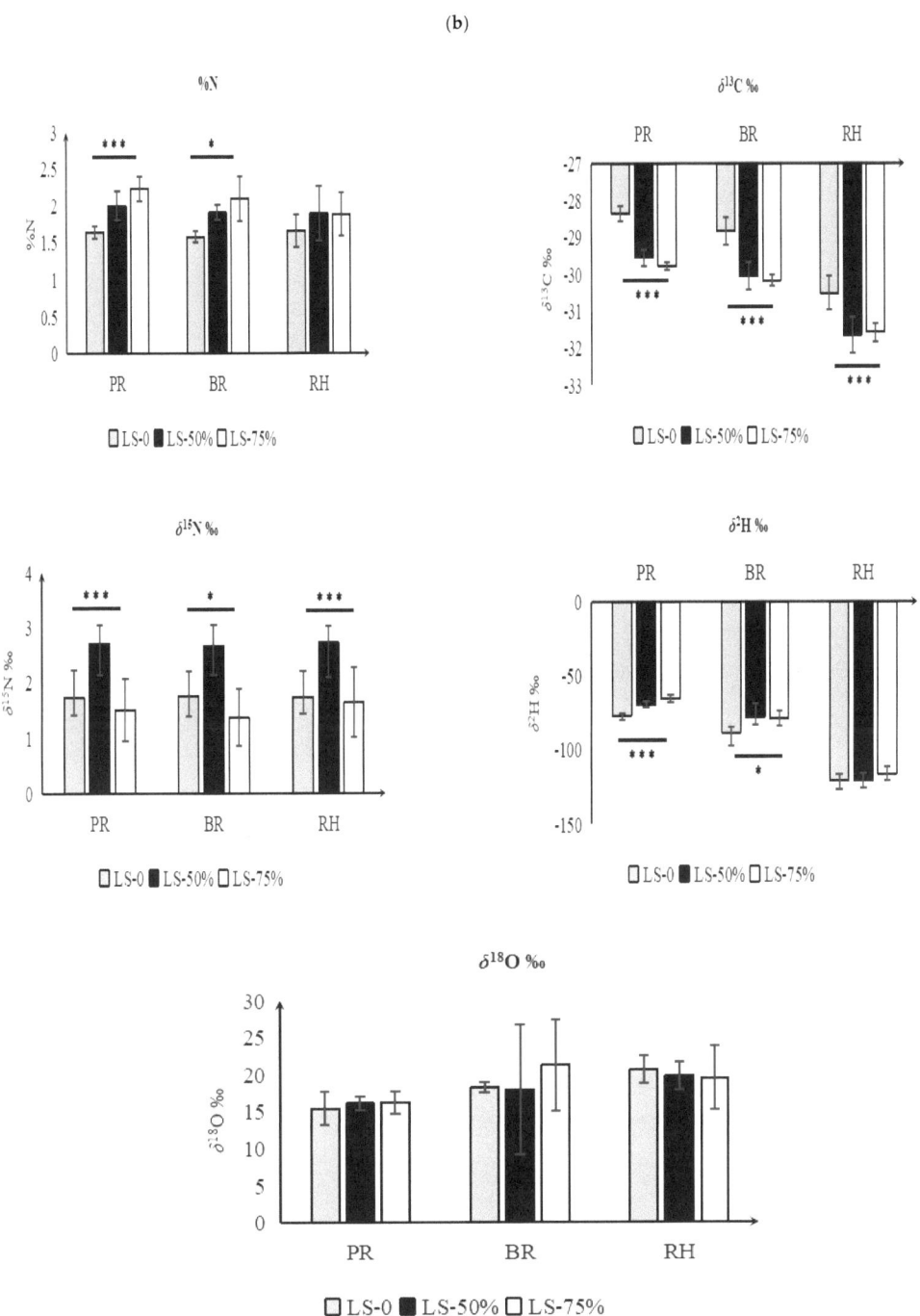

Figure 4. The %N, δ^{13}C, δ^{15}N, δ^{2}H, and δ^{18}O values in rice husk (RH), polished (PR), and brown rice (BR) under (**a**) two different light shading levels and (**b**) three different light shading levels. *** Indicates high significance at $p < 0.001$, ** $p < 0.01$, and * $p < 0.05$ Duncan's test).

The δ^2H values also showed significant variations for PR and BR. In PR, the highest δ^2H value (−65.3‰) was found in LS-75 followed by LS-50 (−69.3‰), and the lowest was observed in LS-0 (−77.0‰), respectively. The same trend was observed for BR and there were significant differences between LS 50/75 and LS-0. Soil water (from groundwater, irrigation water, or precipitation) is the main source of δ^2H in plants, and the present results indicate that different light intensities affect the δ^2H values of soil water, causing the δ^2H signature of rice grains to vary through transpiration. No significant difference was observed for the δ^{18}O values among the different rice fractions at different light intensities.

4. Conclusions

In this study, the effect of cultivar type, fertilizer supply, and light intensity on the distribution of elemental contents and light stable isotopes (C, N, H, and O) in different rice fractions were investigated. Significant variations were observed for δ^{13}C, δ^{15}N, δ^2H, and δ^{18}O values of different rice fractions among different cultivars. Fertilizer application rates showed a strong association with %N, δ^{15}N, δ^2H, and δ^{18}O values, although there was no significant variation in the %C and δ^{13}C values. The light intensity levels also showed a significant influence on isotopic contents among different rice fractions. The δ^{13}C values showed a positive correlation with irradiance. The δ^2H and δ^{15}N values decreased with an increase in the irradiance. It is concluded that all factors mentioned above significantly influence isotopic values and should be considered when addressing the authenticity of rice. Furthermore, care should be taken when selecting the rice fraction for future studies as isotopic signatures vary considerably among different rice fractions. The findings from this study will have a significant impact on understanding different climatic trends (seasonal and annual) and fertilizer effects on rice and allow better understanding of isotopic variability for different geographical regions, farming practices, and environmental conditions.

Author Contributions: Y.Y. and W.Z. conceived the idea. S.A.W. and J.Y. drafted the manuscript, J.N., C.L. and Y.Z. analyzed data. K.M.R. and H.L. edited the manuscript. All authors have read and agreed to the published version of the manuscript.

Funding: This work was supported by Zhejiang Provincial Public Welfare Technology Research Program [Grant No. LGJ20C200003], the Self-design Project from State Key Laboratory for Managing Biotic and Chemical Threats to the Quality and Safety of Agro-products [Grant No. 2010DS700124-ZZ1803]; Crop Varietal Improvement and Insect Pests Control by Nuclear Radiation Project, China; IAEA Coordinated Research Project [Grant No. D52042]; and Special Fund of Discipline Construction for Traceability of Agricultural Product (2022-ZAAS).

Data Availability Statement: The data presented in this study are available on request from the corresponding author.

Acknowledgments: The authors gratefully acknowledge Weigui Zhang, from China National Rice Research Institute, for participating in this field-experimental design and execution, and providing information of materials and methods section.

Conflicts of Interest: The authors declare no conflict of interest.

References

1. Wadood, S.A.; Nie, J.; Li, C.; Rogers, K.M.; Khan, A.; Khan, W.A.; Qamar, A.; Zhang, Y.; Yuwei, Y. Rice Authentication: An Overview of Different Analytical Techniques Combined with Multivariate Analysis. *J. Food Compos. Anal.* **2022**, *112*, 104677. [CrossRef]
2. Maione, C.; Batista, B.L.; Campiglia, A.D.; Barbosa, F.; Barbosa, R.M. Classification of Geographic Origin of Rice by Data Mining and Inductively Coupled Plasma Mass Spectrometry. *Comput. Electron. Agric.* **2016**, *121*, 101–107. [CrossRef]
3. Teye, E.; Amuah, C.L.Y.; McGrath, T.; Elliott, C. Innovative and Rapid Analysis for Rice Authenticity Using Hand-Held NIR Spectrometry and Chemometrics. *Spectrochim. Acta Part A Mol. Biomol. Spectrosc.* **2019**, *217*, 147–154. [CrossRef]
4. Long, N.P.; Lim, D.K.; Mo, C.; Kim, G.; Kwon, S.W. Development and Assessment of a Lysophospholipid-Based Deep Learning Model to Discriminate Geographical Origins of White Rice. *Sci. Rep.* **2017**, *7*, 8552. [CrossRef] [PubMed]

5. Park, J.R.; Yang, W.T.; Kwon, Y.S.; Kim, H.N.; Kim, K.M.; Kim, D.H. Assessment of the Genetic Diversity of Rice Germplasms Characterized by Black-Purple and Red Pericarp Color Using Simple Sequence Repeat Markers. *Plants* **2019**, *8*, 471. [CrossRef]
6. Chung, I.M.; Kim, Y.J.; Moon, H.S.; Chi, H.Y.; Kim, S.H. Long-Term Isotopic Model Study for Ecofriendly Rice (*Oryza sativa* L.) Authentication: Updating a Case Study in South Korea. *Food Chem.* **2021**, *362*, 130215. [CrossRef]
7. Li, C.; Nie, J.; Zhang, Y.; Shao, S.; Liu, Z.; Rogers, K.M.; Zhang, W.; Yuan, Y. Geographical Origin Modeling of Chinese Rice Using Stable Isotopes and Trace Elements. *Food Control* **2022**, *138*, 108997. [CrossRef]
8. Wadood, S.A.; Guo, B.; Liu, H.; Wei, S.; Bao, X.; Wei, Y. Study on the Variation of Stable Isotopic Fingerprints of Wheat Kernel along with Milling Processing. *Food Control* **2018**, *91*, 427–433. [CrossRef]
9. Akamatsu, F.; Okuda, M.; Fujii, T. Long-Term Responses to Climate Change of the Carbon and Oxygen Stable Isotopic Compositions and Gelatinization Temperature of Rice. *Food Chem.* **2020**, *315*, 126239. [CrossRef] [PubMed]
10. Raveh, E.; Cohen, S.; Raz, T.; Yakir, D.; Grava, A.; Goldschmidt, E.E. Increased Growth of Young Citrus Trees under Reduced Radiation Load in a Semi-Arid Climate1. *J. Exp. Bot.* **2003**, *54*, 365–373. [CrossRef] [PubMed]
11. Greer, D.H.; Weedon, M.M. Modelling Photosynthetic Responses to Temperature of Grapevine (*Vitis vinifera* Cv. Semillon) Leaves on Vines Grown in a Hot Climate. *Plant. Cell Environ.* **2012**, *35*, 1050–1064. [CrossRef] [PubMed]
12. Xia, W.; Li, C.; Nie, J.; Shao, S.; Rogers, K.M.; Zhang, Y.; Li, Z.; Yuan, Y. Stable Isotope and Photosynthetic Response of Tea Grown under Different Temperature and Light Conditions. *Food Chem.* **2022**, *368*, 130771. [CrossRef] [PubMed]
13. Rashmi, D.; Shree, P.; Singh, D.K. Stable Isotope Ratio Analysis in Determining the Geographical Traceability of Indian Wheat. *Food Control* **2017**, *79*, 169–176. [CrossRef]
14. Xu, Y.; This, D.; Pausch, R.C.; Vonhof, W.M.; Coburn, J.R.; Comstock, J.P.; McCouch, S.R. Leaf-Level Water Use Efficiency Determined by Carbon Isotope Discrimination in Rice Seedlings: Genetic Variation Associated with Population Structure and QTL Mapping. *Theor. Appl. Genet.* **2009**, *118*, 1065–1081. [CrossRef] [PubMed]
15. Chung, I.M.; Kim, J.K.; Prabakaran, M.; Yang, J.H.; Kim, S.H. Authenticity of Rice (*Oryza sativa* L.) Geographical Origin Based on Analysis of C, N, O and S Stable Isotope Ratios: A Preliminary Case Report in Korea, China and Philippine. *J. Sci. Food Agric.* **2016**, *96*, 2433–2439. [CrossRef]
16. Gómez-Alonso, S.; García-Romero, E. Effect of Irrigation and Variety on Oxygen ($\Delta^{18}O$) and Carbon ($\Delta^{13}C$) Stable Isotope Composition of Grapes Cultivated in a Warm Climate. *Aust. J. Grape Wine Res.* **2010**, *16*, 283–289. [CrossRef]
17. Yuan, Y.; Zhang, W.; Zhang, Y.; Liu, Z.; Shao, S.; Zhou, L.; Rogers, K.M. Differentiating Organically Farmed Rice from Conventional and Green Rice Harvested from an Experimental Field Trial Using Stable Isotopes and Multi-Element Chemometrics. *J. Agric. Food Chem.* **2018**, *66*, 2607–2615. [CrossRef]
18. Wang, J.; Chen, T.; Zhang, W.; Zhao, Y.; Yang, S.; Chen, A. Tracing the Geographical Origin of Rice by Stable Isotopic Analyses Combined with Chemometrics. *Food Chem.* **2020**, *313*, 126093. [CrossRef]
19. Li, C.; Wang, Q.; Shao, S.; Chen, Z.; Nie, J.; Liu, Z.; Rogers, K.M.; Yuan, Y. Stable Isotope Effects of Biogas Slurry Applied as an Organic Fertilizer to Rice, Straw, and Soil. *J. Agric. Food Chem.* **2021**, *69*, 8090–8097. [CrossRef] [PubMed]
20. Fuertes-Mendizábal, T.; Estavillo, J.M.; Duñabeitia, M.K.; Huérfano, X.; Castellón, A.; González-Murua, C.; Aizpurua, A.; González-Moro, M.B. 15N Natural Abundance Evidences a Better Use of N Sources by Late Nitrogen Application in Bread Wheat. *Front. Plant Sci.* **2018**, *9*, 853. [CrossRef]
21. Robinson, D. $\Delta15N$ as an Integrator of the Nitrogen Cycle. *Trends Ecol. Evol.* **2001**, *16*, 153–162. [CrossRef] [PubMed]
22. Kalcsits, L.A.; Buschhaus, H.A.; Guy, R.D. Nitrogen Isotope Discrimination as an Integrated Measure of Nitrogen Fluxes, Assimilation and Allocation in Plants. *Physiol. Plant.* **2014**, *151*, 293–304. [CrossRef] [PubMed]
23. Nehe, A.S.; Misra, S.; Murchie, E.H.; Chinnathambi, K.; Singh Tyagi, B.; Foulkes, M.J. Nitrogen Partitioning and Remobilization in Relation to Leaf Senescence, Grain Yield and Protein Concentration in Indian Wheat Cultivars. *Field Crop. Res.* **2020**, *251*, 107778. [CrossRef] [PubMed]
24. Serret, M.; Ortiz-Monasterio, I.; Pardo, A.; Araus, J. The Effects of Urea Fertilisation and Genotype on Yield, Nitrogen Use Efficiency, δ 15 N and δ 13 C in Wheat. *Ann. Appl. Biol.* **2008**, *153*, 080617165316730. [CrossRef]
25. Liu, H.T.; Gong, X.Y.; Schäufele, R.; Yang, F.; Hirl, R.T.; Schmidt, A.; Schnyder, H. Nitrogen Fertilization and δ 18 O of CO 2 Have No Effect on 18 O-Enrichment of Leaf Water and Cellulose in Cleistogenes Squarrosa (C 4)—Is VPD the Sole Control? *Plant. Cell Environ.* **2016**, *39*, 2701–2712. [CrossRef]
26. Cernusak, L.A.; Barbour, M.M.; Arndt, S.K.; Cheesman, A.W.; English, N.B.; Feild, T.S.; Helliker, B.R.; Holloway-Phillips, M.M.; Holtum, J.A.M.; Kahmen, A.; et al. Stable Isotopes in Leaf Water of Terrestrial Plants. *Plant. Cell Environ.* **2016**, *39*, 1087–1102. [CrossRef]
27. Gao, J. *Effects of Different Light Conditions on Grain Yield and Physiological Characteristics of Summer Maize and Their Regulatory Mechanisation*; Shandong Agricultural University: Taian, China, 2018.
28. Israeli, Y.; Schwartz, A.; Plaut, Z.; Yakir, D. Effects of Light Regime on Delta13C, Photosynthesis and Yield of Field-Grown Banana (*Musa* sp., Musaceae). *Plant Cell Environ.* **1996**, *19*, 225–230. [CrossRef]
29. Cohen, S.; Raveh, E.; Li, Y.; Grava, A.; Goldschmidt, E.E. Physiological Responses of Leaves, Tree Growth and Fruit Yield of Grapefruit Trees under Reflective Shade Screens. *Sci. Hortic.* **2005**, *107*, 25–35. [CrossRef]
30. Gao, J.; Zhao, B.; Dong, S.; Liu, P.; Ren, B.; Zhang, J. Response of Summer Maize Photosynthate Accumulation and Distribution to Shading Stress Assessed by Using 13CO2 Stable Isotope Tracer in the Field. *Front. Plant Sci.* **2017**, *8*, 1821. [CrossRef]

Disclaimer/Publisher's Note: The statements, opinions and data contained in all publications are solely those of the individual author(s) and contributor(s) and not of MDPI and/or the editor(s). MDPI and/or the editor(s) disclaim responsibility for any injury to people or property resulting from any ideas, methods, instructions or products referred to in the content.

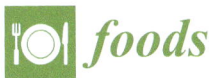

Article

Benchmarking and Validation of a Bioinformatics Workflow for Meat Species Identification Using 16S rDNA Metabarcoding

Grégoire Denay [1,*], Laura Preckel [2], Henning Petersen [3], Klaus Pietsch [4], Anne Wöhlke [5] and Claudia Brünen-Nieweler [2]

1. Chemical and Veterinary Analytical Institute Rhein-Ruhr-Wupper (CVUA-RRW), Deutscher Ring 100, 47798 Krefeld, Germany
2. Chemical and Veterinary Analytical Institute Muensterland-Emscher-Lippe (CVUA-MEL), Joseph-Koenig-Strasse 40, 48147 Muenster, Germany
3. Chemical and Veterinary Analytical Institute Ostwestfalen-Lippe (CVUA-OWL), Westerfeldstrasse 1, 32758 Detmold, Germany
4. State Institute for Chemical and Veterinary Analysis Freiburg (CVUA-FR), Bissierstrasse 5, 79114 Freiburg, Germany
5. Food and Veterinary Institute, Lower Saxony State Office for Consumer Protection and Food Safety (LAVES), Dresdenstrasse 2, 38124 Braunschweig, Germany
* Correspondence: gregoire.denay@cvua-rrw.de

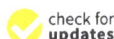

Citation: Denay, G.; Preckel, L.; Petersen, H.; Pietsch, K.; Wöhlke, A.; Brünen-Nieweler, C. Benchmarking and Validation of a Bioinformatics Workflow for Meat Species Identification Using 16S rDNA Metabarcoding. *Foods* 2023, 12, 968. https://doi.org/10.3390/foods12050968

Academic Editors: Hongyan Liu, Hongtao Lei, Boli Guo and Ren-You Gan

Received: 9 December 2022
Revised: 14 February 2023
Accepted: 20 February 2023
Published: 24 February 2023

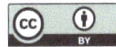

Copyright: © 2023 by the authors. Licensee MDPI, Basel, Switzerland. This article is an open access article distributed under the terms and conditions of the Creative Commons Attribution (CC BY) license (https://creativecommons.org/licenses/by/4.0/).

Abstract: DNA-metabarcoding is becoming more widely used for routine authentication of meat-based food and feed products. Several methods validating species identification methods through amplicon sequencing have already been published. These use a variety of barcodes and analysis workflows, however, no methodical comparison of available algorithms and parameter optimization are published hitherto for meat-based products' authenticity. Additionally, many published methods use very small subsets of the available reference sequences, thereby limiting the potential of the analysis and leading to over-optimistic performance estimates. We here predict and compare the ability of published barcodes to distinguish taxa in the BLAST NT database. We then use a dataset of 79 reference samples, spanning 32 taxa, to benchmark and optimize a metabarcoding analysis workflow for 16S rDNA Illumina sequencing. Furthermore, we provide recommendations as to the parameter choices, sequencing depth, and thresholds that should be used to analyze meat metabarcoding sequencing experiments. The analysis workflow is publicly available, and includes ready-to-use tools for validation and benchmarking.

Keywords: DNA metabarcoding; amplicon sequencing; food authenticity; food adulteration; next generation sequencing; bioinformatics; validation; benchmarking

1. Introduction

Commercial food and feed are subjected to international regulations, ensuring that they are safe and conform to the packaging declarations. Meat products are especially prone to adulteration. This can be the replacement of expensive ingredients with cheaper meat products, misinformation by the addition of undeclared components, or the absence of declared components [1,2]. Classical DNA-based methods such as Polymerase Chain Reaction (PCR) amplification, restriction fragment length polymorphism, or DNA-chips, as well as protein-based methods such as ELISA are limited by their target-based approach. As such, their results are limited to a binary answer regarding a single component and they may not be able to identify all ingredients present in a sample. Sanger sequencing, on the other hand, is a widely used untargeted method for the identification of food ingredients. Unlike targeted methods, untargeted methods do not require prior knowledge of specific targets and can analyze a broader range of ingredients. However, it should be noted that the Sanger sequencing application is limited to pure samples [1]. MALDI-based methods are being developed to overcome these challenges, but the collection of reference spectra is still a work-intensive process [3]. Next-generation sequencing (NGS) methods for food authenticity have been developed in the last decade, taking advantage of the untargeted possibilities of the technology and of existing extensive databases of nucleotide sequences [4,5].

Some NGS methods focus on a metagenomics approach, i.e., sequencing of all DNA-sequences in a sample [6,7]. Other methods use a metabarcoding approach, in which a small conserved DNA fragment is amplified and sequenced, while sequence differences allow for specific taxa identification [8–14]. This method allows untargeted species identification and increased parallelization of sample processing and analysis, while taking advantage of the massive amount of reference sequences available in dedicated databases. The choice of barcode is however non-trivial and can have a strong effect on the method's performance: barcodes should be short enough to still be detectable in highly degraded samples, while still allowing to distinguish between closely related organisms [15]. Metabarcoding presents several advantages over metagenomics: decreased costs, larger reference collections, and less complex analysis, however at the cost of lower taxonomic resolution, being limited to a subset of the taxonomy, and being prone to PCR artifacts [16]. For these reasons, metabarcoding methods are currently widely used for food authenticity determination in a wide-range of matrices [8–12,14,17–19].

Various methods for sample preparation and sequencing of meat products were validated and published, focusing on the two main short-read sequencing technologies [8,10,11,13,14]. While the IonTorrent platform offers proprietary data analysis solutions, a number of alternative bioinformatics workflows are published for Illumina sequencing data [8,9,11,14]. However, currently published workflows present various drawbacks: (1) none of them is freely available beyond the publication; (2) parameter choices in these workflows appear to be arbitrary, with no comparison of different parameters and/or tools, and can widely differ between workflows; (3) most validations were performed using a very limited subset of reference databases, yielding over-optimistic validation performances.

Our goal here is three-fold. Firstly, we aim to assess the possibilities of using large databases such as the NCBI NT database [4] for metabarcoding analysis and compare predicted performances of different metabarcoding methods. Secondly, our goal is to benchmark a selection of algorithms and parameter sets and validate an optimized analysis workflow. To this end, we used a dataset of 79 real samples, spanning 32 individual taxa. We methodically optimized the bioinformatics analysis on this dataset and present a set of parameters for optimal analysis performance. Lastly, we calculate the accuracy of the analysis and formulate recommendations regarding the limit of detection and sequencing depth. Both the dataset and software programs used in this study are made freely available to help future improvement and practical applications in food authenticity analysis laboratories.

2. Materials and Methods

2.1. Reference Material

The 79 reference samples used in the study were acquired from commercial providers DLA Proficiency Tests GmbH (www.dla-lvu.de; accessed on 1 December 2022), Laborvergleichsuntersuchungen Gbr, (www.lvus.de; accessed on 1 December 2022), and LGC Standards (www.lgcstandards.com; accessed on 1 December 2022) were part of interlaboratory ring trials [10], or prepared from certified reference materials or materials whose identity was determined by a certified veterinarian and Sanger sequencing (see Table S1). Some of these samples were used in a previous study [9].

Samples were prepared and sequenced as previously described [9]. Raw sequencing data are deposited to the European Nucleotide Archive with Project accession PRJEB57117.

Down-sampling was performed using the SeqTK 'sample' tool [20]. The sample size and replicate number were concatenated and used as a seed for the random read selection process. The same seed was used on forward and reverse reads.

The BLAST NT database was downloaded on 12 November 2021 and the tax dump files on 19 November 2021 [4].

2.2. In Silico Barcode Analysis

Recovery and analysis of the barcode sequences from the BLAST NT Database [4] was performed using the BaRCoD v1.1.1 pipeline [21]. Briefly, the nucleotide database was filtered to include only Amniote sequences. Primer sequences (Table S2) were searched using the BLAST+ command line tools, with parameters reproducing the implementation of the Primer-BLAST tool. For this, we used a coverage value of 80% and an identity value of 65% [22,23]. Sequences flanked by facing primer sequences were considered barcodes and extracted, and a new BLAST database was created using these sequences. Barcode sequences were then dereplicated in a taxon-wise fashion, primer sequences were removed using cutadapt [24], and global pairwise alignment was performed with VSearch [25]. The pairwise alignments were used to calculate hamming distances. To determine a consensus level for each sequence, we considered all sequences within a given identity level (1-hamming distance/sequence length), the lowest node shared by a majority of taxa was determined as a consensus taxon determined using TaxidTools [26], and the NCBI taxonomy classification [4]. Conspecific probability was calculated as previously described [27].

2.3. Metabarcoding Analysis

Sequencing data analysis was performed with FooDMe v1.6.3 [28]. Parameters indicated thereafter were used if not specified otherwise in the text or figures.

2.3.1. Reads Preprocessing

Primer sequences (Table S2) and their reverse complements were trimmed from the 5′ and 3′ ends of the reads, respectively, using cutadapt [24] with an error rate of 0.1. Trimmed reads were filtered with fastp [29] to discard reads shorter than 50 bp and trim trails using a window of 4 bp with a minimal quality of 25.

2.3.2. De Novo Identity Clustering

Identity clustering was performed with VSearch [25]. Reads were merged with the '–fastq_mergepairs' function, and a quality filter was applied to keep pseudo-reads between 70 and 100 bp and a maximum of 2 expected errors. Pseudo-reads were dereplicated before being clustered with the '–cluster_size' function, using identity levels between 0.97 and 1.0 (dereplication), and OTUs were sorted by size, discarding clusters with less than 2 reads. If required, chimeras were detected and removed using the '–uchime_denovo' function.

2.3.3. Denoising

Denoising was performed with DADA2 [30]. Read pairs were filtered to remove those with more than 2 expected errors using the 'filterAndTrim' function. Forward and reverse error rates were determined with the 'learnError' function, and reads were corrected using the error model in the 'dada' function. Finally, corrected reads were merged with the 'mergePairs' function while allowing for 1 mismatch. If necessary, chimeras were detected and filtered using the 'removeBimeraDenovo' function using the 'per-sample' method.

2.3.4. Taxonomic Assignment

A mask was created for the BLAST NT database [4] by filtering sequence ID corresponding to Vertebrate taxa. Sequences corresponding to extinct taxa were then filtered from this list. OTUs or ASVs were then searched against the masked database using the BLAST+ program [22] using 'megablast' searches with filters for e-value (1.0×10^{-10}), identity (97), and coverage (100). Results were then filtered by applying a bitscore filter [31] of 4, meaning that for each OTU/ASV, matches with a bitscore difference to the best match for this cluster above 4 were discarded. The consensus taxon for each cluster was determined with TaxidTools [26] by applying a majority vote on the matching taxa, with a minimum threshold of 0.51. The consensus corresponds to the lowest node common to at least X fractions of the taxa, X being the consensus level [32].

2.4. Performance Analysis

Run performances were determined using the 'benchmark' module of FooDMe [28]. The observed compositions of each sample were compared to their expected values (Table S1). For this, a concentration threshold of 0.1% was applied and correspondences between expected and predicted values were considered at the genus level. Precision scores, recall scores, average precision scores, and F-scores were calculated using the appropriate functions of the 'scikit-learn' or 'yardstick' libraries [33,34]. Euclidean distance was determined with NumPy's 'linalg.norm' function [35]. Relative error was determined as $E = |predicted - expected| \div expected$.

2.5. Figure Preparation and Statistical Analysis

Figures were prepared in R using the 'tidyverse', 'ggpubr', 'rstatix', 'yardstick', and 'cowplot' libraries [34]. Variations within groups were analyzed using the Kruskal-Wallis test. Variations between groups were analyzed using ANOVA on quantile-normalized values (Average precision) or original values (Distance). Yield, average precision, and distance distribution were compared using the Wilcoxon test and p-values were corrected for multiple comparisons using FDR correction. Different levels of p-values threshold are indicated as follows: n.s. ($p \leq 1$); * ($p < 0.05$); ** ($p < 0.01$); *** ($p < 0.001$); **** ($p < 0.0001$).

3. Results

3.1. Barcode Specificity

Successful identification of the taxon associated with each barcode depends on both the availability of the sequences in the reference database and their differentiability from sequences associated with other taxa. Several distinct methods have been published for birds and mammals barcoding (Table 1 and Table S2) [8,11,14,36–38], targeting different conserved genes: the 16S ribosomal small subunit (16S), Cytochrome B (cytB), or Cytochrome oxidase 1 (COI/COX1). The 16S rDNA-based metabarcoding method published by Dobrovolny et al. in 2019 [11] is currently being adopted as an official method by the German consumer protection authorities and its performances were carefully measured in a recent series of studies [9–11,39]. We, therefore, chose to focus our benchmarking and optimization efforts on this method. Nevertheless, we wanted to compare the predicted performances of this method to other published barcoding methods, as potential shortcomings could be overcome by an alternative barcode.

Table 1. Comparison of barcode number and assignment rank for different targets.

Method	Number of Taxids Retrieved	Median Number of Barcode per Taxid [a]	Median Length of Barcode [bp] [b]	97% Identity Sequences Assigned at Max.		100% Identity Sequences Assigned at Max.	
				Species Level [%]	Genus Level [%]	Species Level [%]	Genus Level [%]
16S_dobrovolny	7701	3	75	66.77	85.36	81.98	93.27
16S_xing	6383	3	204	78.53	95.07	93.29	98.21
cox1_palumbi	2293	5	522	90.16	97.82	97.08	98.63
cytB_meyer	10,909	25	333	91.31	98.47	95.29	98.89
cytB_palumbi	10,078	35	741	94.55	99.17	97.93	99.56
cytB_VDLUFA	18,136	16	220	89.95	98.52	94.38	98.85
miniCOI_palumbo	5482	2	151	82.55	95.46	92.86	97.71

[a] Unique sequences only. [b] Not including primer sequences.

For this purpose, we first extracted all Amniota (the clade grouping birds and mammals taxa, as well as reptiles) barcode sequences for seven different primer sets using a local implementation of the Primer-BLAST algorithm [21,23]. For each different barcode, we determined all other barcodes within 97% identity distance. We then determined the taxonomic assignment consensus that would result in either a 97% or 100% identity clustering for this sequence, based on a strict majority consensus of all barcodes clustering together at the identity level (Table 1).

Of over 35,000 Amniota taxa represented in the BLAST NT database, the methods based on cytochrome B amplification were the ones that yielded barcodes for the most taxa (over 10,000), with the VDLUFA method yielding barcodes for over 18,000. The COX1/COI methods, on the other hand, were the most restricted, yielding barcodes for under 5500 taxa. All methods yielded high assignment quality for both 97% identity and 100% identity, with more than 95% and 97% of barcodes being assigned at the genus level or below, respectively. The 16S-based method published by Dobrovolny et al. (2019) [11] performed significantly worse at the 97% identity level, with 10% fewer barcodes assigned at the genus level or better, and only slightly worse at the 100% identity level. This might be because the amplicon sequence for this method is especially short (~75 bp excluding amplification primers).

Because most taxa in the BLAST NT database are not relevant for food authenticity, we looked closer at a list of food- and feed-stuff-relevant or -adjacent species curated by the German Consumer Protection and Food Safety Office [40,41]. We examined whether each barcoding method could retrieve at least one barcode for each mammal and bird species in this list (Table 2).

Table 2. Food- and feed- relevant and -adjacent species amplifiability predictions for different barcoding methods. A '+' indicates that at least one sequence was retrieved for the given organism using the method in the header, and a grayed '0' indicates that no sequence was retrieved for this organism.

Organism	Taxid	Common Name	16S Dobrovolny	16S Xing	COX1 Palumbi	cytB Meyer	cytB Palumbi	cytB VDLUFA	MiniCOI Palumbo
Addax nasomaculatus	59515	Addax	+	+	+	+	+	+	+
Ailuropoda melanoleuca	9646	Giant panda	+	+	0	+	+	+	+
Alcelaphus buselaphus	59517	Hartebeest	+	+	0	+	+	+	+
Alcelaphus caama	59519	Red hartebeest	+	+	0	+	+	+	+
Alces alces	9852	Eurasian elk	+	+	0	0	0	+	+
Alectoris chukar	9078	Chukar partridge	+	+	+	+	+	+	+
Ammotragus lervia	9899	Barbary sheep	+	+	+	+	+	+	+
Anas platyrhynchos	8839	Duck	+	+	+	+	+	+	+
Anser anser	8843	Greylag goose	+	+	+	+	+	+	+
Anser cygnoides	8845	Chinese goose	+	+	0	+	+	+	+
Anser indicus	8846	Bar-headed goose	+	+	+	+	+	+	+
Anser rossii	56281	Ross' goose	0	0	0	0	0	0	0
Antidorcas marsupialis	59523	Springbok	+	+	+	+	+	+	+
Bison bison	9901	Bison	+	+	0	+	+	+	+
Bison bonasus	9902	Wisent	+	+	+	+	+	+	+
Bos mutus	72004	Yak	+	+	0	+	+	+	+
Bos taurus	9913	Cattle	+	+	+	+	+	+	+
Bubalus bubalis	89462	Water buffalo	+	+	+	+	+	+	+
Cairina moschata	8855	Muscovy duck	+	+	0	+	+	+	+
Canis lupus	9612	Grey wolf, dog	+	+	+	+	+	+	+
Capra aegagrus	9923	Wild goat	+	+	+	+	+	+	+
Capra hircus	9925	Domestic goat	+	+	+	+	+	+	+
Capra ibex	72542	Ibex	+	+	+	+	+	+	+
Capreolus capreolus	9858	Roe deer	+	+	0	+	+	+	+
Cavia porcellus	10141	Guinea pig	+	+	0	+	+	+	+
Cervus elaphus	9860	Red deer	+	+	+	+	+	+	+

Table 2. *Cont.*

Organism	Taxid	Common Name	16S Dobrovolny	16S Xing	COX1 Palumbi	cytB Meyer	cytB Palumbi	cytB VDLUFA	MiniCOI Palumbo
Cervus nippon	9863	Sika deer	+	+	0	+	+	+	+
Columba livia	8932	Domestic pigeon	+	+	0	+	+	+	+
Connochaetes gnou	59528	Black wildebeest	+	+	0	+	+	+	+
Connochaetes taurinus	9927	Blue wildebeest	+	+	+	+	+	+	+
Coturnix coturnix	9091	Common quail	+	+	0	+	+	+	+
Coturnix japonica	93934	Japanese quail	+	+	0	+	+	+	+
Cygnus olor	8869	Mute swan	+	+	0	+	+	+	+
Dama dama	30532	Fallow deer	0	0	0	0	0	+	0
Damaliscus pygargus	9931	Bontebok	+	+	+	+	+	+	+
Equus asinus	9793	Donkey	+	+	+	+	+	+	+
Equus caballus	9796	Horse	+	+	+	+	+	+	+
Equus quagga	89248	Plain zebra	0	0	0	0	0	+	0
Equus zebra	9791	Mountain zebra	+	+	+	+	+	+	+
Felis catus	9685	Cat	+	+	+	+	+	+	+
Gallus gallus	9031	Chicken	+	+	+	+	+	+	+
Gazella dorcas	37751	Dorcas gazelle	+	+	0	+	+	+	+
Gazella subgutturosa	59529	Black-tailed gazelle	+	+	0	+	+	+	+
Glis glis	41261	Fat dormouse	+	+	0	+	+	+	+
Hippotragus niger	37189	Sable antelope	+	+	0	+	+	+	+
Kobus ellipsiprymnus	9962	Waterbuck	+	+	0	+	+	+	+
Lama glama	9844	Llama	+	+	+	+	+	+	+
Lepus europaeus	9983	European hare	+	+	0	+	+	+	+
Macropus fuliginosus	9316	Western gray kangaroo	+	+	0	0	0	+	0
Macropus giganteus	9317	Eastern gray kangaroo	+	+	0	+	+	+	+
Marmota marmota	9993	Alpine marmot	0	0	0	0	0	0	0
Martes martes	29065	European pine marten	+	+	0	+	+	+	+
Meleagris gallopavo	9103	Turkey	+	+	+	+	+	+	+
Muntiacus reevesi	9886	Reeves' muntjac	+	+	0	+	+	+	+
Mus musculus	10090	Mouse	+	+	+	+	+	+	+
Myodes glareolus	447135	Bank vole	+	+	+	+	+	+	+
Numida meleagris	8996	Helmeted guineafowl	+	+	0	+	0	+	+
Oryctolagus cuniculus	9986	Rabbit	+	+	+	+	+	+	+
Oryx dammah	59534	Scimitar-horned oryx	+	+	+	+	+	+	+
Oryx gazella	9958	Gemsbok	+	+	+	+	+	+	+
Osphranter robustus	9319	Common wallaroo	+	+	0	+	+	+	+
Osphranter rufus	9321	Red kangaroo	+	+	+	+	+	+	+
Ovibos moschatus	37176	Musk ox	+	+	0	0	0	+	+
Ovis aries	9940	Sheep	+	+	+	+	+	+	+
Ovis orientalis	469796	Asiatic mouflon	+	+	+	+	+	+	+
Phasianus colchicus	9054	Common pheasant	+	+	0	+	+	+	+
Rangifer tarandus	9870	Reindeer	+	+	+	+	+	+	+
Rattus norvegicus	10116	Rat	+	+	+	+	+	+	+
Struthio camelus	8801	Ostrich	+	+	0	+	+	+	+
Sus scrofa	9823	Pig	+	+	+	+	+	+	+
Syncerus caffer	9970	African buffalo	+	+	+	+	+	+	+
Tragelaphus oryx	9945	Eland	+	+	+	+	+	+	+
Tragelaphus spekii	69298	Sitatunga	+	+	0	+	+	+	+
Vulpes vulpes	9627	Red fox	+	+	+	+	+	+	+

Surprisingly, the 16S and the VDLUFA-cytochrome B methods performed better on the selected species than all other methods. This is likely due to the higher conservation of the primer-binding regions for these methods across the birds and mammals classes. Notably, no methods could find barcodes corresponding to *Anser rossii* (Ross' goose) and

Marmota marmota (alpine marmot), which might reflect the absence or bad quality of mitochondrial sequences for these species in the database. The 16S methods were unable to retrieve barcodes for *Dama dama* (fallow deer) and *Equus quagga* (plains zebra), whereas the VDLUFA method was able to. The inability of the Dobrovolny method to amplify fallow deer was reported before [9] and the method has since then been improved to overcome this problem [42].

Aside from that, the 16-based Dobrovolny method [11] features several advantages. Firstly, the very short amplicons make this method the most suitable for highly processed matrices, where DNA might be heavily degraded [15,43]. Secondly, its ability to amplify most species of interest (Table 2) and a large spectrum of Amniota taxa (Table 1) was shown in silico. Thirdly, there is a growing body of literature on the suitability of this method for metabarcoding experiments, including interlaboratory validation [9–11]. This method also presents some drawbacks, namely comparatively bad predicted performances at 97% identity clustering, and the species rank for 100% identity clustering (Table 1). However, for meat speciation in food and feed, identification at the genus level is usually sufficient for the detection of fraud.

3.2. Workflow Benchmarking and Optimization

The metabarcoding data analysis workflow can be separated into three main phases:
1. Reads preprocessing, where primer sequences are removed, and bad quality bases are trimmed;
2. Clustering, where reads satisfying a given identity level are grouped together;
3. Taxonomic assignment, where clusters of reads are assigned to taxonomic nodes.

Each of these steps can be performed using a variety of different algorithms, each with several parameters, whose values can have a strong impact on the quality of the analysis. Several studies of meat-products metabarcoding have been published in the past years, each using different analysis workflows and reference databases (Table S3). In order to objectively compare different algorithms and parameters, we collected 16S metabarcoding experiments for 79 different samples, totalizing 32 different species (Table S1). The dataset is enriched for taxa at around 1%, which is the threshold commonly used in diagnostic laboratories as a lower limit for legal action in case of undeclared species. For each parameter set, we analyzed all samples assigning reads using the full BLAST NT database. The workflow's performances were determined both qualitatively and quantitatively. Qualitatively, we compared the observed and expected composition of the samples at the genus level, and we calculated the average precision, which is the geometric mean of the precision and recall. Quantitatively, we determined the yield of the analysis as the number of reads retained through to taxonomic assignment and calculated the Euclidean (or L2) distance between the vector of predicted values and the vector of expected values, reflecting how far predictions are from the expected compositions of the samples.

3.2.1. Benchmarking Clustering Parameters

The main bottleneck of the analysis is to obtain read clusters that accurately describe the real composition of the sample. Several clustering methods have been described, amongst which de novo identity clustering and denoising are the main representatives [30,44–46]. We here compared the effects of clustering reads with a 95%, 97%, and 100% (dereplication) identity threshold and using denoising (Figure 1).

While the clustering algorithm choice made no significant difference in the qualitative and quantitative accuracy of the results (Figure 1A,B), the denoising method had a significantly higher yield than de novo clustering with either identity level (Figure 1C). The median yield for denoising was 99%, with most samples above 98%, whereas it fell to a median yield of 97% for dereplication, with samples as low as 93% yield. Additionally, the clusters produced by the denoising algorithm were much closer to the real sample composition, as shown by the splitting level, calculated by taking the log10 of the ratio of cluster number to expected components in each sample (Figure 1D). The splitting level median was close to one for denoising, indicating that each "real" sequence was split between 10 clusters. This level was increasingly high with increasing identity level for the de novo identity clustering method. It reached a median value of 2.5 for the dereplication, indicating that each "real" sequence was split between over 300 clusters. This had a significant impact on the run time of the workflow (Figure 1E). The dereplication method ran over 20 min per sample per core, whereas other methods ran for under 10 min per sample per core. This is consistent with previous work showing a more accurate clustering using denoising [27,45].

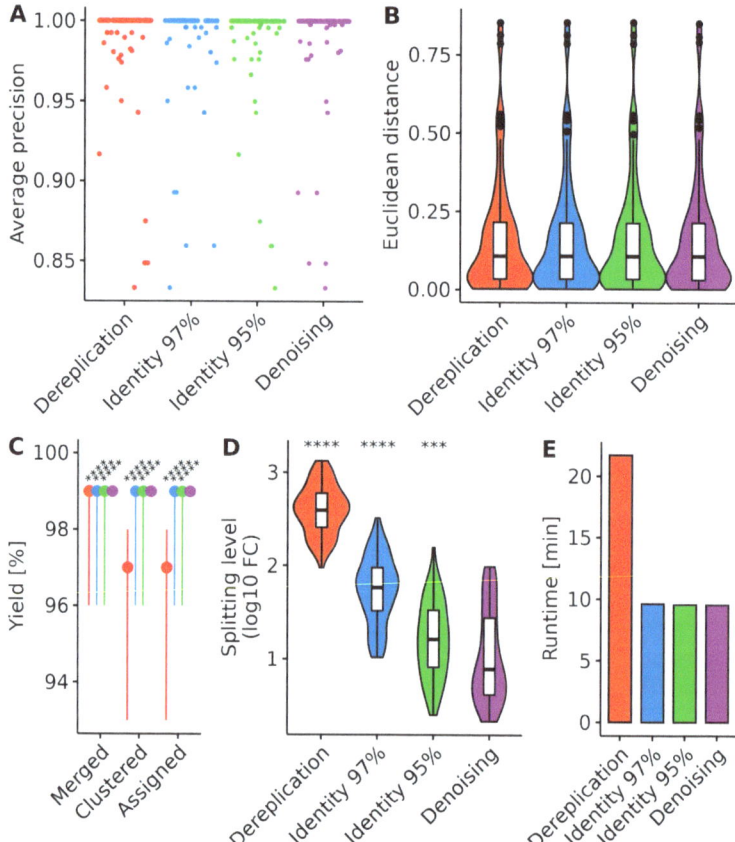

Figure 1. Effects of the clustering method on workflow performances. (**A**) Average precision; (**B**) Euclidean distance between predicted and expected compositions; (**C**) Workflow yields in the number of reads after the read merging step (Merged), after clustering (Clustered), and after taxonomic assignment (Assigned). The dots indicate the median value within each group and the lines represent the range of the distribution. Differences between the groups' means were tested with the Wilcoxon test for paired samples, using Denoising as the reference group. (**D**) Amplicon sequence splitting level is expressed as the log10-fold change between the expected number of taxa in each sample and the number of predicted sequence clusters. (**E**) Average analysis runtime for the 79 samples dataset, expressed in minutes per core per sample. Violin plot outlines represent the kernel density function of the distribution, the included white boxplots represent the range (lines), quartiles (box edges) and median (middle line of the boxes) of the distribution, and outliers are represented by a black point. Different levels of *p*-values threshold are indicated as follows: *** ($p < 0.001$); **** ($p < 0.0001$).

When using denoising, we noticed that it was important to allow for one mismatch for reads merging (Figure S1). Using a strict identity for merging resulted in a considerable yield loss of up to 8%, while allowing one mismatch did not affect the quantitative and qualitative accuracy of the results while maximizing yield. This is due to the short size of the amplicon, which combined with a long read length means that the entire barcode (~75 bp) is used as an overlapping sequence for merging.

We also checked whether detecting and filtering chimeric reads after denoising influenced the results. Although filtering chimera slightly affected yield, in the order of a few percent of the reads, neither the quantitative nor the qualitative performances of the workflow were affected (Figure S2). This likely indicates that very few chimeric sequences are formed during both PCR and sequencing steps using the previously published 16S method [9,11].

In conclusion, we show here that all four tested clustering algorithms yield similar results. However, using denoising while allowing one mismatch in the overlapping sequences during read merging maximizes yield and gives clusters closer to the expected sample composition.

3.2.2. Optimization of Taxonomic Assignment

Consensus sequences for each cluster need to be assigned to a taxonomic node. This was done using the 'megablast' tool by looking for highly similar sequences in the BLAST NT database. As only part of the database is relevant for the identification of birds and mammals, the database was pre-filtered to exclude taxa not belonging to the Vertebrate clade. A BLAST search typically yields many results, most of which are far off the target. In order to narrow the search, several filters are available [31]. We applied a first hard filter consisting of an expect-value (E-value; describes the number of hits one might expect to see by chance in the database) and an identity level (the fraction of identical nucleotides between hit and query) thresholds. Results were then post-filtered using bitscore difference to keep only results within a certain distance to the best result for this query. Finally, each cluster was assigned to a taxonomic node based on a minimal consensus level, between 51% (majority consensus) and 100% (last common ancestor). Using this process, it is possible to assign a taxonomic node to all clusters, even with divergent results, although the consensus may be at the genus or higher rank [32].

The E-value threshold did not influence the assignment accuracy (Figure S3). This is due to the downstream decision of considering only the top results from the BLAST search. It is, however, important to note that using an E-Value threshold lower than 1.0×10^{-20} returned no hits from the BLAST search.

Because the multiple filtering process can have complex synergistic effects, we used a matrix design to test a range of values for each filter: BLAST identity level was varied between 95% and 100%, bitscore difference between 0 and 8 bits, and minimal consensus between 51% and 100%. We then checked if any filter, or combination of filters, had a significant effect on the result's accuracy using analysis of variance (ANOVA).

The ANOVA of average precision values showed a significant effect on each individual filter (Figure 2A). As well as combined effects of the minimal consensus and bitscore filters. However, when omitting the parameter value of 8 for the bitscore filter, which gave significantly worse results than any other (Figure 2C), the interaction effect was not observed anymore. We, therefore, analyzed each effect individually. Average precision improved gradually with improving BLAST identity values, yielding the best results for 100% identity values (Figure 2B). In this context, the bitscore filter was redundant with the identity filter and yielded similar results for any value below 8 (Figure 2C). Consensus gave the best results with values of 80% or below, the value of 100% (last common ancestor) gave significantly worse results (Figure 2D).

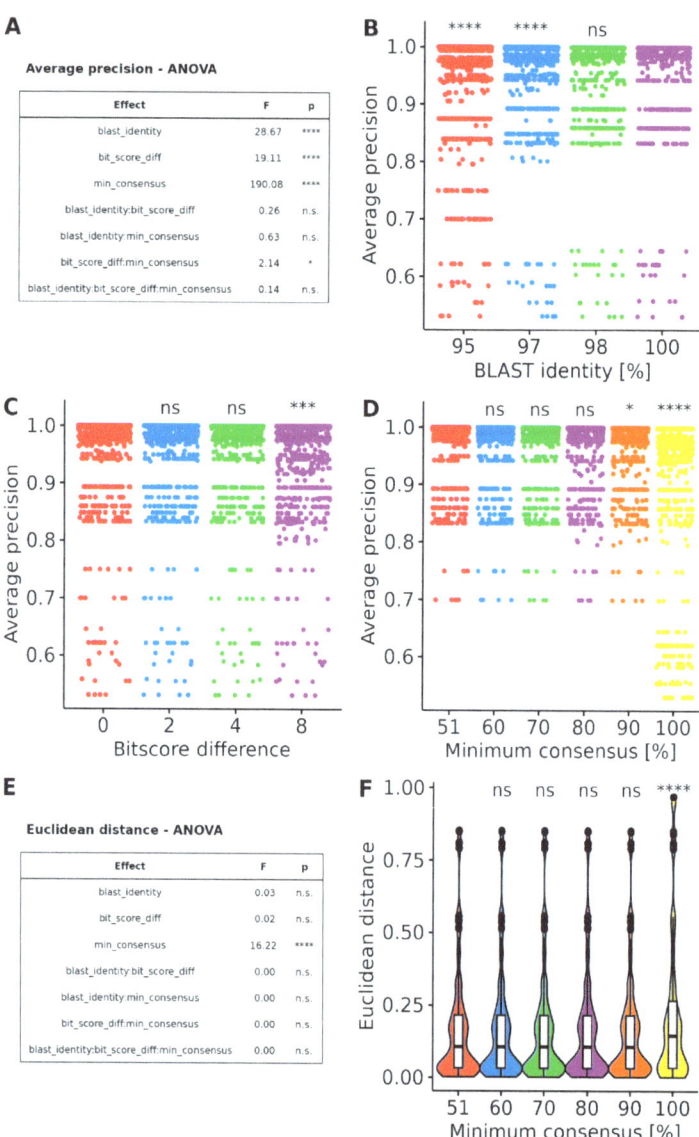

Figure 2. Effects of BLAST filtering parameters on the predictions' accuracy. (**A**) Summary table of the ANOVA on quantile-quantile normalized average precision values showing F statistic and p-value for single effects and their interactions. (**B**) Average precision for different BLAST identity values. (**C**) Average precision for different bitscore-difference values. (**D**) Average precision for different minimum consensus values. (**E**) Summary table of the ANOVA on Euclidean distance values showing F statistic and p-value for single effects and their interactions. (**F**) Euclidean distance for different minimum consensus values. Violin plot outlines represent the kernel density plot of the distribution, the included white boxplots represent the range (lines), quartiles (box edges) and median (middle line of the boxes) of the distribution, and outliers are represented by a black point. Different levels of p-values threshold are indicated as follows: n.s. ($p \leq 1$); * ($p < 0.05$); *** ($p < 0.001$); **** ($p < 0.0001$).

For the Euclidean distance, ANOVA only detected a significant effect of the consensus filter (Figure 2E). Here again, all values below 100% yielded similar results (Figure 2F). The loss of quantitative accuracy at 100% is most likely due to the decrease in qualitative performance at this level, leading to a misassignment of sequences, ultimately resulting in a different predicted composition.

Based on these results, the taxonomic assignment appears very robust to different filtering values within the measured ranges. Best results are observed with a BLAST identity value of 100%, the bitscore difference filter should allow for a maximum of 4 bits difference and consensus should be determined using a majority vote (51%). More stringent parameters (lower bitscore difference and higher minimum consensus level) could be used if necessary to distinguish highly similar sequences, without predicted adverse effects.

3.3. Detection Limit

A common strategy to filter noise from real signals is to set a minimal proportion threshold under which the signal is considered negative. To find the optimal threshold, we calculated precision, and recall in 0.01% of total composition increments (Figure 3A). Recall rapidly decayed after 1%, consistent with the fact that many components were present at a 1% proportion in the dataset. Precision rapidly increased before reaching a plateau at around 0.1%. To find the optimal threshold, we calculated the F2-score, which is the geometric mean of the recall and precision, whereby the recall is considered twice as important as the precision. The F2-score maximum was reached at a threshold value of 0.093%, which can be rounded to 0.1%. This threshold value agrees with the previously published values for small curated databases [10,11].

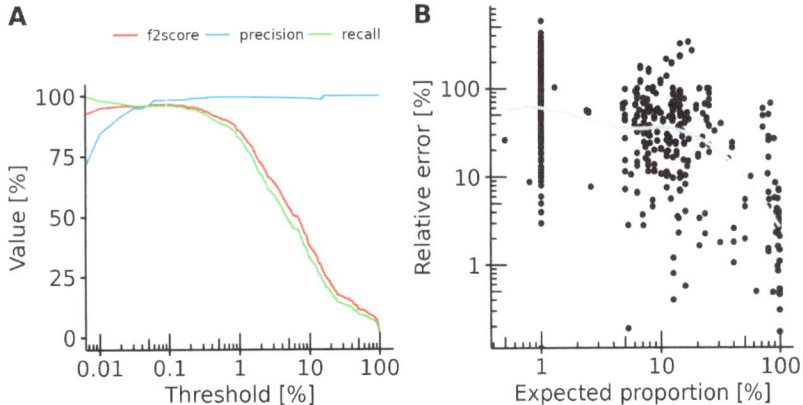

Figure 3. Workflow performances and determination of a minimal composition threshold. (**A**) The precision-recall curve shows the precision (blue), recall (green) and F2-scores (red) over a range of thresholds. The dashed grey line shows the threshold with the maximum F2-score. The X-axis is log10 scaled. (**B**) Relative quantification error in the function of the expected proportion in the sample. Each dot represents a single true positive result. The grey line represents the local estimated scatterplot smoothing. Both axes are log10 scaled.

3.4. Performance Evaluation

Based on the choice of parameters and threshold exposed previously, we calculated various performance metrics for the workflow at both species level, which is the highest resolution that can reasonably be obtained, and genus level, which, although not as resolutive as species, generally yields sufficient information for authenticity determination. At the species and genus levels, respectively, we observed a precision of 90% and 98%, meaning that 10% and 2% of the determined taxa were not expected in the samples. We also observed a recall of 93% and 96%, respectively, meaning that 7% and 4% of the taxa present in the sample were not found (Table 3). These results include 18 samples containing fallow deer (*Dama dama*) to various levels (Table S4). As we showed earlier, and as was previously published, fallow deer is a known miss for the 16S Dobrovolny method used here [9]. When correcting for fallow deer, the precision and recall increased to 90% and 96% at the species level, and 98% and 99% at the genus level. This is slightly lower than the previously reported 100% precision and recall for the method. However, these reports were based on the use of a custom database containing 51 entries at most [9–11]. The database used here contains entries for 16S sequences of over 7700 taxa (Table 1). It should be noted that the performance values reported here are slightly under-estimated. This is due to the fact that some proficiency test samples contain trace amounts of species not added intentionally, e.g., LVU_2018_B, DLA45/2019-2, and DLAptAUS2/2020-3.1, where the majority of participants detected red deer, goat, and horse, respectively, in addition to the expected species [47]. Similarly, several prediction errors are likely linked to incorrect sample compositions: both replicates of the LGC 7244 samples are false negative for chicken, due to chicken being detected under the 0.1% threshold, which was also reported in a previous study with another bioinformatic method [9]. The same study reported a goat positive result for the unintentional traces of goat in sample DLA45/2019-2, which we also observed with our method.

Table 3. Qualitative performance summary of the workflow.

Evaluation Rank	Confusion Matrix			Performance Metrics	
	True Positives	False Positives	False Negatives	Recall	Precision
Species [a]	490 (84%)	56 (10%)	39 (7%)	93%	90%
Species [b]	490 (86%)	56 (10%)	21 (4%)	96%	90%
Genus [a]	494 (95%)	6 (1%)	21 (4%)	96%	99%
Genus [b]	494 (98%)	6 (1%)	3 (1%)	99%	99%

[a] Including 18 *Dama dama* components. [b] Corrected for *Dama dama*.

We also measured the quantitative performance of the workflow by comparing expected vs. predicted proportions of components in the samples. For this, we calculated the absolute value of the difference between expected and predicted proportions and normalized it by the expected proportion (Figure 3B). The relative quantification error peaked at about 60% for components present at 1% in the samples and decreased to a few percent for components making up more than half of the sample. However, a large variance was observed, and the relative error varied to up to five times the expected amount for some low-concentration components. These values are within the variance reported previously, which was shown to be comparable to quantitative real-time PCR assays [9].

In conclusion, the workflow presented here is a very robust screening method for detecting components at 1% or higher. Results should however be interpreted with care and confirmed with a parallel assay such as quantitative or digital PCR, in particular, if quantification is needed.

3.5. Effects of Sequencing Depth on Prediction Recall and Variance

To determine the effects of sequencing depth on the precision and robustness of the results, we selected a subset of 35 samples with at least 350,000 read-pairs each, and whose composition structure was similar to that of the full dataset (Figure S4). We then randomly selected subsets of the samples to produce down-samples with 1000 to 200,000 reads each, in 8 independent replicates. Recall and Euclidean distances were then determined for each down-sample as previously described.

Apart from the sample with 1000 reads, all sampling depths led to comparable results in terms of recall and variance thereof (Figure 4A,B). With only 1000, we could observe a drop in the recall in many samples, which was associated with an increase in the variance of the recall within sample replicates. Only marginal improvements could be observed above 5000 reads, and until 80,000 reads. Above 80,000 reads, no increase in recall could be measured. The Euclidean distance, however, did not vary across the measured range of sampling depths (Figure 4C).

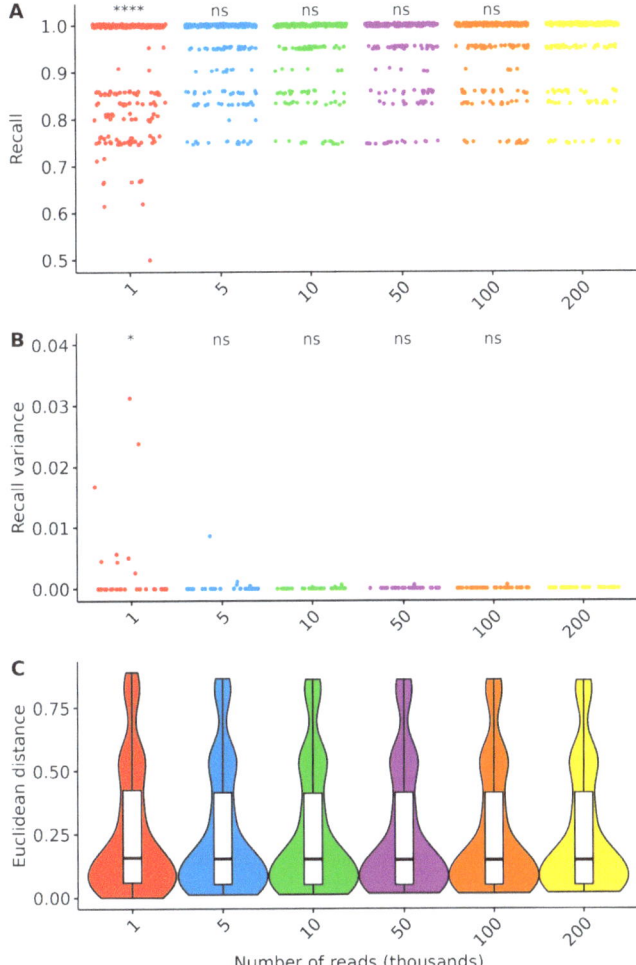

Figure 4. Effects of subsampling of prediction recall and robustness. (**A**) Sample recall across a range of sampling depths from 1000 to 200,000 reads. (**B**) Recall variance across a range of sampling depths. Each dot represents a sample. (**C**) Euclidean distance does not vary in the observed sampling depth range. Violin plots outlines represent the kernel density plot of the distribution, the included white boxplots represent the range (lines), quartiles (box edges) and median (middle line of the boxes) of the distribution, outliers are represented by a black point. Different levels of p-values threshold are indicated as follows: n.s. ($p \leq 1$); * ($p < 0.05$); **** ($p < 0.0001$).

The performance plateau reached at 5000 reads is consistent with a previous study on environmental samples metabarcoding [48], while theoretical calculations for metagenomics experiments proposed 15,000 reads for taxa identification at a 1% threshold [6]. These values are however results of simulations and should be verified experimentally. Most importantly, these do not account for random noise, which might become more visible when sequencing at low depths.

4. Discussion

Our aims here were threefold: (1) Compare the suitability of different published barcode sequences to distinguish mammal and bird species in the full BLAST NT database (2) Optimize the data analysis workflow for Illumina 16S rDNA sequencing using a large dataset of reference samples representative of typical food samples; (3) Validate the workflow and provide minimal input data criteria for accurate and reproducible analysis.

The choice of the barcode for metabarcoding analysis is not trivial and can heavily influence the results of the experiments. One must consider how common this sequence is in the taxa of interests, whether it is specific enough to distinguish different species, and whether it can reliably be amplified from the samples. We here compared a selection of 7 different published barcodes used for either Sanger-based species identification [36–38] or in metabarcoding experiments [8,11,14]. These sequences target either the 16S rDNA, COI/COX1, or cytB genes. For each of these, we determined how many taxa could be retrieved from the BLAST NT database. We measured the taxonomic specificity of each sequence retrieved this way. Finally, we specifically checked whether a set of usual food components or contaminants [40] could be identified using these sequences. We observed that cytB-based methods and especially the VDLUFA method [38], had the best-predicted performances across the Vertebrate clade. The 16S method from Dobrovolny et al. suffered from a lower predicted accuracy but was expected to be able to amplify sequences from most taxa of interest. In addition, it has the advantage of using a very short sequence of ~75 bp, allowing the analysis of highly processed products in which nucleic acids may be degraded [15]. This method is also currently being validated on a large scale and was previously shown to work for a range of food and feed products [9,10]. For these reasons, we chose to focus on this method for the rest of the study. It should however be noted that we predicted the cytB-based VDLUFA method to perform also very well, amplifying and distinguishing a large range of species. It could be a good complement to the Dobrovolny method, provided that the longer sequences of ~220 bp can be amplified from the samples to analyze.

We then set on optimizing the data analysis workflow by comparing different algorithms and parameter combinations on a set of reference samples. These span 32 taxa of interest and are enriched for concentrations at around 1%, which is the limit usually used for legal labeling obligations. The data analysis workflow can be separated into three main steps. Firstly, the reads are checked for quality, amplification primers and sequencing adapters are removed, and bad quality trailing bases are trimmed. Then the reads are grouped into clusters of similar sequences. Finally, each cluster is assigned to a taxonomic node [49]. With the selected method, the barcode is significantly shorter (~75 bp) than the sequencing reads (150 bp). In this case, the sequencing read goes through the amplicon. After primer trimming, the reads are halved, and trailing bad quality bases are already removed. Optimization of the read trimming was, therefore, not necessary here. This should, however, be considered when using a longer barcode, or when sequencing with shorter read lengths available on Illumina platforms.

The clustering step is important as it determines which sequences will be used to interrogate the reference database, and ultimately determine sample composition. Classically, reads are clustered in Operational Taxonomic Units (OTUs) by identity threshold, in general with an identity level of 97%, although it was discussed in recent years that much higher thresholds should be used [27,46]. The accuracy of OTUs is now largely contested, and new statistical methods have been published that aim at determining Amplicon Sequence Variants (ASVs) using denoising procedures [30]. ASVs are expected to better represent the sample composition, whereas OTUs generally overestimate diversity [45]. While OTUs at 97% identity group highly similar sequences and 100% identity would simply dereplicate sequencing reads without filtering noise, ASVs address both issues by determining the correct sequences based on read quality scores. However, several publications nuanced this claim, putting ASVs on par with OTUs [50,51]. Here, we compared the effects of identity clustering at 95%, 97%, 100% (dereplication), and denoising and found no significant differences in terms of prediction accuracy. ASVs did result in a slightly higher yield, and the number of clusters determined was much closer to the true composition of the sample, resulting in a faster processing time than dereplication. For these reasons, we chose to keep working with ASVs, although OTUs led to highly similar results. We expect this result to be generalizable to different barcodes.

Most published meat-metabarcoding methods used reference databases containing only a selected number of entries (between 2 and 500). This has the advantage of ensuring that the database only contains high confidence, high quality sequences and drastically simplifies taxonomic assignment. However, this has the drawback of hiding a large chunk of potential adulteration with species not present in the reference database. Taxonomic assignment using the full BLAST NT database as a reference revealed challenges due to mislabelling of sequences, the presence of low quality sequences, and large heterogeneity in taxa representations. We used a set of filters that enabled us to overcome these hurdles. We restricted the BLAST search by using a mask selecting taxa placed under the Vertebrate node, thus ensuring that no other sequences would contaminate the results. Furthermore, we then applied a coverage threshold of 100%, ensuring that only sequences aligning to the totality of the barcode would be recovered. The minimal identity level required was varied between 95% and 100%, and we determined that it should optimally be 98% or higher. We then used a filter based on the bitscore value of each result, representing the quality of the alignment between the barcode and the reference. Although the E-value is commonly used for filtering BLAST results, this value varies with the size of the database, rendering an E-value filter obsolete as the database grows in size, whereas the bitscore only depends on the alignment and therefore only varies with the barcode used [52]. Therefore, we determined the bitscore of the best alignment for each barcode sequence and kept only these results that were within a certain distance of the best results. We found the optimal value for the bitscore difference to be between 0 and 4. These filtering procedures typically resulted in a few different possible taxa. In order to determine the most likely taxon for each sequence, we used a consensus threshold [32] and found the optimal value of the minimal consensus to be between 51% and 80%. This allowed the assignment of a unique taxon to each barcode sequence in the sample, albeit at a rank depending on the confidence of the BLAST result. Most results were assigned at the species or genus level, allowing for a meaningful interpretation of the results. We expect the parameter choices for the taxonomic assignment step to be highly dependent on both the database and the barcode used. They should therefore be revalidated for each barcode and when the database is updated.

Errors stemming from the PCR-amplification and sequencing processes almost always result in a low amount of wrongly assigned reads that need to be filtered. Fixing a threshold at which results become significant becomes increasingly difficult as the detection limit decreases. We here determined the best threshold to be at around 0.1% to optimally balance precision and recall of the analysis, while ensuring a detection limit at 1% of the true sample composition. The optimized workflow resulted in 1% of both false-positive and false-negative results, while the quantification accuracy was comparable to that of other DNA-based methods [9]. Moreover, the results were identical to those of a previously published analysis of part of this dataset using a different bioinformatics workflow and a database consisting of only 51 entries [9]. These validation values indicate that the workflow allows for robust screening methods. The cost-effectiveness of NGS-based methods is an important consideration for laboratories. It was previously calculated that metabarcoding can be more cost-efficient than PCR when parallelizing enough samples [9]. In order to estimate the number of reads required for a robust analysis, we down-sampled a part of our dataset and calculated the recall and variability of the analysis for a range of 1000 to 200,000 reads. We determined that the results did not significantly improve beyond 5000 reads. This is far below the previous recommendations of 120,000 to 200,000 reads [9,11]. There is therefore a potential for further decreasing the costs of metabarcoding analysis. This result is in line with previous calculations [48], but should be verified experimentally.

The use of the full BLAST NT database allows us to take full advantage of the untargeted aspect of metabarcoding methods, however, it comes with its own set of limitations as the database contains some doubtful sequences and annotations and is highly biased towards commercially interesting and model species. One could consider using the BOLD database, which is more tightly curated than BLAST [5]. This database is, however, largely incomplete for 16S rDNA sequences, and more suitable for cytB or COI/COX1 sequences. Several publications have tried to address this problem directly, either by selecting sequences with trustful metadata and setting some quality filters [27], or by assigning quality scores to each sequence and using them to either filter the database or assign confidence scores to metabarcoding results [53]. These approaches should be explored in future works, with the aim of optimizing food authentication methods.

In order to improve reproducible analysis and ease the dissemination of the metabarcoding methods in laboratories, we packaged the analysis workflow in a free open-source software [28]. The workflow is implemented using Snakemake [54] and runs on UNIX platforms. It allows for scalable and reproducible automated analysis of amplicon sequencing runs on Illumina platforms. It also contains a module comparing the workflow's results to the theoretical composition of the samples, making the validation process straightforward. Another module allows us to run the same analysis using different sets of parameters and compare the results with each other, significantly simplifying the process of finding the optimal set of parameters for new barcodes or matrices.

5. Conclusions

The results of the present study demonstrate the accuracy and robustness of the 16S metabarcoding method as a tool for meat authenticity testing. This study proposes standardization of the data analysis and shows that it can be used with non-curated nucleotide databases such as the BLAST NT database, thereby expanding the detection range. Furthermore, the workflow presented here is versatile and can be adapted to other food matrices, such as plants, seafood, insects, or spice mixtures, making it a valuable tool for a wide range of products. With the increasing demand for transparency and traceability in the food supply chain, this method has the potential to play a significant role in helping to ensure that consumers can trust the food they are eating.

Supplementary Materials: The following supporting information can be downloaded at: https://www.mdpi.com/article/10.3390/foods12050968/s1. Table S1. Sample composition; Table S2. Published methods for mammals and birds barcoding; Table S3. Published meat-metabarcoding studies and workflow parameters; Table S4. Optimized workflow results at the genus level; Figure S1. Performance metrics for different number of authorized mismatch in the overlapping sequence when using denoising. (A) Yield of the analysis in proportion of retained reads; (B) Average precision (recall-weighted) of the analysis; (C) Euclidian distance between predicted and expected values; Figure S2. Effects of chimeras detection and filtering on the analysis performances. (A) Yield of the analysis in proportion of retained reads; (B) Average precision (recall-weighted) of the analysis; (C) Euclidian distance between predicted and expected values; Figure S3. Effects of E-value thresholds on the analysis performances. (A) Average precision (recall-weighted) of the analysis; (B) Euclidian distance between predicted and expected values; Figure S4. Creation of down-samples. (A) Read counts in the full dataset. (B) Composition structure in the full dataset. (C) Composition structure in the samples selected for subsampling.

Author Contributions: Conceptualization, formal analysis, data curation, software, visualization, and original draft: G.D.; funding acquisition: C.B.-N.; resources and investigation: A.W., C.B.-N., H.P., K.P. and L.P.; review and editing: all authors. All authors have read and agreed to the published version of the manuscript.

Funding: We gratefully acknowledge funding for metabarcoding analyses of CVUA-MEL by the Ministry for Environment, Agriculture, Conservation and Consumer Protection of the State of North Rhine-Westphalia (2020; AZ: 8.80.01.02.07).

Data Availability Statement: The FooDMe and BaRCoD workflows are openly available from github and referenced on Zenodo at: github.com/CVUA-RRW/FooDMe (DOI: 10.5281/zenodo.7078595) and github.com/CVUA-RRW/BaRCoD (DOI: 10.5281/zenodo.6976282). The dataset used for the analysis is openly available from the European Nucleotide Archive (ENA) at ebi.ac.uk/ena/browser/home, under Project accession PRJEB57117. The NCBI NT database is available from ftp.ncbi.nlm.nih.gov/blast/db/. Additional code used for figure preparation and detailed analysis results for all samples and parameter combinations are available upon request.

Acknowledgments: The authors thank in no particular order: LVU Lippold Gbr for releasing data on sample composition ahead of the official date. CVUA-RRW's IT department for their continuous technical support. Past and present members of the §64-LFGB working group "species identification" for fruitful discussions.

Conflicts of Interest: The authors declare no conflict of interest.

References

1. Ballin, N.Z. Authentication of Meat and Meat Products. *Meat Sci.* **2010**, *86*, 577–587. [CrossRef] [PubMed]
2. Montowska, M.; Pospiech, E. Authenticity Determination of Meat and Meat Products on the Protein and DNA Basis. *Food Rev. Int.* **2010**, *27*, 84–100. [CrossRef]
3. Rau, J.; Hiller, E.; Männig, A.; Dyk, M.; Wenninger, O.; Stoll, P.; Wibbelt, G.; Schreiter, P. Animal Species Identification of Meat Using MALDI-TOF Mass Spectrometry. *ChemRxiv* **2021**. [CrossRef]
4. NCBI Resource Coordinators Database Resources of the National Center for Biotechnology Information. *Nucleic Acids Res.* **2016**, *44*, D7–D19. [CrossRef]
5. Ratnasingham, S.; Hebert, P.D.N. Bold: The Barcode of Life Data System. *Mol. Ecol. Notes* **2007**, *7*, 355–364. [CrossRef]
6. Haiminen, N.; Edlund, S.; Chambliss, D.; Kunitomi, M.; Weimer, B.C.; Ganesan, B.; Baker, R.; Markwell, P.; Davis, M.; Huang, B.C.; et al. Food Authentication from Shotgun Sequencing Reads with an Application on High Protein Powders. *Npj Sci. Food* **2019**, *3*, 24. [CrossRef]
7. Ripp, F.; Krombholz, C.F.; Liu, Y.; Weber, M.; Schäfer, A.; Schmidt, M.; Köppel, R.; Hankeln, T. All-Food-Seq (AFS): A Quantifiable Screen for Species in Biological Samples by Deep DNA Sequencing. *BMC Genom.* **2014**, *15*, 639. [CrossRef]
8. Xing, R.-R.; Wang, N.; Hu, R.-R.; Zhang, J.-K.; Han, J.-X.; Chen, Y. Application of next Generation Sequencing for Species Identification in Meat and Poultry Products: A DNA Metabarcoding Approach. *Food Control* **2019**, *101*, 173–179. [CrossRef]
9. Preckel, L.; Brünen-Nieweler, C.; Denay, G.; Petersen, H.; Cichna-Markl, M.; Dobrovolny, S.; Hochegger, R. Identification of Mammalian and Poultry Species in Food and Pet Food Samples Using 16S RDNA Metabarcoding. *Foods* **2021**, *10*, 2875. [CrossRef]
10. Dobrovolny, S.; Uhlig, S.; Frost, K.; Schlierf, A.; Nichani, K.; Simon, K.; Cichna-Markl, M.; Hochegger, R. Interlaboratory Validation of a DNA Metabarcoding Assay for Mammalian and Poultry Species to Detect Food Adulteration. *Foods* **2022**, *11*, 1108. [CrossRef]
11. Dobrovolny, S.; Blaschitz, M.; Weinmaier, T.; Pechatschek, J.; Cichna-Markl, M.; Indra, A.; Hufnagl, P.; Hochegger, R. Development of a DNA Metabarcoding Method for the Identification of Fifteen Mammalian and Six Poultry Species in Food. *Food Chem.* **2019**, *272*, 354–361. [CrossRef] [PubMed]
12. Ribani, A.; Schiavo, G.; Utzeri, V.J.; Bertolini, F.; Geraci, C.; Bovo, S.; Fontanesi, L. Application of next Generation Semiconductor Based Sequencing for Species Identification and Analysis of Within-Species Mitotypes Useful for Authentication of Meat Derived Products. *Food Control* **2018**, *91*, 58–67. [CrossRef]
13. Bertolini, F.; Ghionda, M.C.; D'Alessandro, E.; Geraci, C.; Chiofalo, V.; Fontanesi, L. A Next Generation Semiconductor Based Sequencing Approach for the Identification of Meat Species in DNA Mixtures. *PLoS ONE* **2015**, *10*, e0121701. [CrossRef] [PubMed]
14. Palumbo, F.; Scariolo, F.; Vannozzi, A.; Barcaccia, G. NGS-Based Barcoding with Mini-COI Gene Target Is Useful for Pet Food Market Surveys Aimed at Mislabelling Detection. *Sci. Rep.* **2020**, *10*, 17767. [CrossRef]
15. Gryson, N. Effect of Food Processing on Plant DNA Degradation and PCR-Based GMO Analysis: A Review. *Anal. Bioanal. Chem.* **2010**, *396*, 2003–2022. [CrossRef]
16. Piombo, E.; Abdelfattah, A.; Droby, S.; Wisniewski, M.; Spadaro, D.; Schena, L. Metagenomics Approaches for the Detection and Surveillance of Emerging and Recurrent Plant Pathogens. *Microorganisms* **2021**, *9*, 188. [CrossRef]
17. Bruno, A.; Sandionigi, A.; Agostinetto, G.; Bernabovi, L.; Frigerio, J.; Casiraghi, M.; Labra, M. Food Tracking Perspective: DNA Metabarcoding to Identify Plant Composition in Complex and Processed Food Products. *Genes* **2019**, *10*, 248. [CrossRef]
18. Raclariu-Manolică, A.C.; Anmarkrud, J.A.; Kierczak, M.; Rafati, N.; Thorbek, B.L.G.; Schrøder-Nielsen, A.; de Boer, H.J. DNA Metabarcoding for Quality Control of Basil, Oregano, and Paprika. *Front. Plant Sci.* **2021**, *12*, 665618. [CrossRef]
19. Gense, K.; Peterseil, V.; Licina, A.; Wagner, M.; Cichna-Markl, M.; Dobrovolny, S.; Hochegger, R. Development of a DNA Metabarcoding Method for the Identification of Bivalve Species in Seafood Products. *Foods* **2021**, *10*, 2618. [CrossRef]
20. Li, H. Lh3/Seqtk. Available online: https://github.com/lh3/seqtk (accessed on 24 October 2022).
21. Denay, G. CVUA-RRW/BaRCoD: BaRCoD v1.1.1. Available online: https://zenodo.org/record/6976282 (accessed on 24 October 2022).
22. Camacho, C.; Coulouris, G.; Avagyan, V.; Ma, N.; Papadopoulos, J.; Bealer, K.; Madden, T.L. BLAST+: Architecture and Applications. *BMC Bioinform.* **2009**, *10*, 421. [CrossRef]

23. Ye, J.; Coulouris, G.; Zaretskaya, I.; Cutcutache, I.; Rozen, S.; Madden, T.L. Primer-BLAST: A Tool to Design Target-Specific Primers for Polymerase Chain Reaction. *BMC Bioinform.* **2012**, *13*, 134. [CrossRef] [PubMed]
24. Martin, M. Cutadapt Removes Adapter Sequences from High-Throughput Sequencing Reads. *EMBnet. J.* **2011**, *17*, 10–12. [CrossRef]
25. Rognes, T.; Flouri, T.; Nichols, B.; Quince, C.; Mahé, F. VSEARCH: A Versatile Open Source Tool for Metagenomics. *PeerJ* **2016**, *4*, e2584. [CrossRef] [PubMed]
26. Denay, G. CVUA-RRW/TaxidTools: 2.2.3. Available online: https://zenodo.org/record/5556006 (accessed on 26 August 2022).
27. Edgar, R.C. Updating the 97% Identity Threshold for 16S Ribosomal RNA OTUs. *Bioinformatics* **2018**, *34*, 2371–2375. [CrossRef] [PubMed]
28. Denay, G. CVUA-RRW/FooDMe: Foodme v1.6.3. Available online: https://zenodo.org/record/7078595 (accessed on 14 September 2022).
29. Chen, S.; Zhou, Y.; Chen, Y.; Gu, J. Fastp: An Ultra-Fast All-in-One FASTQ Preprocessor. *Bioinformatics* **2018**, *34*, i884–i890. [CrossRef] [PubMed]
30. Callahan, B.J.; McMurdie, P.J.; Rosen, M.J.; Han, A.W.; Johnson, A.J.A.; Holmes, S.P. DADA2: High-Resolution Sample Inference from Illumina Amplicon Data. *Nat. Methods* **2016**, *13*, 581–583. [CrossRef]
31. Bazinet, A.L.; Ondov, B.D.; Sommer, D.D.; Ratnayake, S. BLAST-Based Validation of Metagenomic Sequence Assignments. *PeerJ* **2018**, *6*, e4892. [CrossRef]
32. Bokulich, N.A.; Kaehler, B.D.; Rideout, J.R.; Dillon, M.; Bolyen, E.; Knight, R.; Huttley, G.A.; Gregory Caporaso, J. Optimizing Taxonomic Classification of Marker-Gene Amplicon Sequences with QIIME 2's Q2-Feature-Classifier Plugin. *Microbiome* **2018**, *6*, 90. [CrossRef]
33. Pedregosa, F.; Varoquaux, G.; Gramfort, A.; Michel, V.; Thirion, B.; Grisel, O.; Blondel, M.; Prettenhofer, P.; Weiss, R.; Dubourg, V.; et al. Scikit-Learn: Machine Learning in Python. *J. Mach. Learn. Res.* **2011**, *12*, 2825–2830.
34. Wickham, H.; Averick, M.; Bryan, J.; Chang, W.; McGowan, L.D.; François, R.; Grolemund, G.; Hayes, A.; Henry, L.; Hester, J.; et al. Welcome to the Tidyverse. *J. Open Source Softw.* **2019**, *4*, 1686. [CrossRef]
35. Harris, C.R.; Millman, K.J.; van der Walt, S.J.; Gommers, R.; Virtanen, P.; Cournapeau, D.; Wieser, E.; Taylor, J.; Berg, S.; Smith, N.J.; et al. Array Programming with NumPy. *Nature* **2020**, *585*, 357–362. [CrossRef] [PubMed]
36. Meyer, R.; Höfelein, C.; Lüthy, J.; Candrian, U. Polymerase Chain Reaction-Restriction Fragment Length Polymorphism Analysis: A Simple Method for Species Identification in Food. *J. AOAC Int.* **1995**, *78*, 1542–1551. [CrossRef] [PubMed]
37. Palumbi, S.R.; Martin, A.; Romano, S.; McMillan, W.O.; Stice, L.; Grabowski, G. *The Simple Fool's Guide to PCR*, 2nd ed.; University of Hawaii at Manoa, Kewalo Marine Laboratory, Dept. of Zoology and Kewalo Marine Laboratory; University of Hawaii: Honolulu, HI, USA, 2002; pp. 25–37.
38. Verband Deutscher Landwirtschaftlicher Untersuchungs-und Forschungsanstalten MB3-29.1 Molekularbiologischer Nachweis von tierischen Bestandteilen (PCR-Methode). In *125 Jahre Verband Deutscher Landwirtschaftlicher Untersuchungs-und Forschungsanstalten e.V: Eine Dokumentation*; VDLUFA-Schriftenreihe; VDLUFA-Verl: Darmstadt, Germany, 2013; ISBN 978-3-941273-14-6.
39. Szabo, K.; Malorny, B.; Stoyke, M. Etablierung der § 64 LFGB Arbeitsgruppen "NGS—Bakteriencharakterisierung" und "NGS—Speziesidentifizierung". *J. Consum. Prot. Food Saf.* **2020**, *15*, 85–89. [CrossRef]
40. Matthes, N.; Pietsch, K.; Rullmann, A.; Näumann, G.; Pöpping, B.; Szabo, K. The Barcoding Table of Animal Species (BaTAnS): A New Tool to Select Appropriate Methods for Animal Species Identification Using DNA Barcoding. *Mol. Biol. Rep.* **2020**, *47*, 6457–6461. [CrossRef]
41. BVL—Amtliche Sammlung von Untersuchungsverfahren—Barcoding-Tabelle Für Die Tierartenbestimmung (Barcoding Table of Animal Species—BaTAnS). Available online: https://www.bvl.bund.de/SharedDocs/Downloads/07_Untersuchungen/Barcoding-Tabelle%20f%C3%BCr%20die%20Tierartenbestimmung.html?nn=11009496 (accessed on 26 August 2022).
42. Dobrovolny, S.; Austrian Agency for Health and Food Safety (AGES), Institute for Food Safety, Vienna, Austria. Fallow Deer Primers. Personal communication, 2022.
43. Karlsson, A.O.; Holmlund, G. Identification of Mammal Species Using Species-Specific DNA Pyrosequencing. *Forensic Sci. Int.* **2007**, *173*, 16–20. [CrossRef]
44. Blaxter, M.; Mann, J.; Chapman, T.; Thomas, F.; Whitton, C.; Floyd, R.; Abebe, E. Defining Operational Taxonomic Units Using DNA Barcode Data. *Philos. Trans. R. Soc. B Biol. Sci.* **2005**, *360*, 1935–1943. [CrossRef]
45. Callahan, B.J.; McMurdie, P.J.; Holmes, S.P. Exact Sequence Variants Should Replace Operational Taxonomic Units in Marker-Gene Data Analysis. *ISME J.* **2017**, *11*, 2639–2643. [CrossRef]
46. Westcott, S.L.; Schloss, P.D. De Novo Clustering Methods Outperform Reference-Based Methods for Assigning 16S RRNA Gene Sequences to Operational Taxonomic Units. *PeerJ* **2015**, *3*, e1487. [CrossRef]
47. DLA Proficiency Tests Gmbh. Ring-Trials Reports for PtAUS3.2 and 45/2019. Private communication, 2020.
48. Dully, V.; Balliet, H.; Frühe, L.; Däumer, M.; Thielen, A.; Gallie, S.; Berrill, I.; Stoeck, T. Robustness, Sensitivity and Reproducibility of EDNA Metabarcoding as an Environmental Biomonitoring Tool in Coastal Salmon Aquaculture—An Inter-Laboratory Study. *Ecol. Indic.* **2021**, *121*, 107049. [CrossRef]
49. Staats, M.; Arulandhu, A.J.; Gravendeel, B.; Holst-Jensen, A.; Scholtens, I.; Peelen, T.; Prins, T.W.; Kok, E. Advances in DNA Metabarcoding for Food and Wildlife Forensic Species Identification. *Anal. Bioanal. Chem.* **2016**, *408*, 4615–4630. [CrossRef]

50. García-López, R.; Cornejo-Granados, F.; Lopez-Zavala, A.A.; Cota-Huízar, A.; Sotelo-Mundo, R.R.; Gómez-Gil, B.; Ochoa-Leyva, A. OTUs and ASVs Produce Comparable Taxonomic and Diversity from Shrimp Microbiota 16S Profiles Using Tailored Abundance Filters. *Genes* **2021**, *12*, 564. [CrossRef] [PubMed]
51. Chiarello, M.; McCauley, M.; Villéger, S.; Jackson, C.R. Ranking the Biases: The Choice of OTUs vs. ASVs in 16S RRNA Amplicon Data Analysis Has Stronger Effects on Diversity Measures than Rarefaction and OTU Identity Threshold. *PLoS ONE* **2022**, *17*, e0264443. [CrossRef] [PubMed]
52. Altschul, S.F.; Gish, W.; Miller, W.; Myers, E.W.; Lipman, D.J. Basic Local Alignment Search Tool. *J. Mol. Biol.* **1990**, *215*, 403–410. [CrossRef] [PubMed]
53. Neto, L.; Pinto, N.; Proença, A.; Amorim, A.; Conde-Sousa, E. 4SpecID: Reference DNA Libraries Auditing and Annotation System for Forensic Applications. *Genes* **2021**, *12*, 61. [CrossRef] [PubMed]
54. Mölder, F.; Jablonski, K.P.; Letcher, B.; Hall, M.B.; Tomkins-Tinch, C.H.; Sochat, V.; Forster, J.; Lee, S.; Twardziok, S.O.; Kanitz, A.; et al. Sustainable Data Analysis with Snakemake. *F1000Research* **2021**, *10*, 33. [CrossRef] [PubMed]

Disclaimer/Publisher's Note: The statements, opinions and data contained in all publications are solely those of the individual author(s) and contributor(s) and not of MDPI and/or the editor(s). MDPI and/or the editor(s) disclaim responsibility for any injury to people or property resulting from any ideas, methods, instructions or products referred to in the content.

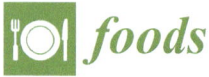

Communication

Development of Non-Targeted Mass Spectrometry Method for Distinguishing Spelt and Wheat

Kapil Nichani [1,2], Steffen Uhlig [3], Bertrand Colson [1], Karina Hettwer [1], Kirsten Simon [1], Josephine Bönick [4], Carsten Uhlig [5], Sabine Kemmlein [6], Manfred Stoyke [6,†], Petra Gowik [6], Gerd Huschek [7] and Harshadrai M. Rawel [2,*]

1. QuoData GmbH, Prellerstr. 14, D-01309 Dresden, Germany
2. Institute of Nutritional Science, University of Potsdam, Arthur-Scheunert-Allee 114-116, D-14558 Nuthetal, Germany
3. QuoData GmbH, Fabeckstr. 43, D-14195 Berlin, Germany
4. Bundesinstitut für Risikobewertung, Max-Dohrn-Str. 8-10, D-10589 Berlin, Germany
5. Akees GmbH, Ansbacher Str. 11, D-10787 Berlin, Germany
6. Bundesamt für Verbraucherschutz und Lebensmittelsicherheit, Diedersdorfer Weg. 1, D-12277 Berlin, Germany
7. IGV-Institut für Getreideverarbeitung GmbH, Arthur-Scheunert-Allee 40/41, D-14558 Nuthetal, Germany
* Correspondence: rawel@uni-potsdam.de
† Currently independent researcher.

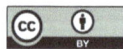

Citation: Nichani, K.; Uhlig, S.; Colson, B.; Hettwer, K.; Simon, K.; Bönick, J.; Uhlig, C.; Kemmlein, S.; Stoyke, M.; Gowik, P.; et al. Development of Non-Targeted Mass Spectrometry Method for Distinguishing Spelt and Wheat. *Foods* 2023, *12*, 141. https://doi.org/10.3390/foods12010141

Academic Editor: Maria Castro-Puyana

Received: 21 November 2022
Revised: 13 December 2022
Accepted: 21 December 2022
Published: 27 December 2022

Copyright: © 2022 by the authors. Licensee MDPI, Basel, Switzerland. This article is an open access article distributed under the terms and conditions of the Creative Commons Attribution (CC BY) license (https://creativecommons.org/licenses/by/4.0/).

Abstract: Food fraud, even when not in the news, is ubiquitous and demands the development of innovative strategies to combat it. A new non-targeted method (NTM) for distinguishing spelt and wheat is described, which aids in food fraud detection and authenticity testing. A highly resolved fingerprint in the form of spectra is obtained for several cultivars of spelt and wheat using liquid chromatography coupled high-resolution mass spectrometry (LC-HRMS). Convolutional neural network (CNN) models are built using a nested cross validation (NCV) approach by appropriately training them using a calibration set comprising duplicate measurements of eleven cultivars of wheat and spelt, each. The results reveal that the CNNs automatically learn patterns and representations to best discriminate tested samples into spelt or wheat. This is further investigated using an external validation set comprising artificially mixed spectra, samples for processed goods (spelt bread and flour), eleven untypical spelt, and six old wheat cultivars. These cultivars were not part of model building. We introduce a metric called the D score to quantitatively evaluate and compare the classification decisions. Our results demonstrate that NTMs based on NCV and CNNs trained using appropriately chosen spectral data can be reliable enough to be used on a wider range of cultivars and their mixes.

Keywords: non-targeted methods; LC-MS; fingerprinting; machine learning; convolutional neural networks; wheat; spelt; food fraud

1. Introduction

Public awareness around food fraud and food authenticity is mainly driven by high-visibility media discussions, e.g., in connection with public health consequences or when a large-scale operation is uncovered and the ensuing scandal brings disrepute to companies or regulatory authorities [1,2]. However, even when not topical, food fraud is widespread and exacts considerable economic costs [3,4]. Its manifold manifestations include adulteration, mislabeling, dilution, substitution, etc. [5]. Establishing procedures and quality indicators to detect food fraud, therefore, continues to be an important and urgent task [4].

Being one of the most important food crops in the world, wheat, its varieties, and derived products are defenseless against rampant fraud [6]. Analytical testing for determination of authenticity and detection of fraud is an important control measure to identify, monitor, and act—to ensure consumer safety and punish the perpetrators [7]. The testing can range from differentiating grain types, e.g., durum, einkorn, spelt, etc. [8], tracing geographic identity [9], especially protected geographic identity, e.g., that of Fränkischer Grünkern (a spelt product) [10], testing the presence of adulterants [11,12], and checking crop growing or harvesting conditions (e.g., organic wheat) [13], among others.

It is reported that spelt (*Triticum spelta*) is one of the three ancient wheats that are considered to be the ancestors of modern wheat. The other two are emmer and einkorn. Genetic data suggests that spelt can occur from the hybridization of bread wheat and emmer wheat, but only after the first *Aegilops*-tetraploid wheat hybridization. The considerably later development of spelt in Europe might be attributed to a later, second hybridization between emmer and bread wheat [14]. Hence, for centuries, spelt (or *"Dinkel"* in German) has remained a major grain in the DACH region (Germany, Switzerland, and Austria) [15]. They are very resilient to austere irrigation conditions while having favorable digestive and nutritional values [16]. As a consequence, its demand and market price are on the rise. Lately, spelt has become part of many bakery products, pasta, noodles, and even beer [17]. In light of accelerating demand and consumption of spelt and spelt-derived products, it is hard to ignore the possibility of market-driven fraudulent practices. As these grains command a premium price, there is an economic benefit to devising new tactics for adulteration, tampering, substitution, etc. Thus, there is a need to address this through the development of new methods for distinguishing spelt and wheat [18,19]. At this point, it is necessary to mention that addressing the economic or nutritional benefits of spelt over wheat is outside the scope of this work.

Spelt is mostly referred to by its phylogenetic and morphological characteristics, but in practice, unequivocal identification of spelt based on physiological properties is non-trivial [20–23]. Perhaps this is because of its close botanical relationship with wheat and crossbreeding over hundreds of years. Consequently, determining whether a cultivar can be classified as spelt is challenging [22]. Switzerland maintains guidelines laid out through IP-SUISSE and Bio-Suisse in cooperation with IG Dinkel to regulate the growing and selling of certain old spelt species (Urdinkel in German) [24]. Thus, the questions arise: which cultivars are true spelt, and how can they be determined?—the latter being the more challenging question. The general European Union (EU) legal framework, as put forward in regulations such as 2017/625 and 1169/2011, aims to ensure food safety and consumer protection by compelling producers to correctly label ingredients and their sources [25,26]. In this case, product labeling must be combined with an authentication analysis of grain ingredients and additives. Under the circumstances of the lack of consensus on which cultivars are truly spelt, the challenge of performing an authentication analysis is formidable. The challenges of discerning species only snowball when it comes to processed goods, such as bakery items. In Germany, there is a guideline (Leitsätze des Deutschen Lebensmittelbuchs für Brot und Kleingebäck) that serves as a guiding principle for the manufacture and sale of spelt bread [27]. It states that spelt bread must contain at least 90% spelt. Thereby, processed goods will certainly contain wheat along with spelt, which only further complicates the process of identifying or detecting spelt for authenticity testing. Adding newer cultivars of spelt to the mix, such as "pre-spelt," or "wheat-spelt" crossed cultivars (together referred to in this work as "untypical spelts"), only increases the challenge to unequivocally define what is spelt and what is not.

Non-targeted methods (NTMs) are being increasingly developed and deployed in the detection of food fraud and ratifying the authenticity of food substances [28–30]. An NTM encompasses analytical measurement, resulting in, e.g., a highly resolved fingerprint (referred to herein as the wet lab procedure), followed by mathematical modeling and data evaluation (referred to as the dry lab procedure), without laying a special spotlight on predetermined analytes of interest [31].

In the wet lab part, mass spectrometry (MS) based testing is a dominant and useful kind of NTM [32]. Coupling with liquid chromatographic (LC) separation and connection to a high-resolution (HR) mass analyzer like the time of flight (TOF) enables precise mass determination at different retention times (Rt) [33]. The resulting LC-HRMS spectra are useful to capture the slightest differences between sample populations, which arise because peptides and proteins in food substances are expressed differentially, not only due to inherent genetic composition but also due to external factors that might have their genesis in nature (such as soil type and quality, climatic conditions) or be caused by humans (agricultural practices, adulteration, mixing, etc.) [34].

The other important component of an NTM is the dry lab, which includes statistical modeling [31]. Given the complexity and size of the measurement data that is generated with LC-HRMS, there is a need to resort to contemporary machine learning methods like neural networks [35,36]. Neural networks have become increasingly popular in different application areas, including MS, because several studies have been reported in the literature exploiting neural networks for MS data. The strategies in the reported studies can be essentially grouped by the different tasks undertaken, for instance, (1) peak pre-processing such as normalization [37] and peak alignment [38], (2) evaluation of peak features [39–42], (3) spectra prediction [43], (4) spectral annotation and molecular structure prediction [44,45], and (5) classification of samples based on the associated spectra. The fifth strategy can be divided into two types: one that utilizes a peak list or feature list, and the other that uses the entire spectrum. With the latter, a few reports have explored using 1-d MS spectra with convolutional neural networks (CNN) [46–48].

CNNs are a type of neural network that have been shown to be powerful for image processing tasks like face classification and recognition [49,50]. Herein, we aim to apply these capabilities to parse HR mass spectra with normalized mass windows (SWATH acquisition) [51] and, thereby, classify spelt or wheat (as illustrated in Figure 1A). An image can be formed from the 2-d spectral data using the peak height intensities for each mass/charge (m/z) and Rt (see Figure 1B,C). The combination of 2-D spectral data with CNNs as an NTM for the classification of spelt and wheat has not been previously reported, to the best of our knowledge. To this end, in this work, we describe an NTM in which the wet lab component captures the food fingerprint (peptide marker profile) using LC-HRMS and the dry lab component uses CNN to learn the differences between the fingerprints and eventually classify the tested sample. The predicted outcomes are compared using a new metric that we call the D score.

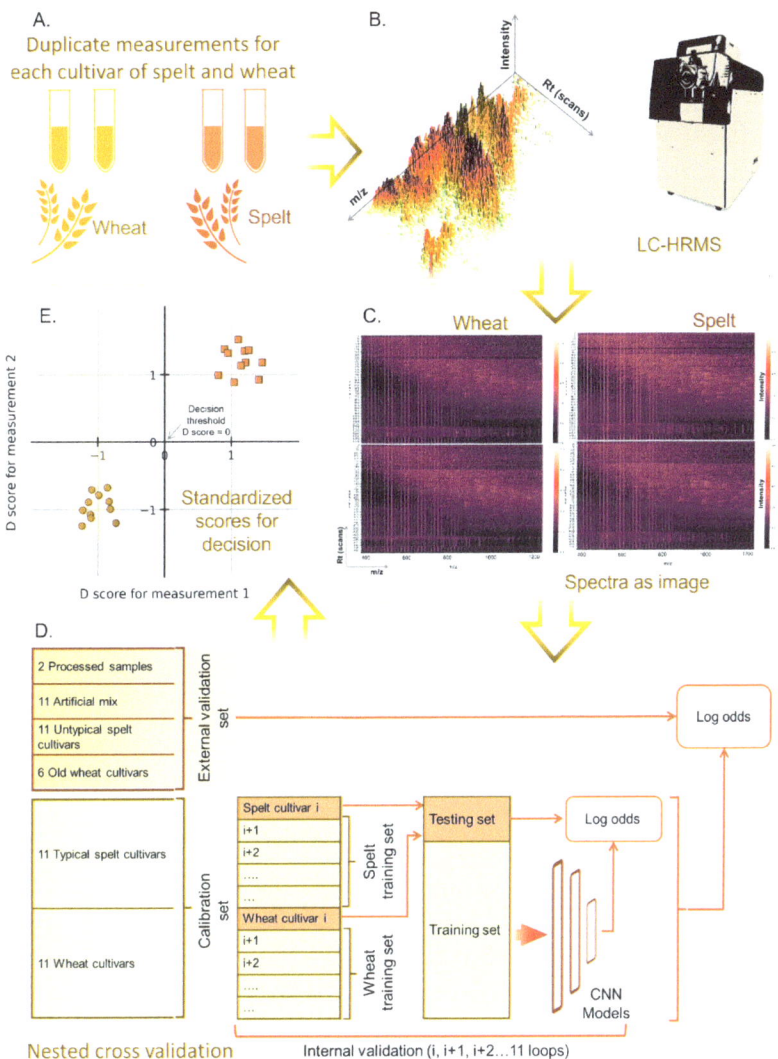

Figure 1. Schematic illustration showing the high-resolution liquid chromatography mass spectrometry (LC-HRMS) based non-targeted method (NTM) proposed and developed in this work to distinguish spelt and wheat. (**A**) Duplicate samples for each cultivar of spelt and wheat were prepared, and (**B**) measured using a SCIEX ESI-TripleTOF 5600 with SWATH acquisition. (**C**) The 2-D spectra are depicted as an image with mass by charge (m/z) as the x-axis, retention time (Rt) as the y-axis, and intensity as the z-axis. The exemplary images shown are the duplicate measurement spectra for Bernstein wheat and Badekrone spelt. (**D**) A nested cross validation (NCV) approach was adopted with a separate calibration and external validation set. Convolutional neural network (CNN) models trained with 11-fold internal validation. The log odds values are calculated using the output probabilities of the CNN models. (**E**) Using the log odds, a standardized value called the D score is calculated and plotted on a Youden plot. The scores help in the identification of the tested sample. A decision threshold score of zero is used in this case. The plot shows exemplary point clouds for the spelt (orange squares) and wheat (brown circles) cultivars.

2. Materials and Methods

2.1. Description of Spelt and Wheat Samples

Samples for all spelt and wheat cultivars were kindly sourced and provided by the Institut für Getreideverarbeitung (IGV) GmbH, Nuthetal, Germany. Eleven cultivars each of typical spelt and wheat were used to train the CNN models. The distinction of whether it is spelt or wheat was made according to investigations of their marker peptide profiles, as previously described elsewhere [52]. For the list of eleven cultivars each for spelt and wheat, see supplementary Table S1. Each of the cultivars was measured in duplicate on different days (different runs). Together, 44 MS1 spectra constitute the "calibration dataset," i.e., all the spectra that were used to train the CNN models. In this communication, we choose to refer to this as the calibration dataset in accordance with other reports [46,53]. For each of the internal validation folds, the calibration set was split into the training and testing sets (see Figure 1D). The term "training of models" refers to obtaining the weights and biases of the neural network through a process of back propagation [54]. Further details are described in Section 2.3.

Two processed samples were prepared to keep in mind commonly available processed spelt goods. The first sample was a mixture of spelt flour made of *Oberkulmer Rotkorn* with 10% wheat flour T405. The second sample was a spelt bread baked using spelt flour T630 with 10% soft wheat flour T550. To simulate the flour and bread samples, an artificial spectral mix was generated by the weighted addition of two spectra. Duplicate measurements for each of the eleven wheat cultivars were 10% down-weighted and added to 90% of the spectral intensities of one spectrum of *Oberkulmer Rotkorn* spelt to yield eleven pairs of artificial mix spectra. As per the guiding principle for the manufacture and sale of spelt bread [27], which states that the spelt bread must contain at least 90% spelt, the maximum possible wheat content of 10% was chosen.

Additionally, eleven cultivars of untypical spelt were sourced. These cultivars of spelt are known to be either "newer" cultivars of spelt or wheat-spelt crosses; hence, they are collectively referred to herein as "untypical spelt." Furthermore, six wheat cultivars were also sourced whose pedigrees can be be traced to the late 18th to early 19th centuries, hence being referred to herein as "old wheat" cultivars. For a list of untypical spelt and old wheat cultivars, see supplementary Table S1. Together, these constitute the "external validation dataset," which consists of unseen data used to test the trained models. Just like the calibration set, for each of the mixture samples and cultivars, duplicate measurements were performed.

2.2. Wet Lab Procedure

This section briefly describes the sample preparation and LC-HRMS measurements as part of the wet lab procedure. The detailed MS procedure has been reported as part of previously conducted targeted studies [51,52].

2.2.1. Sample Preparation, Protein Digestion and Purification

All buffer solutions and dilutions were prepared with water suitable for LC-MS analysis. Each sample was weighed to 1.0 ± 0.001 g in a 50 mL centrifuge tube, to which 10 mL of extraction buffer was added. Extraction buffer was prepared with 100 mM ammonium bicarbonate, 4 M urea, and 5 mM 1,4-Dithiothreitol (DTT) (all from Carl Roth GmbH, Karlsruhe, Germany). The tube was shaken at room temperature for 1 h using an overhead shaker, after which it was centrifuged at 4000 g for 5 min. 2 mL of the supernatant was transferred to a 15 mL centrifuge tube and centrifuged again at 7000× g for 5 min. 1 mL of the supernatant was removed and transferred to another 15 mL centrifuge tube, to which 30 µL of 0.5 M Iodoacetamide (IAA) solution was added. 0.5 M IAA solution was prepared fresh, as it is light sensitive, by dissolving 11.55 mg of IAA (Sigma-Aldrich, Taufkirchen, Germany) in 1.25 mL water. The resulting solution was incubated for 20 min by shaking at 50 °C, after which (a) 3000 µL of digestion buffer and (b) 100 µL of chymotrypsin solution (from bovine pancreas for enzymatic digestion purchased from Sigma Aldrich,

Taufkirchen, Germany) were added. This is followed by incubation of the reaction mixture overnight at 25 °C. The (a) digestion buffer was prepared by dissolving 1.304 g ammonium bicarbonate in 25 mL Acetonitrile (ACN) (both from Carl Roth GmbH, Karlsruhe, Germany) and diluting with 140 mL of water. The (b) chymotrypsin solution was freshly prepared using activated chymotrypsin (>1000 USP-U/mg) (Carl Roth GmbH, Karlsruhe, Germany) at a concentration of 8 mg /mL. The digestion reaction was stopped by adding 100 μL of 40% formic acid (FA) (Carl Roth GmbH, Karlsruhe, Germany). The extract obtained was stored for at least 1 h in the freezer at −20 °C, so that most of the fat or wax components precipitated. The reaction tubes were then centrifuged at $7000 \times g$ for 2 min.

The sample extract was desalted and concentrated using an SPE column (Carl Roth GmbH, Karlsruhe, Germany). For this purpose, the SPE columns were conditioned with 6 mL of buffer A followed by 6 mL water. Buffer A was made by mixing 100 mL water, 100 mL can, and 200 μL FA. Then the entire sample extract was added to the column and unbound components were washed out by subsequent rinsing with 6 mL of buffer B. Buffer B was prepared by mixing 200 μL water with 200 μL FA. The eluted peptides were then concentrated to dryness under nitrogen at 30 °C and resuspended in a mixture of 450 μL buffer B and 50 μL buffer A. Lastly, the mix was centrifuged for 2 min at $7000 \times g$. The supernatant was diluted with buffer B in a ratio of 1:100 and then measured.

2.2.2. Liquid Chromatography Mass Spectrometry (LC-MS)

Data were acquired using ultra-high performance liquid chromatography triple time of flight mass spectrometry (UHPLC Triple ToF) (MS/MS) consisting of a micro-flow UHPLC expert microLC 200 with an autosampler CTC Pal system and a SCIEX electrospray ionization (ESI) TripleTOF 5600 with SWATH (sequential window acquisition of all theoretical fragment-ion spectra) acquisition. HRMS data acquisition of MS/MS data was done using data-independent acquisition (DIA-SWATH) [55]. Although MS2 SWATH data was also acquired, it was not utilized for the analysis shown in this work. As mentioned earlier, every measurement was performed in duplicate.

2.3. Dry Lab Pipeline

2.3.1. Spectral Data Preparation

The acquired data were first converted to the mzXML file format from the WIFF and WIFFSCAN formats using ProteoWizard [56]. All MS datasets were used without undergoing any preprocessing (e.g., peak alignment, baseline correction) or feature selection steps. The mzXML file was read in the Python programming language (python.org), and the MS1 spectra were aggregated to integer mass accuracy. The resulting data was a matrix of size 1375 (number of scans) and 801 (values of m/z ranging from 400 to 1200 Da). The aggregation of spectra was performed to make it manageable for CNN model training on a personal computer. The data matrices were obtained for all the samples in the calibration set and external validation set, which were then used as input to the CNN models. Each scan was z-normalized, i.e., subtract the mean of a scan from every peak intensity value and divide by the standard deviation (SD) of the scan.

2.3.2. Nested Cross Validation (NCV)

Central to the analysis pipeline was the NCV approach shown in Figure 1D. The calibration set comprised eleven cultivars each for typical spelt and wheat as the two classes for the CNN model classifier. In this, separate models were trained with a training set comprising duplicate spectra for (randomly chosen) ten cultivars each of typical spelt and wheat (totaling forty spectra) and tested on the spectra for the remaining eleventh cultivar for typical spelt and wheat (totaling four spectra). For instance, in the first fold, spectra for *Badekrone* spelt and *Bernstein* wheat cultivars were kept aside for testing the model trained on the remaining spectra of the cultivars. In the next fold, spectra for *Badensonne* spelt and *Brilliant* wheat cultivars were kept aside for testing the model trained on the spectra for the remaining cultivars. In this way, eleven models were trained, corresponding to each fold of the internal validation loop. In other words, every cultivar in the calibration set was used once to test the trained models. The NCV procedure is advantageous because it can deal with the availability of a limited number of distinct samples (cultivars), each having a large number of features (peaks). For the external validation dataset, every spectrum was run through models for each fold of the NCV to obtain a classification outcome in the form of a probability. The final classification probability for the external validation spectra was obtained by averaging across all the model outcomes (i.e., the average of eleven models' outcomes).

2.3.3. Neural Network Analysis

In this communication, a short description is provided for how the neural network was constructed, assuming that the reader is aware of terms used in the field. The reader is referred to rich literature available elsewhere for (a) the theoretical fundamentals behind neural networks and (b) an exhaustive review on the types of neural network architectures [57–61]. A shallow CNN architecture was used with convolutional layers and pooling layers, each of which was setup using standard settings [62]. All programming was done in Python (python.org) using the Keras and Tensorflow libraries [63,64]. Four convolution layers were stacked together to hierarchically capture the inherent patterns within the spectra. The convolution layers were interspersed with "maximum pooling" layers, which help reduce the effect of spectral noise in the learned features and emphasize the larger peak intensities [65]. Together, the above-described apparatus tries to automatically extract the "features"—which, in this context, are the spectral peaks (or their combinations). We hypothesize that the features learned by the CNNs directly help to identify a particular class (spelt or wheat), which otherwise would have been done by a human expert.

For each fold of internal validation, the calibration set was split into a training and a testing set. According to the NCV approach, CNN models were trained on the training set and then checked using the testing set. The CNN was trained using gradient descent, which minimizes a loss function by calculating its partial derivative with respect to the learnable parameters through backpropagation and iteratively updating them until they converge for each layer [46,47,54]. The output of the CNN was a probability value (used for the D score calculation as described in the next section), based on which a binary classification was obtained (spelt or wheat). The performance of the classifier was tracked by looking at the confusion matrix, i.e., counts of true positives (TP), true negatives (TN), false negatives (FN), and false positives (FP). Using these values, Matthew's correlation coefficient (MCC) was calculated according to Equation (1). MCC = 1 means a perfect prediction, whereas MCC = -1 means completely flipped (incorrect) predictions.

$$MCC = \frac{TP \times TN - FP \times FN}{\sqrt{(TP+FP)(TP+FN)(TN+FP)(TN+FN)}} \tag{1}$$

In this study, the features available to train the CNNs were ample, i.e., ~1 million per measurement, while the number of cultivars per class was limited (11 each). Hence, it was important to keep the models "simple" and avoid extensive hyperparameter tuning. Hyperparameters can be thought of as knobs and dials available to design CNNs and determine how they are trained. For instance, the number of layers in a CNN, the learning rate of the gradient descent algorithm, the number of epochs, etc. [40,57]. Tuning these parameters can result in model predictions being overly dependent on the underlying training data, i.e., lead to overfitting. This means that when models are trained for a set of cultivars, they may not perform very well on other types of cultivars.

2.4. Decision Based on D Scores

The newly proposed quantitative score, called the D score, is a measure of the classification outcome that can be easily compared for different types of samples, experimental runs, models, or even laboratories. The classification outcome from the CNN models was extracted in the form of probabilities (p_i). The probabilities were converted to log odds ratios. A linear transformation was then performed on the log odds ratio values to scale the values such that the mean values of the spelt and wheat classes are +1 and −1, respectively (Equations (2)–(4)). The resultant values are referred to as "D scores." The linear transformation parameters (λ, θ) were obtained based on the calibration set of samples, i.e., using the means of log odds for spelt ($\overline{\mu}_{spelt}$) and wheat ($\overline{\mu}_{wheat}$). The calculated D scores for the duplicate measurements were then plotted on a Youden plot, as shown in Figure 1E. A Youden plot is essentially a scatter plot that helps to visualize and analyze data when two measurement runs on the same type of sample (in this case, the cultivar).

$$D_i = ln\left(\frac{p_i}{1-p_i}\right) \times \lambda + \theta; \text{ for } i^{th} \text{ measured sample} \quad (2)$$

$$\text{where, } \lambda = \frac{2}{\overline{\mu}_{spelt} - \overline{\mu}_{wheat}} \text{ and} \quad (3)$$

$$\theta = 1 - \lambda \times \overline{\mu}_{spelt} \quad (4)$$

The decision for classification would be based on a decision threshold, which is chosen to be zero in this study. Hence, when the D score is positive ($D_i > 0$), then spelt, and when it is negative ($D_i < 0$), then wheat. In comparison to a qualitative binary classification (yes/no) outcome, D scores offer three main advantages. First, the distribution of D scores allows one to evaluate the performance of the model or the method as a whole by calculating the variation of the scores within a class. This is further discussed in Section 3.3. Secondly, it allows direct comparison of samples and informs about the relationship between the compared samples. For instance, 2 samples with D scores of 0.8 and 1 are expected to be closely related (from their prediction classification) compared to samples with D scores of +0.8 and −0.8. This is further illustrated in Section 3.2. Finally, D scores are model- and class-agnostic. Hence, the procedure for calculation and interpretation of D scores will not change on (a) replacing the neural network model with another (type of) classifier and (b) when the classes are changed from spelt or wheat to any other generic class A or B (for example, a white wine from Germany and a white wine from France).

3. Results

3.1. Wet Lab LC-HRMS Measurements

With the purpose of utilizing complete and raw spectra from the LC-MS measurements, the 2-D spectra for each sample were obtained. The 2-D spectrum can be visualized as an image. Figure 1C shows exemplary heatmap images for duplicate measurements of spelt and wheat. The x-axis of the image shows the m/z and the y-axis shows the scans corresponding to different retention times, and the intensity of the values is indicated by the color map. The heatmaps are plotted with power-law normalization of the intensity for better visual contrast. Even on closer inspection, distinction between the patterns (or fingerprints) is hard to make only with the human eye. Hence, the need for devising suitable models that are able to parse the data, capture the underlying patterns, and help distinguish the food items (here, spelt and wheat) is apparent. These images were used as input for the dry lab model.

3.2. Internal Validation: Youden Plot with the D Scores for Calibration Set

After going through the NCV procedure for internal validation, D scores were obtained for each of the spectra in the calibration set. Recall, two extracted samples were measured, hence, two sets of spectra are available for each cultivar, and each cultivar is tested once with a model trained on cultivars other than itself. Hence, this gives us a D score for the entire calibration set. The λ and θ values calculated according to Equations (2) and (3) are −0.13 and −0.02, respectively (see supplementary results Section S2.1). Figure 2A shows a list of spelt cultivars, where each cultivar is indicated by a point in the magnified cluster of the plot shown in Figure 2B. Figure 2C shows a Youden plot with point clouds for the spelt (orange squares) and wheat (brown circles) cultivars in the calibration set. Figure 2D shows a magnified cluster of points where each point on the plot represents a wheat cultivar that is listed in Figure 2E. The Youden plot allows us to intuitively establish the extent of discrimination (a) between the samples of the two classes (spelt and wheat) and (b) among the samples of the same class.

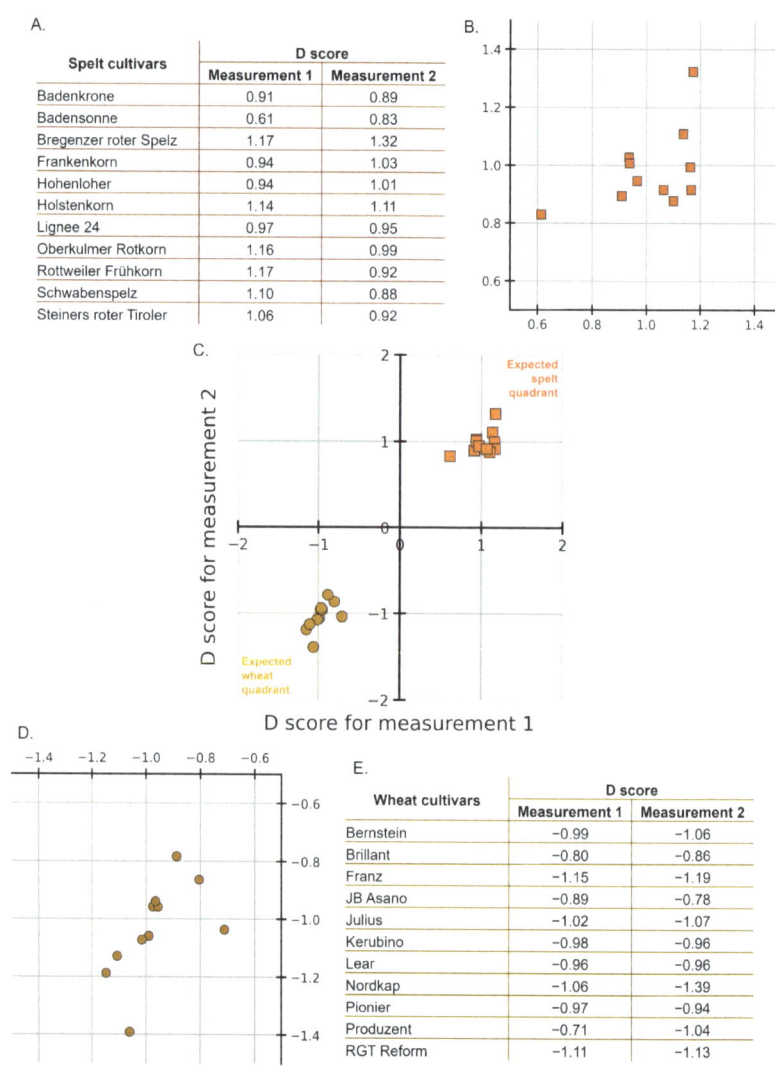

Figure 2. The D scores for the spelt cultivars (orange squares) and for wheat cultivars (brown circles) in the calibration set are plotted. (**A**) List of spelt cultivars along with their D scores. (**B**) A magnified view of the Youden plot for spelt cultivars. (**C**) Youden plot with the D scores. (**D**) A magnified view of the Youden plot for wheat cultivars. (**E**) List of wheat cultivars along with their D scores.

The lack of any overlap between the point clouds directly shows the high discriminatory power of the trained models. Considering zero as the decision threshold for the D scores, when a D score is positive for both measurements, it lies in the first quadrant (top right) and is predicted to be spelt. Likewise, when it is negative for both D scores, it lies in the third quadrant (lower left) and is predicted to be wheat. Here, the advantage of the D score is evident in being able to immediately identify if the classification outcome is spelt or wheat (for a list of D scores for the calibration set, see Supplementary Table S2A,B). If visual proof is insufficient, the classification performance can be summarized using the Matthews correlation coefficient (MCC), which is suggested to be the most informative of all the different classification metrics [66]. MCC of +1 is obtained, which shows complete agreement between the true and predicted classes, making the high classification performance very evident. The separation in the D score point clouds shows that CNNs prove effective in learning visual representations of 2-D spectral data that are passed as images. It is expected that convolution layers are able to capture the local shifts in the peaks (that are typically then aligned, corrected, etc. in spectral preprocessing).

3.3. Precision Parameters

It is essential to ensure that the discriminatory power remains adequate (a) when applied to other sets of data than the training set, covering the entire population falling under the scope of the method, and (b) under all in-house testing conditions or when applied to data from different laboratories. Using the D scores, various precision estimates can be obtained based on concepts laid out in ISO 5725-3 [67]. Note that the standard describes precision parameters that are given for a sample, but in this context the parameters are provided for the class (e.g., spelt or wheat and not for a specific cultivar). Here we calculate the classification SD (the variation of D scores for cultivars within a class) and intermediate SD (the average variation of D scores for several measurements (at least 2) of the same cultivar under intermediate conditions, averaged across cultivars of the same class). The precision estimates for the D score can be obtained by using the approach described in previous reports [68,69] (see supplementary Table S3).

The single laboratory classification SD is used to check whether the decision threshold can be considered reliable for the whole population falling within the scope of the classification method. SD values of 0.393 and 0.391 are obtained for spelt and wheat, respectively. If we assume that D scores are normally distributed within each of the two classes, then with a mean value of 1 and SD of 0.393, the risk of misclassification for spelt, i.e., a value below zero, would have a probability of $\Phi\left(\frac{-1}{0.393}\right) \approx 0.5\%$. Similarly, the risk of misclassification for wheat, would be $1 - \Phi\left(\frac{1}{0.391}\right) \approx 0.5\%$. Here, Φ denotes the cumulative distribution function of the standard normal distribution. There is no indication that the point clouds of D scores for each class are not normally distributed. Thus, the risk of misclassification is very low (<1%).

With the intermediate SD, the in-house reproducibility of the D score can be described. We obtained an intermediate SD of 0.075 and 0.074 for spelt and wheat, respectively, which means that the analytical variability is almost equal to the variability between different cultivars. It can, therefore, be stated that the analytical variability is more than sufficient for the purpose of classification between wheat and spelt; on the other hand, the differences within the spelt cultivars studied are very small and cannot be precisely measured with the D score. The next section describes how the trained models perform on external validation samples. Predictions on external validation samples were performed using all the models trained in the internal validation NCV loops.

3.4. External Validation Set: Processed Goods and Artificial Mixes

Even with the limited number of distinct cultivars used for training a CNN model, the present study was designed to determine whether successful classification models can be built using LC-HRMS spectra, and thereby laying the groundwork for an NTM that can be used in routine (e.g., for official control). The models trained with typical spelt and wheat varieties are put to the test by using real-world processed goods. Remember that each of the eleven internal validation models provided an output prediction, which was then averaged to get an average D score for each external validation sample. Figure 3A shows spelt bread (orange square) and spelt flour mix (orange diamond) in the expected spelt quadrant, hence showing the correct classification. Figure 3B shows a magnified view of the points (for a list of D scores, see Supplementary Table S4). The resulting D scores for both measurements of spelt bread are around 0.79 and the scores for the duplicate measurements of spelt flour mix are around 0.78 and 0.75. Together, the D scores for processed goods indicate a correct prediction.

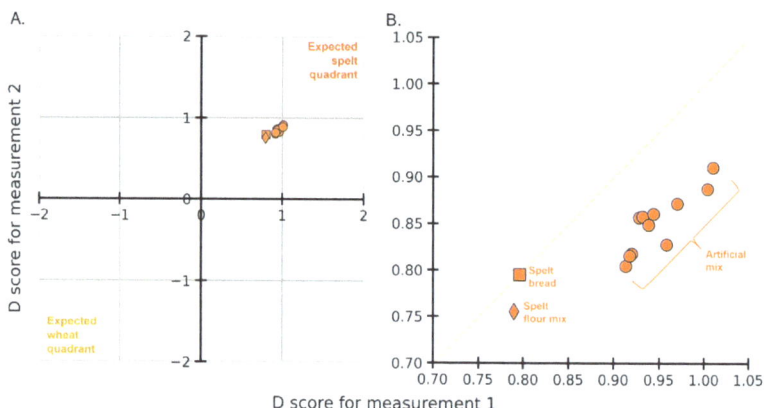

Figure 3. Youden plot showing the D scores for processed goods and artificial mix in the external validation set in (**A**) and a magnified section in (**B**). Spelt bread (orange square), spelt flour mix (orange diamonds), and artificial spectral mix (orange circles) are shown to be correctly predicted as spelt.

Turning now to predicting the artificially generated spectral mixes, Figure 3 shows the D scores (orange circles) for each of the eleven wheat cultivars whose spectra were 10% downweighed and added to 90% of the spectral intensities of *Oberkulmer Rotkorn* spelt. The average D score for these eleven points is around 0.9. Interestingly, the point cloud for the artificial mix is further away (top right) from the actual processed goods. In other words, the predictions from CNN models are relatively (and marginally) more confident about the artificial mix being spelt than the spelt bread and flour. Perhaps this is because the spectra for bread and flour have a more complex fingerprint than the one resulting from the linear combination of their constituents. In summary, the predictions on the external validation set show that successful distinction can be made even on processed spelt samples.

3.5. External Valdiation with Untypical Spelt Cultivars

The next question was to check if other spelt cultivars (that were not used in the calibration set) could be correctly identified as spelt. Figure 4A shows the cluster of eleven cultivars (brown squares) lying in the spelt quadrant of the Youden plot, indicating correct classification. Figure 4B is the zoomed-in section of the plot showing the distribution of D scores with the corresponding cultivar name (see Supplementary Table S5 for a list of D scores for untypical spelt). The point cloud is in the first quadrant, showing the correct classification for spelt. The average D score is 0.57. Comparing this to the average of 1 for the spelt cultivars in the calibration set (Figure 2B), there is a difference in the prediction outcome of these untypical (for external validation) and typical (for the calibration set) spelt. This suggests that the fingerprints, as learned by the CNNs through the spectra of typical spelt, are dissimilar to those of untypical spelt. This could be linked to the evolving proteomic fingerprints of older cultivars of spelt (used in the calibration set) compared to the newer ones in untypical spelt. The larger spread of the points in the Youden plot for untypical spelt (Figure 4) in comparison to the spread of typical spelt (Figure 2) is a remarkable result. This can be owing to the dissimilarities between the learned and predicted fingerprints of typical and untypical spelt cultivars.

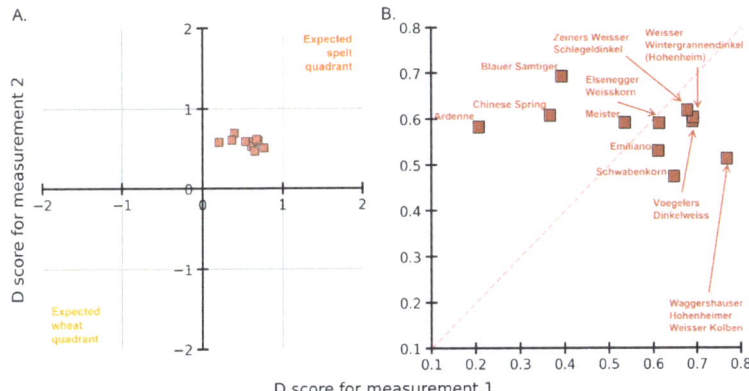

Figure 4. Youden plot showing the D scores for untypical spelt cultivars (**A**) with the magnified section in (**B**). Untypical spelt (brown squares) with their corresponding names, shown to be correctly predicted as spelt.

3.6. External Validation with Other Wheat Cultivars (Old Wheat Cultivars)

On a similar line of inquiry, further investigations were made to determine whether old wheat cultivars, which were not part of the model building, can be distinguished from spelt (or wheat). Figure 5A shows the D scores for six cultivars with the zoomed view in Figure 5B (brown circles) (see Supplementary Table S6 for a list of D scores for old wheat). We see that even though five of the six cultivars lie in the wheat quadrant, i.e., D scores for five of the six cultivars are negative. However, for one cultivar, *Ackermanns Bayernkoenig*, it is positive. With zero as the decision threshold, it can be said that one cultivar is misclassified. However, all six cultivars are very close to the decision threshold. The mean D score for the other five is −0.1. Comparing this to the mean value of −1 for the wheat cultivars in the calibration set, there is a clear distancing from it.

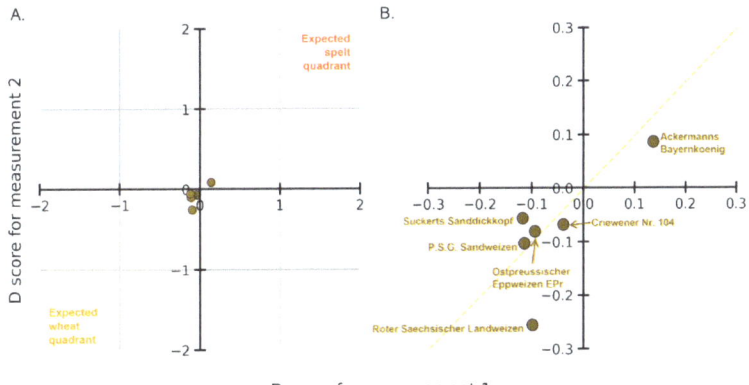

Figure 5. Youden plot showing the D scores for old wheat cultivars (**A**) with the magnified section in (**B**). The cultivars (brown circles) are shown to be not unambiguously classified as spelt or wheat.

By connecting these results to the pedigree of the cultivar, it may be possible to explain why they have either positive or close to zero D scores. For instance, *Ackermanns Bayernkoenig* an old cultivar, is a cross between wheat and spelt wheat, which could explain why CNN identifies it as being closer to spelt than wheat. Overall, these samples proved to be "challenging samples" for the method with the CNN models in their current form [31].

4. Discussion

This paper describes an NTM comprising LC-HRMS data acquisition as the wet lab component and using the 2-D MS1 spectral data as inputs for the CNN for classification tasks as the dry lab component. Note that the wet lab part involves duplicate measurements, which proves advantageous in capturing the variation due to sample preparation and measurement. In the dry lab part, the model development employs an NCV approach that relies on a calibration data set that is split into training and validation sets for each iteration. The study shows the merits of appropriately (and carefully) choosing datasets to train classification models. The classification probabilities obtained at the output layer of the CNN are transformed into a set of standardized numerical values that we call D scores. D scores provide a quantitative appraisal of the discrimination of two classes, and the results show how they also provide a visual representation of how clusters of samples are "related" to each other.

Catering to the question of differentiating spelt from wheat, the distribution of D scores shows that the CNN models are able to completely distinguish typical spelt and wheat cultivars with a very low risk of misclassification (<1%). The developed models were then put to the test to classify processed goods (spelt bread, spelt flour mix) and artificial mixes. These were correctly identified in all instances tested. We foresee the use of such an NTM on-site by laboratories of food production companies and official control, to aid with testing food authenticity and ensuring correct labeling of spelt products. After the labs have obtained the spectral measurement, it can be run through the models accessed by means of a suitable application interface, which will provide the D score. We believe this method adds to the battery of methods that have been reported thus far that utilize electrophoresis or molecular methods to distinguish spelt and wheat [12,15,19,21]. LC-HRMS measurements give a vast, high resolution, and high-fidelity database for the cost trade-off. However, when utilized appropriately by training CNNs using NCV, as described herein, it provides rapid, accurate and cost-effective results.

The CNN models developed as part of the dry lab procedure were further challenged with cultivars of spelt and wheat that were not part of the training. The untypical spelt were all correctly classified. D scores for old wheat cultivars were close to the decision, proving to be challenging samples for the NTM, with one out of six cultivars being misclassified. Systematic inclusion of such challenging cultivars along with additional ones that were not considered in the study would indeed help to upgrade the NTM. The discriminatory power of the method can be further improved by mobilizing the complete fragment-ion MS/MS spectrum.

An initial objective of the project was to make use of raw aggregated spectra without any alignment or peak picking, and this work describes a procedure to fulfill that objective. This is increasingly beneficial when (a) there is no a priori knowledge of which peaks to focus on, or (b) a combination pattern of several peaks is contributing to the identification or discrimination of the measured entity (in this case, spelt and wheat), or (c) processed food samples and matrix effects make it hard to detect the presence of specific marker peaks.

As previously discussed, bucketing of cultivars into spelt, wheat-spelt, and spelt-wheat are subjective with overlapping boundaries. All this leads to an unclear definition of spelt for both consumers and producers, which can be taken advantage of by the latter for economic benefits. Thus, raising questions about "what is true spelt?" As well as when does an untypical spelt cultivar stop being referred to as spelt? The NTM described here can help answer those questions by quantifying (using D scores) the deviations in characteristics (captured through the LC-MS fingerprint). The results described in Sections 3.5 and 3.6 attest to the potential of the approaches described in this work to help get to a definition of spelt buckets. A further study involving the utilization of D scores to define what can be regarded as spelt (or not) is therefore proposed. For example, subjective buckets with diffused boundaries for spelt can be replaced by well-defined buckets by establishing suitable quantitative criteria (e.g., a D score greater than 0.5 results in true spelts).

A variety of NTMs involving proteomic- or metabolomic-based approaches are being developed to keep pace with new ways of deception with food substances. It is the view of the authors that NTMs in food testing clearly stand at a crossroads—with great promise for wide applicability and adoption that can be ushered in by establishing method validation schemes. Method validation schemes allow for the evaluation of the method's performance, which can help standardize the method and bring it into routine use [31]. The provision of a complete method validation scheme is outside the scope of this work. However, a suitable scheme can be contemplated to utilize the quantitative D scores to evaluate the precision parameters. Consequently, performance characteristics like sensitivity and specificity, false-positive and false-negative rates can also be evaluated based on a chosen threshold score (D score of zero). The advantages of the proposed procedure of transforming the classification probabilities into standardized D scores become more evident when measurements across different laboratories can be directly compared in a validation study (single- or multi-laboratory).

From one perspective, the study is limited by the small dataset for training neural networks (calibration set). In such a scenario, one has to be careful with over-fitting issues. To alleviate these issues, the NCV approach was used, which helps achieve greater generalization on unseen data. This can be seen in the results for the external validation samples. Firstly, all processed goods were correctly classified. Secondly, untypical cultivars and old wheat cultivars were also meaningfully identified. The reader should bear in mind that this work does not aim and claim to provide the "best" models for classification of spelt vs. wheat with matchless classification metrics. Rather, the study aims to establish effective approaches and, thereby, contribute to the growing area of NTMs for food fraud.

In food fraud testing, one can imagine that data corresponding to "authentic" food samples will always be "limited," as obtaining truly authentic samples might be burdensome or impractical. As in this study, knowledge about the real identity of the cultivar relies on elaborate biochemical tests and known cross-breeding histories. There is an increased role for the means by which the dataset is obtained or generated to reduce reliance on large datasets for model building. (a) Conducting duplicate measurements of cultivars, (b) selecting suitable cultivars as the two classes for the training, and (c) designing folds of the NCV approach are some of the procedures for systematic curation proposed in this work.

Overall, the described method can be easily (a) extended to include more cultivars and their mixes and (b) adapted for other application areas, such as the prediction of geographical identity. Furthermore, the modular nature of the method (wet lab + dry lab) means alternative approaches (e.g., different LC-MS instruments) can be used. The procedures, including duplicate measurements, NCV, and calculation of D scores, would still be applicable, as stated here.

5. Conclusions

This study describes a new NTM in which the wet lab component records the food fingerprint using LC-HRMS and the dry lab component utilizes CNN to identify the tested sample. The D score results show correct identification of relevant cultivars, with very low risk of misclassification. We see promise in the method's usefulness not only in connection with the question of the authenticity of different food items and matrices but also, e.g., in characterizing blood plasma in connection with diagnostic, prognostic, and therapeutic research.

Supplementary Materials: The following supporting information can be downloaded at: https://www.mdpi.com/article/10.3390/foods12010141/s1, Table S1: List of spelt and wheat varieties used in the study; Table S2A: Log odds and D scores for spelt cultivars in the calibration set; Table S2B: Log odds and D scores for wheat cultivars in the calibration set; Table S3: Summary of precision parameters for spelt and wheat; Table S4: Log odds and D scores for processed goods and artificial mixes; Table S5: Log odds and D scores for untypical spelt cultivars; Table S6: Log odds and D scores for old wheat cultivars.

Author Contributions: Conceptualization, K.N., S.U., B.C., K.H., C.U., S.K., M.S., P.G. and H.M.R.; methodology, K.N., S.U., B.C., K.H., C.U., G.H. and H.M.R.; software, K.N., S.U. and C.U.; validation, K.N., S.U., B.C., K.H. and H.M.R.; formal analysis, K.N. and S.U.; investigation, K.N., S.U., J.B. and G.H.; resources, K.S., G.H. and H.M.R.; data curation, K.N., S.U., J.B. and G.H.; writing—original draft preparation, K.N. and S.U.; writing—review and editing, K.N., S.U., B.C., K.H., S.K., M.S. and H.M.R.; visualization, K.N.; supervision, K.S., S.K., M.S., P.G. and H.M.R.; project administration, K.N., S.U., K.S., G.H. and H.M.R.; funding acquisition, K.S., S.K., M.S., P.G., G.H. and H.M.R. All authors have read and agreed to the published version of the manuscript.

Funding: This research received no external funding.

Data Availability Statement: Not applicable.

Acknowledgments: We acknowledge the support of the Deutsche Forschungsgemeinschaft (DFG, German Research Foundation—Projektnummer 491466077) and Open Access Publishing Fund of the University of Potsdam.

Conflicts of Interest: The authors and in case of being affiliated to a company, than both declare no conflict of interest.

References

1. Barrere, V.; Everstine, K.; Théolier, J.; Godefroy, S. Food Fraud Vulnerability Assessment: Towards a Global Consensus on Procedures to Manage and Mitigate Food Fraud. *Trends Food Sci. Technol.* **2020**, *100*, 131–137. [CrossRef]
2. Marvin, H.J.; Hoenderdaal, W.; Gavai, A.K.; Mu, W.; van den Bulk, L.M.; Liu, N.; Frasso, G.; Ozen, N.; Elliott, C.; Manning, L. Global Media as an Early Warning Tool for Food Fraud; an Assessment of MedISys-FF. *Food Control* **2022**, *137*, 108961. [CrossRef]
3. Johnson, R. *Food Fraud and "Economically Motivated Adulteration" of Food and Food Ingredients*; Congressional Research Service: Washington, DC, USA, 2018.
4. Ulberth, F. Tools to Combat Food Fraud–a Gap Analysis. *Food Chem.* **2020**, *330*, 127044. [CrossRef]
5. Robson, K.; Dean, M.; Haughey, S.; Elliott, C. A Comprehensive Review of Food Fraud Terminologies and Food Fraud Mitigation Guides. *Food Control* **2021**, *120*, 107516. [CrossRef]
6. Faller, A.C.; Kesanakurti, P.; Arunachalam, T. Fraud in Grains and Cereals. In *Food Fraud*; Elsevier: msterdam, The Netherlands, 2021; pp. 281–308.
7. Liu, H.-Y.; Wadood, S.A.; Xia, Y.; Liu, Y.; Guo, H.; Guo, B.-L.; Gan, R.-Y. Wheat AuthenticatioN: An Overview on Different Techniques and Chemometric Methods. *Crit. Rev. Food Sci. Nutr.* **2021**, *63*, 1–24. [CrossRef]
8. Righetti, L.; Rubert, J.; Galaverna, G.; Folloni, S.; Ranieri, R.; Stranska-Zachariasova, M.; Hajslova, J.; Dall'Asta, C. Characterization and Discrimination of Ancient Grains: A Metabolomics Approach. *nt. J. Mol. Sci.* **2016**, *17*, 1217. [CrossRef]
9. Cavanna, D.; Loffi, C.; Dall'Asta, C.; Suman, M. A Non-Targeted High-Resolution Mass Spectrometry Approach for the Assessment of the Geographical Origin of Durum Wheat. *Food Chem.* **2020**, *317*, 126366. [CrossRef]
10. EU Commision. Commission implementing regulation (EU) 2015/550—Of 24 March 2015—Entering a Name in the Register of Protected Designations of Origin and Protected Geographical Indications [Fränkischer Grünkern (PDO)]. *Off. J. Eur. Union* **2015**.
11. De Girolamo, A.; Arroyo, M.C.; Cervellieri, S.; Cortese, M.; Pascale, M.; Logrieco, A.F.; Lippolis, V. Detection of Durum Wheat Pasta Adulteration with Common Wheat by Infrared Spectroscopy and Chemometrics: A Case Study. *LWT* **2020**, *127*, 109368. [CrossRef]
12. Von Büren, M.; Stadler, M.; Lüthy, J. Detection of Wheat Adulteration of Spelt Flour and Products by PCR. *Eur. Food Res. Technol.* **2001**, *212*, 234–239. [CrossRef]
13. Bonte, A.; Neuweger, H.; Goesmann, A.; Thonar, C.; Mäder, P.; Langenkämper, G.; Niehaus, K. Metabolite Profiling on Wheat Grain to Enable a Distinction of Samples from Organic and Conventional Farming Systems. *J. Sci. Food Agric.* **2014**, *94*, 2605–2612. [CrossRef] [PubMed]
14. Faris, J.D. Wheat Domestication: Key to Agricultural Revolutions Past and Future. In *Genomics of Plant Genetic Resources*; Springer: Berlin/Heidelberg, Germany, 2014; pp. 439–464.
15. Mayer, F.; Haase, I.; Graubner, A.; Heising, F.; Paschke-Kratzin, A.; Fischer, M. Use of Polymorphisms in the γ-Gliadin Gene of Spelt and Wheat as a Tool for Authenticity Control. *J. Agric. Food Chem.* **2012**, *60*, 1350–1357. [CrossRef] [PubMed]
16. Kohajdová, Z.; Karovicova, J. Nutritional Value and Baking Application of Spelt Wheat. *Acta Sci. Pol. Technol. Aliment.* **2008**, *7*, 5–14.
17. Muñoz-Insa, A.; Selciano, H.; Zarnkow, M.; Becker, T.; Gastl, M. Malting Process Optimization of Spelt (*Triticum Spelta* L.) for the Brewing Process. *LWT* **2013**, *50*, 99–109. [CrossRef]
18. Tsagkaris, A.S.; Kalogiouri, N.; Hrbek, V.; Hajslova, J. Spelt Authenticity Assessment Using a Rapid and Simple Fourier Transform Infrared Spectroscopy (FTIR) Method Combined to Advanced Chemometrics. *Eur. Food Res. Technol.* **2022**. [CrossRef]
19. Köppel, R.; Guertler, P.; Waiblinger, H.-U. Duplex Droplet Digital PCR (DdPCR) Method for the Quantification of Common Wheat (Triticum Aestivum) in Spelt (*Triticum Spelta*). *Food Control* **2021**, *130*, 108382. [CrossRef]
20. Campbell, K.G. Spelt: Agronomy, Genetics, and Breeding. *Plant Breed. Rev.* **2010**, *15*, 187–213.

21. Koenig, A.; Konitzer, K.; Wieser, H.; Koehler, P. Classification of Spelt Cultivars Based on Differences in Storage Protein Compositions from Wheat. *Food Chem.* **2015**, *168*, 176–182. [CrossRef]
22. Wieser, H. Comparison of Genuine Spelt with Spelt/Wheat Crossbreeds. *Getreidetechnologie* **2006**, *60*, 223.
23. Abrouk, M.; Athiyannan, N.; Müller, T.; Pailles, Y.; Stritt, C.; Roulin, A.C.; Chu, C.; Liu, S.; Morita, T.; Handa, H. Population Genomics and Haplotype Analysis in Spelt and Bread Wheat Identifies a Gene Regulating Glume Color. *Commun. Biol.* **2021**, *4*, 375. [CrossRef]
24. Das Wertvollste Getreide. Available online: https://www.urdinkel.ch/de/urdinkel/marke (accessed on 21 October 2022).
25. Regulation (EU) 2017/625 of the European Parliament and of the Council of 15 March 2017 on Official Controls and Other Official Activities Performed to Ensure the Application of Food and Feed Law, Rules on Animal Health and Welfare, Plant Health and Plant Protection Products, Amending Regulations (EC) No 999/2001, (EC) No 396/2005, (EC) No 1069/2009, (EC) No 1107/2009, (EU) No 1151/2012, (EU) No 652/2014, (EU) 2016/429 and (EU) 2016/2031 of the European Parliament and of the Council, Council Regulations (EC) No 1/2005 and (EC) No 1099/2009 and Council Directives 98/58/EC, 1999/74/EC, 2007/43/EC, 2008/119/EC and 2008/120/EC, and Repealing Regulations (EC) No 854/2004 and (EC) No 882/2004 of the European Parliament and of the Council, Council Directives 89/608/EEC, 89/662/EEC, 90/425/EEC, 91/496/EEC, 96/23/EC, 96/93/EC and 97/78/ EC and Council Decision 92/438/EEC (Official Controls Regulation); European Union: Brussels, Belgium, 2017.
26. Regulation (EU) no 1169/2011 of the European Parliament and of the Council of 25 Oct 2011 on the Provision of Food Information to Consumers, Amending Regulations (EC) No 1924/2006 and (EC) No 1925/2006 of the European Parliament and of the Council, and Repealing Commission Directive 87/250/EEC, Council Directive 90/496/EEC, Commission Directive 1999/10/EC, Directive 2000/13/EC of the European Parliament and of the Council, Commission Directives 2002/67/EC and 2008/5/EC and Commission Regulation (EC) No 608/2004; European Union: Brussels, Belgium, 2011.
27. Leitsätze des Deutschen Lebensmittelbuchs für Brot und Kleingebäck. Available online: https://www.bmel.de/SharedDocs/Downloads/DE/_Ernaehrung/Lebensmittel-Kennzeichnung/LeitsaetzeBrot.pdf?__blob=publicationFile&v=4 (accessed on 1 November 2022).
28. Medina, S.; Pereira, J.A.; Silva, P.; Perestrelo, R.; Câmara, J.S. Food Fingerprints–A Valuable Tool to Monitor Food Authenticity and Safety. *Food Chem.* **2019**, *278*, 144–162. [CrossRef] [PubMed]
29. Gao, B.; Holroyd, S.E.; Moore, J.C.; Laurvick, K.; Gendel, S.M.; Xie, Z. Opportunities and Challenges Using Non-Targeted Methods for Food Fraud Detection. *J. Agric. Food. Chem.* **2019**, *67*, 8425–8430. [CrossRef] [PubMed]
30. McGrath, T.F.; Haughey, S.A.; Patterson, J.; Fauhl-Hassek, C.; Donarski, J.; Alewijn, M.; van Ruth, S.; Elliott, C.T. What Are the Scientific Challenges in Moving from Targeted to Non-Targeted Methods for Food Fraud Testing and How Can They Be Addressed?–Spectroscopy Case Study. *Trends Food Sci. Technol.* **2018**, *76*, 38–55. [CrossRef]
31. Nichani, K.; Uhlig, S.; Stoyke, M.; Kemmlein, S.; Ulberth, F.; Haase, I.; Döring, M.; Walch, S.G.; Gowik, P. Essential Terminology and Considerations for Validation of Non-Targeted Methods. *Food Chem. X* **2022**, *17*, 100538. [CrossRef]
32. Esteki, M.; Shahsavari, Z.; Simal-Gandara, J. Food Identification by High Performance Liquid Chromatography Fingerprinting and Mathematical Processing. *Food Res. Int.* **2019**, *122*, 303–317. [CrossRef] [PubMed]
33. Holewinski, R.J.; Parker, S.J.; Matlock, A.D.; Venkatraman, V.; Eyk, J.E.V. Methods for SWATH^{TM}: Data Independent Acquisition on TripleTOF Mass Spectrometers. In *Quantitative Proteomics by Mass Spectrometry*; Springer: Berlin/Heidelberg, Germany, 2016; pp. 265–279.
34. Guo, J.; Huan, T. Comparison of Full-Scan, Data-Dependent, and Data-Independent Acquisition Modes in Liquid Chromatography–Mass Spectrometry Based Untargeted Metabolomics. *Anal. Chem.* **2020**, *92*, 8072–8080. [CrossRef]
35. Jimenez-Carvelo, A.M.; Cuadros-Rodríguez, L. Data Mining/Machine Learning Methods in Foodomics. *Curr. Opin. Food Sci.* **2021**, *37*, 76–82. [CrossRef]
36. Sen, P.; Lamichhane, S.; Mathema, V.B.; McGlinchey, A.; Dickens, A.M.; Khoomrung, S.; Orešič, M. Deep Learning Meets Metabolomics: A Methodological Perspective. *Brief. Bioinform.* **2021**, *22*, 1531–1542. [CrossRef]
37. Rong, Z.; Tan, Q.; Cao, L.; Zhang, L.; Deng, K.; Huang, Y.; Zhu, Z.-J.; Li, Z.; Li, K. NormAE: Deep Adversarial Learning Model to Remove Batch Effects in Liquid Chromatography Mass Spectrometry-Based Metabolomics Data. *Anal. Chem.* **2020**, *92*, 5082–5090. [CrossRef]
38. Li, M.; Wang, X.R. Peak Alignment of Gas Chromatography–Mass Spectrometry Data with Deep Learning. *J. Chromatogr. A* **2019**, *1604*, 460476. [CrossRef]
39. Risum, A.B.; Bro, R. Using Deep Learning to Evaluate Peaks in Chromatographic Data. *Talanta* **2019**, *204*, 255–260. [CrossRef] [PubMed]
40. Kantz, E.D.; Tiwari, S.; Watrous, J.D.; Cheng, S.; Jain, M. Deep Neural Networks for Classification of LC-MS Spectral Peaks. *Anal. Chem.* **2019**, *91*, 12407–12413. [CrossRef]
41. Gloaguen, Y.; Kirwan, J.A.; Beule, D. Deep Learning-Assisted Peak Curation for Large-Scale LC-MS Metabolomics. *Anal Chem.* **2022**, *94*, 4930–4937. [CrossRef] [PubMed]
42. Melnikov, A.D.; Tsentalovich, Y.P.; Yanshole, V.V. Deep Learning for the Precise Peak Detection in High-Resolution LC–MS Data. *Anal Chem.* **2019**, *92*, 588–592. [CrossRef] [PubMed]
43. Wei, J.N.; Belanger, D.; Adams, R.P.; Sculley, D. Rapid Prediction of Electron–Ionization Mass Spectrometry Using Neural Networks. *ACS Cent. Sci.* **2019**, *5*, 700–708. [CrossRef]

44. Dührkop, K.; Nothias, L.-F.; Fleischauer, M.; Reher, R.; Ludwig, M.; Hoffmann, M.A.; Petras, D.; Gerwick, W.H.; Rousu, J.; Dorrestein, P.C. Systematic Classification of Unknown Metabolites Using High-Resolution Fragmentation Mass Spectra. *Nat. Biotechnol.* **2021**, *39*, 462–471. [CrossRef]
45. Kim, H.W.; Wang, M.; Leber, C.A.; Nothias, L.-F.; Reher, R.; Kang, K.B.; Van Der Hooft, J.J.; Dorrestein, P.C.; Gerwick, W.H.; Cottrell, G.W. NPClassifier: A Deep Neural Network-Based Structural Classification Tool for Natural Products. *J. Nat. Prod.* **2021**, *84*, 2795–2807. [CrossRef]
46. Uhlig, S.; Colson, B.; Hettwer, K.; Simon, K.; Uhlig, C.; Wittke, S.; Stoyke, M.; Gowik, P. Valid Machine Learning Algorithms for Multiparameter Methods. *Accredit. Qual. Assur.* **2019**, *24*, 271–279. [CrossRef]
47. Malek, S.; Melgani, F.; Bazi, Y. One-dimensional Convolutional Neural Networks for Spectroscopic Signal Regression. *J. Chemom.* **2018**, *32*, e2977. [CrossRef]
48. Seddiki, K.; Saudemont, P.; Precioso, F.; Ogrinc, N.; Wisztorski, M.; Salzet, M.; Fournier, I.; Droit, A. Cumulative Learning Enables Convolutional Neural Network Representations for Small Mass Spectrometry Data Classification. *Nat. Commun.* **2020**, *11*, 5595. [CrossRef]
49. Lawrence, S.; Giles, C.L.; Tsoi, A.C.; Back, A.D. Face Recognition: A Convolutional Neural-Network Approach. *IEEE Trans. Neural Netw.* **1997**, *8*, 98–113. [CrossRef] [PubMed]
50. Gu, J.; Wang, Z.; Kuen, J.; Ma, L.; Shahroudy, A.; Shuai, B.; Liu, T.; Wang, X.; Wang, G.; Cai, J. Recent Advances in Convolutional Neural Networks. *Pattern Recognit.* **2018**, *77*, 354–377. [CrossRef]
51. Huschek, G.; Bönick, J.; Merkel, D.; Huschek, D.; Rawel, H. Authentication of Leguminous-Based Products by Targeted Biomarkers Using High Resolution Time of Flight Mass Spectrometry. *LWT* **2018**, *90*, 164–171. [CrossRef]
52. Bönick, J.; Huschek, G.; Rawel, H.M. Determination of Wheat, Rye and Spelt Authenticity in Bread by Targeted Peptide Biomarkers. *J. Food Compost Anal.* **2017**, *58*, 82–91. [CrossRef]
53. Mialon, N.; Roig, B.; Capodanno, E.; Cadiere, A. Untargeted Metabolomic Approaches in Food Authenticity: A Review That Showcases Biomarkers. *Food Chem.* **2022**, *398*, 133856. [CrossRef] [PubMed]
54. Curry, B.; Rumelhart, D.E. MSnet: A Neural Network Which Classifies Mass Spectra. *Tetrahedron Comput. Methodol.* **1990**, *3*, 213–237. [CrossRef]
55. Doerr, A. DIA Mass Spectrometry. *Nat. Methods* **2015**, *12*, 35. [CrossRef]
56. Kessner, D.; Chambers, M.; Burke, R.; Agus, D.; Mallick, P. ProteoWizard: Open Source Software for Rapid Proteomics Tools Development. *Bioinformatics* **2008**, *24*, 2534–2536. [CrossRef]
57. Mendez, K.M.; Broadhurst, D.I.; Reinke, S.N. The Application of Artificial Neural Networks in Metabolomics: A Historical Perspective. *Metabolomics* **2019**, *15*, 142. [CrossRef]
58. Creydt, M.; Fischer, M. Food Phenotyping: Recording and Processing of Non-Targeted Liquid Chromatography Mass Spectrometry Data for Verifying Food Authenticity. *Molecules* **2020**, *25*, 3972. [CrossRef]
59. Brereton, R.G. Pattern Recognition in Chemometrics. *Chemometr. Intell. Lab. Syst.* **2015**, *149*, 90–96. [CrossRef]
60. Paul, A.; de Boves Harrington, P. Chemometric Applications in Metabolomic Studies Using Chromatography-Mass Spectrometry. *TrAC Trends Anal. Chem.* **2021**, *135*, 116165. [CrossRef]
61. Huang, Y.; Kangas, L.J.; Rasco, B.A. Applications of Artificial Neural Networks (ANNs) in Food Science. *Crit. Rev. Food Sci. Nutr.* **2007**, *47*, 113–126. [CrossRef]
62. Lei, F.; Liu, X.; Dai, Q.; Ling, B.W.-K. Shallow Convolutional Neural Network for Image Classification. *SN Appl. Sci.* **2020**, *2*, 97. [CrossRef]
63. Chollet, F. Keras. 2015. Available online: https://github.com/fchollet/keras (accessed on 10 November 2022).
64. Abadi, M.; Barham, P.; Chen, J.; Chen, Z.; Davis, A.; Dean, J.; Devin, M.; Ghemawat, S.; Irving, G.; Isard, M.; et al. TensorFlow: A System for Large-Scale Machine Learning. In Proceedings of the 12th USENIX Symposium on Operating Systems Design and Implementation, Savannah, GA, USA, 2–4 November 2016; p. 21.
65. Guo, D.; Föll, M.C.; Volkmann, V.; Enderle-Ammour, K.; Bronsert, P.; Schilling, O.; Vitek, O. Deep Multiple Instance Learning Classifies Subtissue Locations in Mass Spectrometry Images from Tissue-Level Annotations. *Bioinformatics* **2020**, *36*, i300–i308. [CrossRef] [PubMed]
66. Chicco, D.; Jurman, G. The Advantages of the Matthews Correlation Coefficient (MCC) over F1 Score and Accuracy in Binary Classification Evaluation. *BMC Genom.* **2020**, *21*, 6. [CrossRef] [PubMed]
67. ISO 5725-3; Accuracy (Trueness and Precision) of Measurement Methods and Results. Part 3: Intermediate Measures of the Precision of a Standard Measurement Method. International Organization for Standardization: Geneva, Switzerland, 1994.
68. Uhlig, S.; Nichani, K.; Colson, B.; Hettwer, K.; Simon, K.; Uhlig, C.; Stoyke, M.; Steinacker, U.; Becker, R.; Gowik, P. Performance Characteristics and Criteria for Non-Targeted Methods. In Proceedings of the Eurachem Workshop, Tartu, Estonia, 20–21 May 2019.
69. Uhlig, S.; Nichani, K.; Stoyke, M.; Gowik, P. Validation of Binary Non-Targeted Methods: Mathematical Framework and Experimental Designs. *bioRxiv* **2021**. [CrossRef]

Disclaimer/Publisher's Note: The statements, opinions and data contained in all publications are solely those of the individual author(s) and contributor(s) and not of MDPI and/or the editor(s). MDPI and/or the editor(s) disclaim responsibility for any injury to people or property resulting from any ideas, methods, instructions or products referred to in the content.

MDPI AG
Grosspeteranlage 5
4052 Basel
Switzerland
Tel.: +41 61 683 77 34

Foods Editorial Office
E-mail: foods@mdpi.com
www.mdpi.com/journal/foods

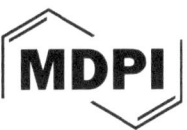

Disclaimer/Publisher's Note: The title and front matter of this reprint are at the discretion of the Guest Editors. The publisher is not responsible for their content or any associated concerns. The statements, opinions and data contained in all individual articles are solely those of the individual Editors and contributors and not of MDPI. MDPI disclaims responsibility for any injury to people or property resulting from any ideas, methods, instructions or products referred to in the content.

www.ingramcontent.com/pod-product-compliance
Lightning Source LLC
LaVergne TN
LVHW072356090526
838202LV00019B/2558